Intraoperative Neuromonitoring

Josef Zentner • David B. MacDonald
Celine Wegner

Editors

Intraoperative Neuromonitoring

Fundamentals, Possibilities, Limitations

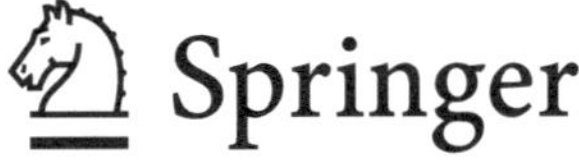

Editors
Josef Zentner
Department of Neurosurgery
University Medical Center
Freiburg, Germany

David B. MacDonald
ARKANA Forum GmbH
Emmendingen, Germany

Celine Wegner
ARKANA Forum GmbH
Emmendingen, Germany

ISBN 978-3-031-46127-9   ISBN 978-3-031-46125-5   (eBook)
https://doi.org/10.1007/978-3-031-46125-5

Translation from the German language edition: "Intraoperatives Neuromonitoring" by Josef Zentner et al., © Arkana Forum GmbH 2020. Published by Medizinisch Wissenschaftliche Verlagsgesellschaft. All Rights Reserved.

This Springer imprint is published by the registered company Springer Nature Switzerland AG
The registered company address is: Gewerbestrasse 11, 6330 Cham, Switzerland

Paper in this product is recyclable.

Preface

Intraoperative neurophysiological monitoring (IONM) has gained increasing interest during the past decades and is now an integral part of various surgical disciplines, especially in neurosurgery, but also in otolaryngology, orthopedics, vascular surgery, and general surgery. With expanding applications and evolving techniques, the monitoring team is faced with increasingly complex tasks and responsibilities. Despite its importance and significance in modern surgical medicine and the expectations associated with it, IONM is still not a regular part of the training program of medical professionals. Although knowledge on monitoring is imparted in basic courses offered by a few professional societies, systematic training of medical and non-medical staff according to a standardized curriculum is still lacking.

This handbook aims to contribute to closing this gap. It provides a practical guide to help medical, nursing, and technical personnel get familiar with intraoperative neuromonitoring. The basic tenor is to combine theoretical and practical knowledge and thus to systematically convey essential skills about fundamentals, possibilities, but also limitations of IONM to a broad circle of readers. In order to achieve this goal, the text has been reduced to the absolutely necessary length in favor of numerous illustrations and tables.

After an introduction to the tasks, the significance, and the historical development of IONM, the anatomical, physiological, and physical basics are presented. This is followed by a presentation of various modalities as well as stimulation and recording techniques. The intraoperative part begins with some information on the organizational processes in the operating room, and a description of the influences of anesthesia on monitoring, including the special aspects of awake surgery. This is followed by a rough overview of the application fields of IONM in various disciplines including representative case examples. The manual concludes with remarks on the efficiency and safety of monitoring and practical recommendations for the detection and elimination of intraoperative sources of error. Self-tests in individual chapters are intended to give readers the opportunity to determine their level of knowledge.

Since this manual has been designed for a wide range of readers, it is unavoidable that various explanations may appear superfluous for some readers due to corresponding prior knowledge, while the respective information is essential for a better understanding of the matter for others. Accordingly, it is left to the individual readers to set their own priorities in studying this book. In line with the character of a user-friendly manual, generally known and accepted information is deliberately not supported by literature. References are limited to some specific aspects. For further information, we refer to the relevant literature.

To achieve the goal of a comprehensive multidisciplinary presentation, various authors with medical and technical backgrounds have collaborated on this book. Our special thanks are due to all authors for their valuable contributions, which were reviewed and brought into a coherent structure by the editors. We would also like to thank Lisa Disch for her initiative in this book project as well as Kathleen Seidel for her vestibular schwannoma case example and Andrea Szelényi for her material and constructive comments. Moreover, we owe gratitude to all those unnamed individuals who have contributed to this manual by their critical discussion.

This book was written in cooperation with inomed Medizintechnik GmbH. For over 10 years experts and users have been sharing their knowledge in IONM courses and trainings. The resulting contributions and discussions have shaped the content of this book. Originally designed as training material for application specialists of the company, this book has been systematically developed toward a comprehensive work for the practice of Intraoperative Neuromonitoring. For this reason, the accessories shown in this book are mainly products of inomed Medizintechnik. However comparable accessories are available from other manufacturers as well.

Freiburg im Breisgau, Germany
Emmendingen, Germany
Emmendingen, Germany

Josef Zentner
David B. MacDonald
Celine Wegner

Contents

Editors and Contributors

Editors

Josef Zentner Department of Neurosurgery, University Medical Center, Freiburg, Germany

David B. MacDonald ARKANA Forum GmbH, Emmendingen, Germany

Celine Wegner ARKANA Forum GmbH, Emmendingen, Germany

Contributors

Barbara Bischoff Department of Neurosurgery, Sozialstiftung Bamberg, Bamberg, Germany

Kristin Block Medizinelektronik Kuttner GmbH & Co. KG, Halle (Saale), Germany

Hanna Burdich inomed Medizintechnik GmbH, Emmendingen, Germany

Marianella Campos Friz ARKANA Forum GmbH, Emmendingen, Germany

Carolin Gierschner Department of Epileptology, University Medical Center, Freiburg, Germany

Ludwig Kuttner Medizinelektronik Kuttner GmbH & Co. KG, Halle (Saale), Germany

David B. MacDonald ARKANA Forum GmbH, Emmendingen, Germany

Theresia Maik iNCU GmbH, Emmendingen, Germany

Michael Malcharek Praxisklinik Leipzig, Leipzig, Germany

Hans-Joachim Priebe Department of Anesthesiology and Critical Care, University Medical Center, Freiburg, Germany

Claudia Seibold inomed Medizintechnik GmbH, Emmendingen, Germany

René Tamba inomed Medizintechnik GmbH, Emmendingen, Germany

Celine Wegner ARKANA Forum GmbH, Emmendingen, Germany

Anika Wipfler inomed Medizintechnik GmbH, Emmendingen, Germany

Josef Zentner Department of Neurosurgery, University Medical Center, Freiburg, Germany

Figures and Illustrations

Maike Jacobi

List of Figures

List of Tables

Introduction

1

Josef Zentner

Contents

1.1 Why Neuromonitoring?

Surgical interventions in the nervous system are associated with considerable risks due to the vulnerability of nervous structures. For example, the morbidity rate of neurosurgical operations in critical brain areas was almost 100% in the first half of the last century along with a high mortality rate. At that time, the primary concern was to **preserve life**.

This situation has changed significantly with the availability of new imaging techniques and the introduction of microsurgery. Computed tomography and in particular magnetic resonance imaging facilitated exact localization and delineation of the lesion to be removed and its topographic relationships to brain areas of high functionality, thus rendering precise surgical planning possible. Surgical microscope and microsurgical instrumentation allowed gentle removal of even deep lesions using natural clefts (cisterns). Microsurgery and modern imaging have led to a decisive reduction in mortality and morbidity. As a result, surgical interventions on the brain could be performed with calculable risks. Neurosurgery was no longer so much a matter of preserving life, but rather of **preserving function** in the sense of **functionally oriented surgery**.

Despite these technical advances, there remained a significant risk of neurological complications during interventions in critical areas. This is particularly true since with further development of surgical techniques the indication for surgical interventions was also extended. In addition, risks of neurological deficits affect not only neurosurgical but also ears nose and throat (ENT), orthopedic, vascular, or even general surgical procedures whenever nervous structures are involved. Since these procedures are usually performed under general anesthesia, the neurological status can be assessed only after awakening, i.e., at a time when the surgical measures have been completed and can no longer be corrected.

J. Zentner (✉)
Department of Neurosurgery, University Medical Center, Freiburg, Germany

© The Author(s), under exclusive license to Springer Nature Switzerland AG 2024
J. Zentner et al. (eds.), *Intraoperative Neuromonitoring*,
https://doi.org/10.1007/978-3-031-46125-5_1

Thus, in order to achieve a further reduction in neurological morbidity, a new approach is needed that allows monitoring of the vulnerable nervous structures during the surgical procedure under general anesthesia.

This is where intraoperative neuromonitoring (IONM) comes in: With the help of nerve and muscle action potentials as well as evoked potentials, neural structures can be monitored during operations under general anesthesia in order to reduce and minimize the risk of neurological deterioration. Furthermore, monitoring during surgical dissection should provide information about the spatial relationships to critical neural structures to avoid damage. It is of particular importance that the surgeon incorporates the results of monitoring into operative measures and is willing to be guided by monitoring and adjust operative strategy to the potential findings. Coming from the demand of preserving function, IONM now intends to usher in a new era, the era of **functionally guided surgery**.

1.2 Historical Aspects

Intraoperative neuromonitoring started in **neurosurgery** with **spinal cord monitoring** using **somatosensory evoked potentials (SEPs)** in the 1970s. However, it became apparent early on that the value of spinal cord monitoring with SEPs in neurosurgery is noticeably limited. This is particularly true because in neurosurgical patients, function is usually already impaired preoperatively, so that SEPs are often of low quality or not available at all. Furthermore, SEPs that are purely sensory cannot detect selective motor injury. Consequently, although especially in spinal patients with neurological deficits the relevance of SEP monitoring is high, its validity is low. For these reasons, spinal cord monitoring with SEPs lost importance in neurosurgery.

Subsequently, SEP spinal cord monitoring was increasingly used in **orthopedics**, particularly in **scoliosis surgery**. In these patients, function is usually intact preoperatively. Accordingly, well-defined SEPs are available. Therefore, the validity of monitoring is high in these cases. The effectiveness of SEP spinal cord monitoring in reducing neurological complications in scoliosis surgery has been demonstrated in a multicenter study.

After the introduction of electrical and magnetic transcranial stimulation in the 1980s, spinal cord monitoring in neurosurgery focused on intraoperative recording of **motor evoked potentials (MEPs)**. Initial difficulties in generating usable muscle action potentials intraoperatively under general anesthesia were overcome with the availability of the technique of brief high-frequency pulse train stimulation, which found general acceptance.

In parallel, intraoperative monitoring of **cranial nerves** VII (facial nerve) and VIII (vestibulocochlear nerve) found widespread use in the 1980s. In **ENT surgery**, monitoring of the facial nerve was applied with great success during surgical procedures in the area of the parotid gland. In **neurosurgery**, monitoring cranial nerves VII and VIII found great interest during interventions in the cerebellopontine angle (e.g., for acoustic neuromas). This is particularly true since controlled studies have demonstrated the value of monitoring cranial nerves VII and VIII both in ENT surgery and neurosurgery with statistical significance. Thus, monitoring of those cranial nerves has become standard practice in neurosurgery and ENT surgery since the 1990s.

Later, monitoring was extended to cranial nerves III to XII during **skull base surgery**, whereas intraoperative monitoring of the optic nerve (II) by means of visual evoked potentials found less acceptance due to difficulties in generating reliable potentials without patient cooperation. In addition, recurrent nerve monitoring has found widespread use in **thyroid surgery**. At the same time, SEPs and MEPs have been increasingly applied in neurosurgical procedures for **vascular malformations** (aneurysms, angiomas) and **tumors** (low-grade gliomas). Moreover, SEP and MEP monitoring of spinal cord function has gained interest in the surgical treatment of thoracic and abdominal aneurysms. Finally, techniques for monitoring sphincter function during **colorectal surgery** have been developed.

Currently, IONM is part of the standard repertoire in various disciplines: **neurosurgery, orthopedic surgery, ENT surgery, vascular surgery, and general surgery**. The IONM is based on the monitoring concept.

1.3 Monitoring Concept

The decisive prerequisite for successful electrophysiological monitoring is that potential deterioration occurs at the earliest possible stage of impending functional impairment, i.e., at a stage at which correction of the surgical measures is still possible in order to avoid neurological deficits. Impending functional disorders must therefore be detectable by signal deterioration at a reversible stage. The surgeon must be able to react to adverse changes in order to reverse both signal deterioration and the associated neurological impairment. Such responses may include reducing retraction of neural structures by spatula, reducing manipulation of nerves and vessels, changing the site of dissection, or simply pausing preparation. On the other hand, stable potentials should validly reassure the surgeon that the surgical course so far is harmless and that no additional neurological deficits of the monitored structures are likely.

Overall, all modalities (nerve and muscle action potentials, evoked potentials) used for IONM must be shown to fulfill the requirements of the monitoring concept: **Deteriorated potentials** must indicate **impending neurologic dysfunction** in the **reversible stage**, while **unchanged potentials** should provide **reassurance** to the surgeon regarding the **safety** of the surgical steps undertaken so far. This places special demands on the monitoring team and the interpretation of IONM results.

1.4 Monitoring Team

The monitoring team has many different tasks. **First**, depending on the preoperative neurological status and the type and extent of the surgical procedure, the **technique** to be used (pathways to be examined, modalities, stimulation and recording techniques, etc.) must be defined. This is done in consultation with the surgeon. Likewise, collaboration with the anesthesiologist is required to select the most appropriate anesthetic regime to minimize deleterious effects of anesthesia on the monitored potentials. **Second,** after induction of anesthesia and positioning of the patient in the operating room, the **electrodes** are securely attached to the patient and connected to the monitoring device. Subsequently, the connections are checked. **Third,** after stabilization of the anesthesia and before surgical measures are commenced, the initial **baselines** are registered.

During the surgical procedure, neurophysiological testing is done at regular intervals, the recordings are observed and **interpreted**, and the surgeon is informed of **critical adverse changes**. It is of particular importance that the monitoring team is oriented about the operative processes and the essential surgical steps to ensure a close monitoring of the structures at risk, especially during the critical phases. The surgeon must be in a position to rely on critical deterioration of potentials being detected and communicated in a timely manner. **After completion of the surgical measures** and before termination of the anesthesia, the last recordings are done. Finally, the electrodes are removed, and the intraoperative records are documented.

In order to meet these diverse tasks, solid **training** is required, which includes not only electrophysiological expertise but also medical aspects. Usually, monitoring is performed by a **medical technical assistant (MTA)** with electrophysiological qualification. Supervision by an electrophysiologically trained **physician** is generally required. The necessary extent of medical supervision depends on the experience and qualification of the MTA. The numerical size of the monitoring team largely varies depending on the frequency to use IONM (number and duration of monitored surgical procedures, number of monitoring systems to be supervised simultaneously, etc.) at the respective institution.

Anatomical and Physiological Basics

2

Marianella Campos Friz and Barbara Bischoff

Contents

2.1 Positional and Directional Designations

Positional and directional designations are necessary for **orientation** on the human body. Terms such as "up" and "down" are misleading because they depend on the current position of the body. The anatomical designations for position and direction refer to the main planes and the main axis of the body and are therefore unambiguous because they are independent of its current position.

The human body can be described with three **main planes** (Fig. 2.1): The transverse plane

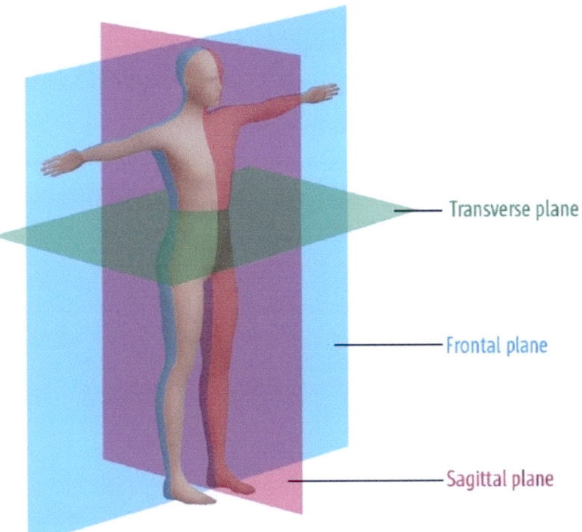

Fig. 2.1 Main planes of the human body. © ARKANA Forum GmbH 2022. All Rights Reserved

M. C. Friz (✉)
ARKANA Forum GmbH, Emmendingen, Germany
e-mail: m.campos@arkana-forum.com

B. Bischoff
Department of Neurosurgery, Sozialstiftung Bamberg, Bamberg, Germany

© The Author(s), under exclusive license to Springer Nature Switzerland AG 2024
J. Zentner et al. (eds.), *Intraoperative Neuromonitoring*,
https://doi.org/10.1007/978-3-031-46125-5_2

shown in green describes a horizontal area perpendicular to the longitudinal axis of the body. The blue frontal plane divides the body into front and back, the red sagittal plane into right and left (in each case from the patient's perspective).

The directions are given relative to the **neural axis** (Figs. 2.2 and 2.3). This is an imaginary axis that runs along the central nervous system from the front of the brain to the end of the spinal cord. In the brain, this axis describes a kink at the level

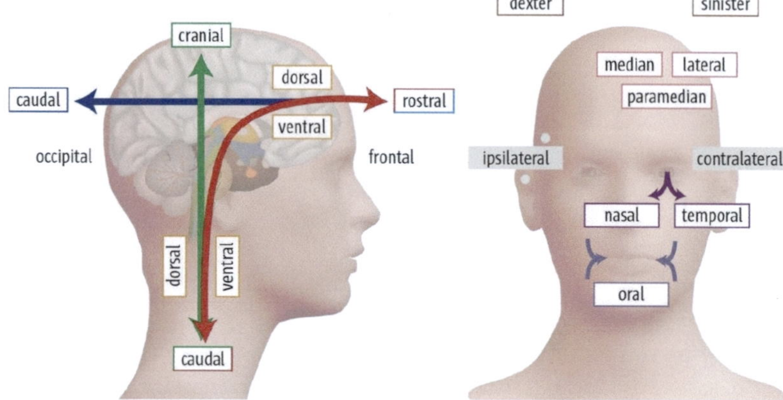

Fig. 2.2 Positional and directional designations on the skull and brain. © ARKANA Forum GmbH 2022. All Rights Reserved

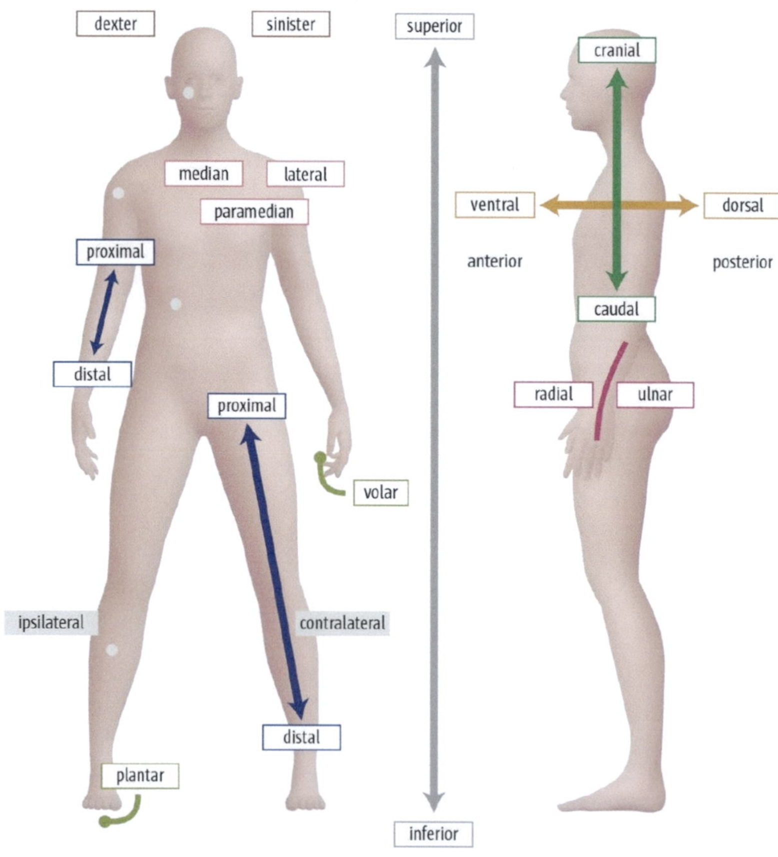

Fig. 2.3 Positional and directional designations on the body. © ARKANA Forum GmbH 2022. All Rights Reserved

of the thalamus, so that the directional designations shift. For example, while in the periphery of the body the term "caudal" translates as "toward the bottom," this term means in the brain "toward the back." In practice, directional designations in the brain are based on the names of brain lobes, e.g., occipital (located toward the occipital lobe), temporal (located toward the temporal lobe), and frontal (located toward the frontal lobe).

The most important **positional and directional designations** are listed below:

- Anterior: Lying in the front, identical with ventral
- Posterior: Lying in the back, identical with dorsal
- Ventral: Toward the belly, identical with anterior
- Dorsal: Toward the back, identical with posterior
- Cranial: Toward the cranium
- Caudal: Toward the cauda equina (ponytail)
- Superior: Lying at the top
- Inferior: Lying at the bottom
- Distal: Away from the body center
- Proximal: Toward the body center
- Ipsilateral: On the same side
- Contralateral: On the opposite side
- Lateral: Sideways
- Median: In the middle
- Paramedian: Beside the middle
- Frontal: Toward the frontal lobe (front of head)
- Occipital: Toward the occipital lobe (back of head)
- Temporal: Toward the temporal lobe (temple region)
- Rostral: Toward the front of head
- Nasal: Toward the nose
- Oral: Toward the mouth
- Radial: Toward the radius bone of the forearm
- Ulnar: Toward the ulna bone of the forearm
- Plantar: Toward the foot sole
- Volar: Toward the palm

- Dexter: On the right side (from patient's perspective)
- Sinister: On the left side (from patient's perspective)

2.2 The Nervous System

The nervous system represents the **control center** of the body. Its basic principles of operation can best be described with the terms **"perception-processing-reaction."** Signals from the environment and from inside the body are received by the sensory receptors and transmitted via afferent pathways with various intermediate stations to the regulatory centers in the spinal cord and brain. From here, appropriate responses run through efferent pathways to the executing target organs (effectors). This control system allows the body to respond adequately to stimuli and changes in the environment or within itself.

From an anatomical and functional point of view, the human nervous system can be divided as follows:

- **Anatomically**, a distinction is made between the central nervous system (CNS) and the peripheral nervous system (PNS).
- **Functionally**, one can distinguish between the somatic nervous system and the vegetative/autonomic nervous system.

The **CNS** consists of the brain and spinal cord, while the **PNS** comprises the nerves leaving the brain and spinal cord.

The **somatic/voluntary nervous system** includes parts of the CNS and PNS. It is responsible for the conscious perception of external stimuli and voluntary actions (e.g., via the muscles).

The **vegetative/autonomic nervous system** works involuntarily (autonomously) and regulates vital functions such as breathing, circulation, digestion, and water balance. It is primarily responsible for the activity of the internal organs.

The two essential parts of the vegetative/autonomic nervous system are the **sympathetic** and **parasympathetic systems**, which act as counterparts in their function. While the sympathetic system prepares the organism for "escape," the parasympathetic system dampens the external body activities and stimulates the function of the internal organs.

2.2.1 The Nerve Cell (Neuron)

Microscopically, the brain and spinal cord consist of the **nerve cells** or **neurons** with their processes and the **glial cells,** the latter accounting for about 90% of the cells in the CNS.

The **nerve cells** (**neurons**) are responsible for signal processing (Fig. 2.4). Each neuron receives information from other nerve cells via its branched processes, the dendrites. From the dendrites, the information is transmitted to the cell body (soma). Here, the stimuli are processed by the nucleus and the cell organelles in a complex process. Subsequently, the nerve cell transmits the signals via its axon and its terminals to the dendrites of other nerve cells or to its target organ, such as a muscle cell.

The **glial cells** are not directly involved in signal processing but perform a variety of other functions. They support the structural integrity of neurons ("supporting cells") and perform protective and metabolic functions. In addition, the glial cells form myelin sheaths around axons in the CNS and PNS and thereby provide an insulating cover for controlled signal transmission.

Myelinated **axons** together form a bundle of nerve fibers that in turn join together to form a nerve (Fig. 2.5). Individual nerves, for example, in the legs, can reach a length of up to 1 m.

2.2.2 Signal Conduction and Transmission

2.2.2.1 Axon and Synapse

As already described, signal conduction and transmission are effected via axons and nerve cells. To understand these processes, a closer look at the functioning of the axons is necessary.

The **axon** or **nerve fiber** represents the outgoing element of the nerve cell. It divides at its distal end into several branches called telodendria. Each telodendron terminates in an axon terminal (synaptic bouton or terminal bouton). Signaling substances that have been formed and "packaged" in the cell body are transported along the axon to its end. There they are stored in the terminal boutons. Transport toward the end of the axon is called anterograde or orthodromic. In contrast, retrograde or antidromic transport means that substances are transported back to the cell body.

The axon is covered by the **myelin sheath**. In the CNS, this myelin sheath is formed by oligodendrocytes and in the PNS by Schwann cells. At

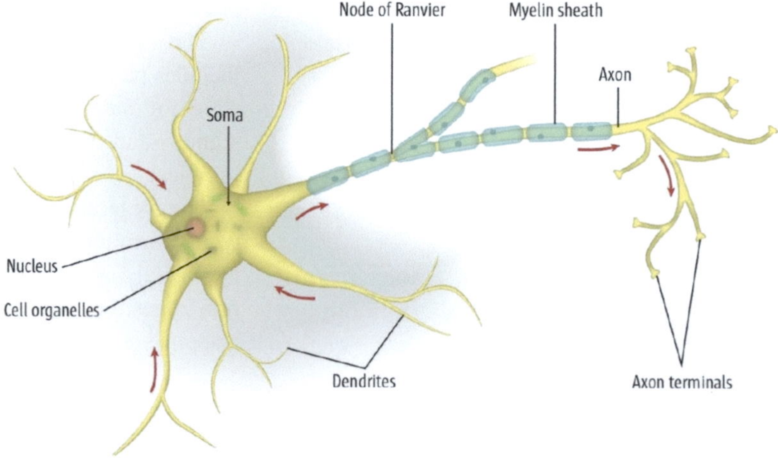

Fig. 2.4 Structure of a nerve cell (neuron). © ARKANA Forum GmbH 2022. All Rights Reserved

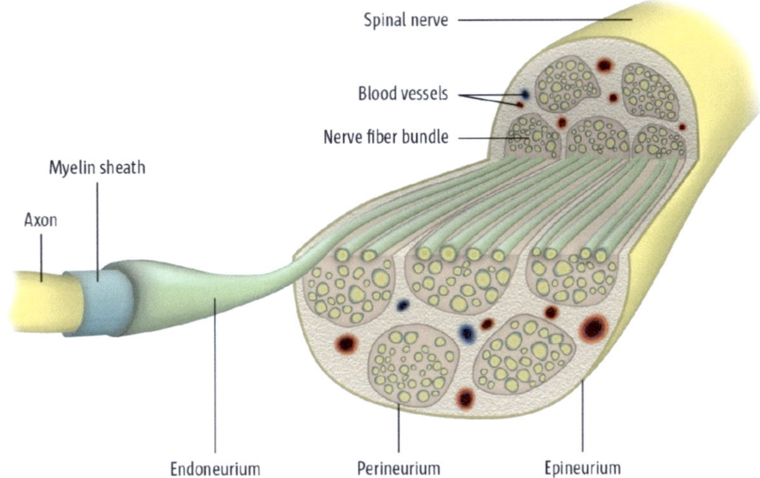

Fig. 2.5 Structure of a peripheral nerve consisting of nerve fibers and nerve fiber bundles. © ARKANA Forum GmbH 2022. All Rights Reserved

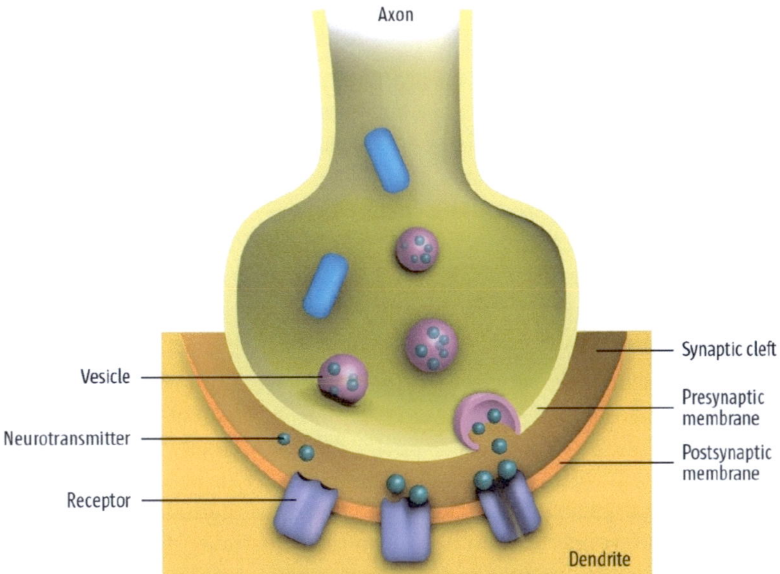

Fig. 2.6 Structure of a synapse. © ARKANA Forum GmbH 2022. All Rights Reserved

certain intervals between the individual cells, there are unmyelinated axonal segments, called nodes of Ranvier. These structures are essential for fast signal conduction along an axon.

The connection between the end of an axon and its corresponding target, e.g., the dendrite of another nerve cell, is called a **synapse** (Fig. 2.6). This is where the signal transmission from one nerve cell to the next takes place. At the terminal boutons of the axons, the signaling substances, the neurotransmitters, are stored in vesicles. The membrane at the end of the boutons is called the presynaptic membrane, and the membrane of the adjacent nerve cell is termed the postsynaptic membrane. Between both membranes, there is the synaptic cleft.

2.2.2.2 Action Potential

When the stimulus excites a nerve cell, an action potential (Fig. 2.7) is generated at the axon hillock, that is, the junction between the nerve cell and its axon, provided that a certain threshold voltage is exceeded. Thereby sodium channels are opened that allow positively charged sodium ions to enter the cell due to a high concentration difference. This process is called **depolarization**.

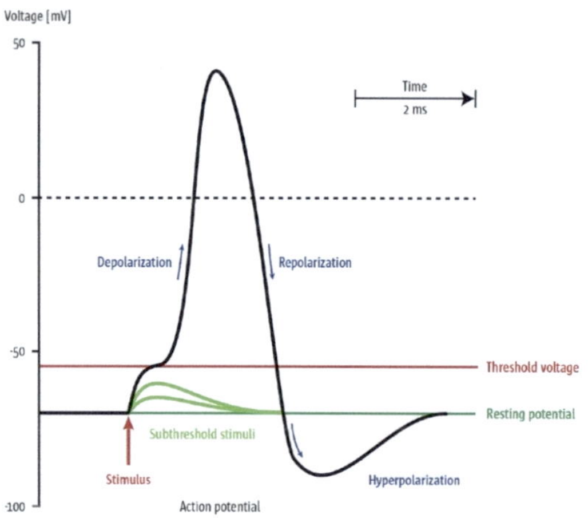

Fig. 2.7 Time course of an action potential. © ARKANA Forum GmbH 2022. All Rights Reserved

Subsequently, **repolarization** of the membrane occurs. Other positive particles, including positively charged potassium ions, flow out of the cell via potassium channels, and the sodium channels are closed. In addition, sodium ions from the cell are exchanged with potassium ions via the sodium-potassium pump. In this way, the resting potential is reached again. Only thereafter can a new action potential be triggered.

The **myelin sheath** insulates the membranes of the axons, and electrical resistance is increased. Thus, transmission of signals takes place only at the nodes of Ranvier. Here, the electric field of the respective preceding depolarization leads to a renewed depolarization of the next node of Ranvier. This results in **saltatory conduction** which leads to a substantial increase in conduction velocity. If the insulating myelin sheath is missing, as in the case of unmyelinated nerve fibers, the signal is conducted continuously along the axon and thus more slowly (Fig. 2.8).

The signal that arrives at the axon terminal causes depolarization of the presynaptic membrane, thus opening calcium channels. The calcium influx results in the release of signals to fuse the vesicles to the presynaptic membrane. This releases **neurotransmitters** into the synaptic cleft. At the postsynaptic membrane, the neurotransmitters bind to transmitter-specific **receptors**. Depending on the type of neurotrans-

mitter, this causes an excitatory (depolarizing) or inhibitory (hyperpolarizing) **postsynaptic potential** of the postsynaptic membrane. If several excitatory postsynaptic potentials sum to **firing threshold**, then the postsynaptic neuron discharges an action potential.

In the **sensory system**, the signals originate at the receptors in the periphery, which are able to excite corresponding nerve cells, thus generating an action potential. In the **motor system**, the action potential in the periphery reaches the motor end plate, where depolarization of the muscle cells takes place, resulting in contraction of the muscles (Fig. 2.9).

2.2.3 Central Nervous System

The CNS includes the **brain** and **spinal cord**. Both are surrounded by bones (skull and spinal column, respectively) and three connective tissue membranes (**meninges**) and "float" in a clear fluid, the cerebrospinal fluid (CSF).

The outer meninx is called **dura mater** (meninx fibrosa or pachymeninx) and consists of two layers. The space between the dura and the bone is termed the epidural space, but this space is present in the cranial region only under pathological conditions, e.g., epidural hemorrhage. Otherwise, the two dura layers adhere closely to the bone. At different locations, they separate in a physiological manner and form dural duplications, the **sinuses**, which act as venous blood vessels, collecting the blood and carrying it back toward the heart via the jugular veins (venae jugulares). In contrast to the cranium, an epidural space containing loose connective tissue, fat tissue, and vessels is physiologically present in the spinal region. The dura mater is supplied by sensory branches of the trigeminal nerve, the vagus nerve, and the spinal nerves and is thus algesic (pain sensitive).

The middle meninx, the **arachnoid mater** (spider web), is a thin membrane composed of fibrous tissue. It is connected to the inner meninx, called the **pia mater**, by fine filaments, the arachnoid trabeculae. The pia mater represents a soft

Fig. 2.8 Signal propagation in myelinated (top) and unmyelinated (bottom) nerve fibers (axons). © ARKANA Forum GmbH 2022. All Rights Reserved

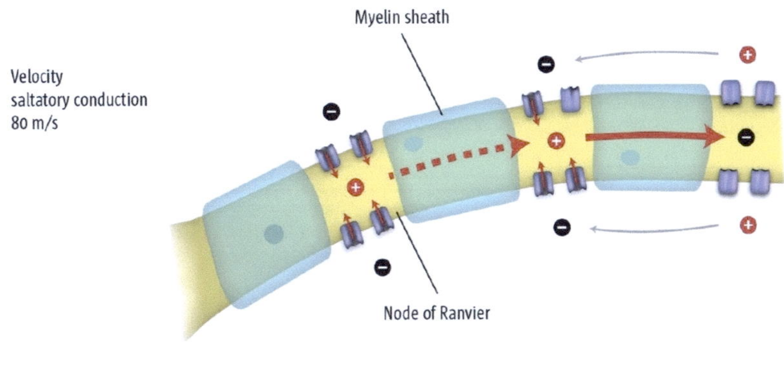

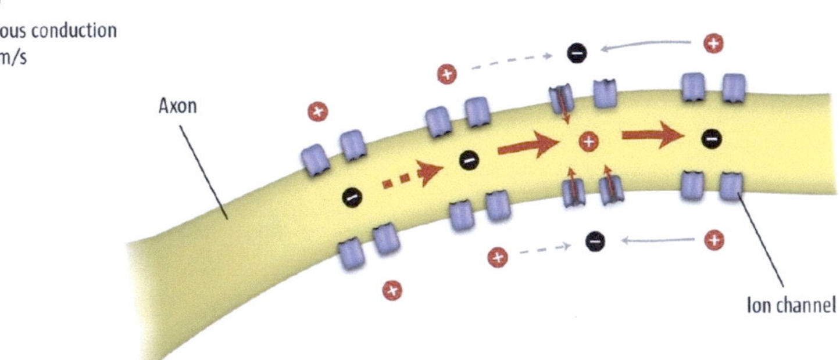

Fig. 2.9 The motor end plate. © ARKANA Forum GmbH 2022. All Rights Reserved

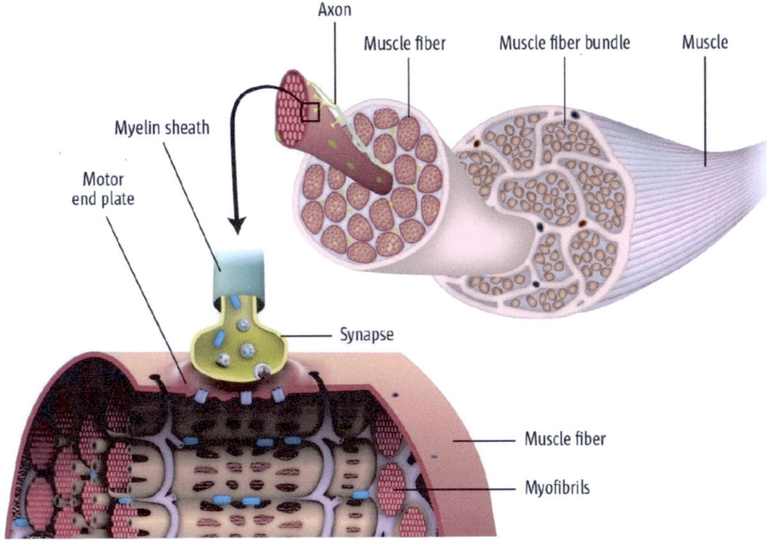

membrane that firmly adheres to the brain and spinal cord. It contains small arteries and veins (Figs. 2.10 and 2.11). Between the dura and arachnoid lies the very narrow subdural space. The space between the arachnoid and the pia mater is named the subarachnoid space. This is where the CSF circulates.

The **CSF** fills the internal (ventricular system, central canal) and external (cisterns, subarachnoid space) cavities of the brain and spinal cord. It is produced in the ventricles by small vascular convolutions called the choroid plexus, circulates throughout the ventricular system and the subarachnoid space (Fig. 2.12), and is reabsorbed via

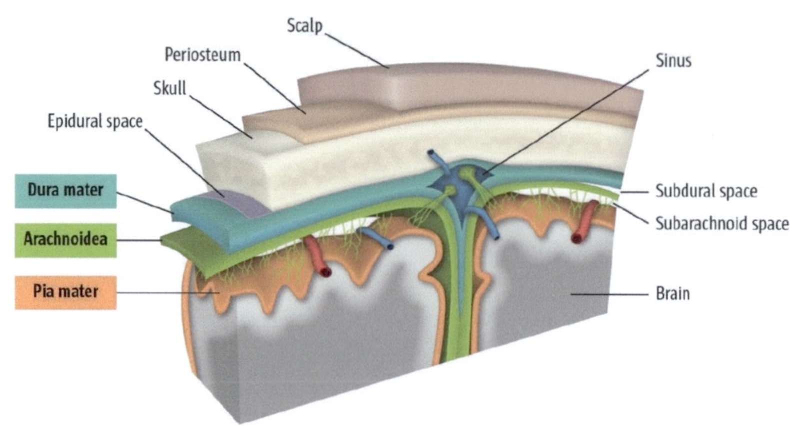

Fig. 2.10 Structure of the cranial meninges. © ARKANA Forum GmbH 2022. All Rights Reserved

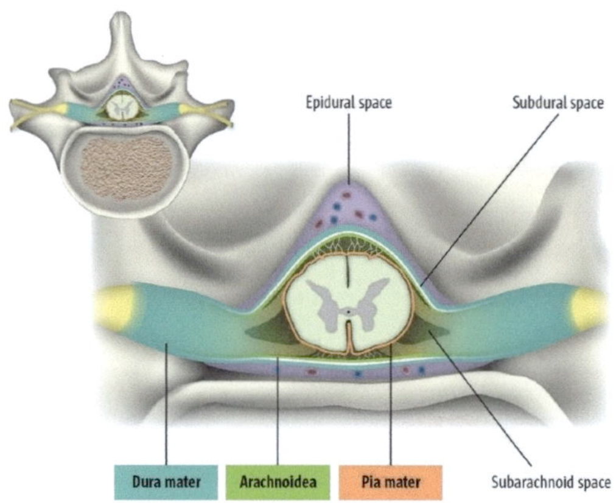

Fig. 2.11 Structure of the spinal meninges (meninges medullae spinalis). © ARKANA Forum GmbH 2022. All Rights Reserved

the arachnoid granulations (pacchionian granulations or bodies) in the area of the sinuses and through the cranial and spinal nerve sheaths. Its total volume is about 150 ml, and it is replaced several times a day by new production (about 300–500 ml per day). Its main function is that of a fluid buffer to protect the pressure- and shock-sensitive brain and spinal cord from mechanical injury.

Looking at a macroscopic section through the CNS, the brain and spinal cord each show a gray and a white layer (gray and white matter) (Figs. 2.13 and 2.14).

While the **gray matter** forms the surface in the brain (cerebral cortex), it is located inside the spinal cord. Viewed in transversal section, it appears there in the shape of an H or a butterfly (Fig. 2.14). In the brain, the **white matter** lies inside the gray cortex, whereas in the spinal cord it surrounds the gray matter.

The gray matter contains mainly the nerve cells with their dendrites and glial cells. The white matter consists primarily of myelinated nerve fibers. The white color is due to the high content of fatty substances in the myelin sheath.

2.2.3.1 Brain

In descending (cranial-caudal) order, the brain is anatomically divided into the following parts: **Telencephalon** (cerebrum), **diencephalon** (inter-brain), **mesencephalon** (midbrain), and **rhomben-cephalon** (rhomboid brain). The rhombencephalon includes the pons with transition into the medulla oblongata and the cerebellum (Fig. 2.15).

The **cerebrum** comprises the cerebral cortex, the subcortical white matter, and the basal ganglia. The basal ganglia represent a part of the motor system and consist of different nuclei (e.g., caudate nucleus, putamen, and globus pallidus) (Fig. 2.16). They are involved in complex circuits. Basal ganglia dysfunction can lead to severe neurological abnormalities, such as for example, Parkinson's syndrome.

The surface of the cerebrum is strongly folded in the form of convolutions (**gyri**). These gyri noticeably enlarge the surface of the brain. The gyri are separated from each other by fissures (**fissurae and sulci**).

The **cerebrum** is divided into two halves (**hemispheres**). Within the two hemispheres, different brain lobes (**lobi**) are distinguished (Figs. 2.17 and 2.18):

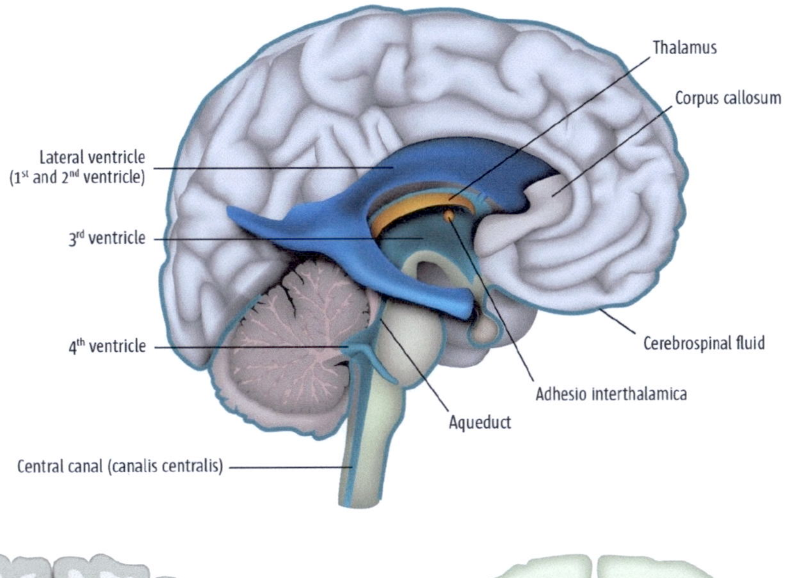

Fig. 2.12 Internal and external cerebrospinal fluid cavities. © ARKANA Forum GmbH 2022. All Rights Reserved

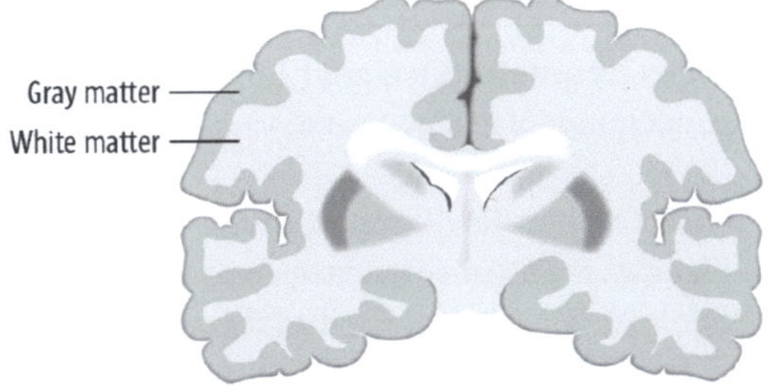

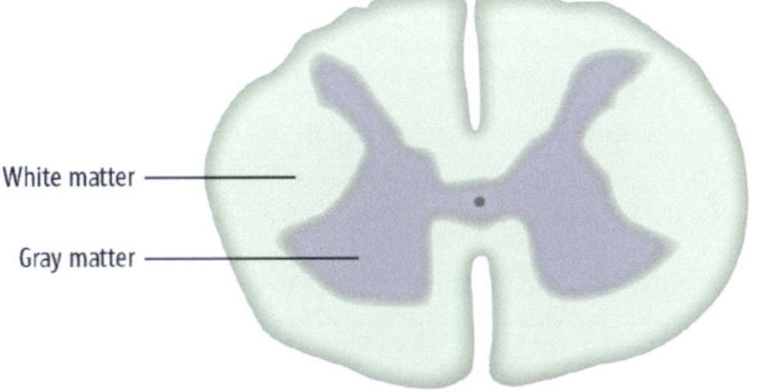

Fig. 2.13 Coronal section through the brain showing gray and white matter. © ARKANA Forum GmbH 2022. All Rights Reserved

Fig. 2.14 Transversal section through spinal cord with gray and white matter. © ARKANA Forum GmbH 2022. All Rights Reserved

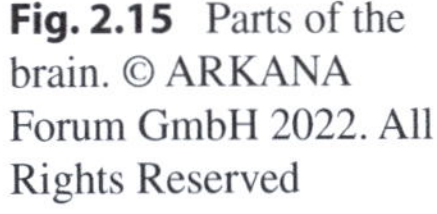

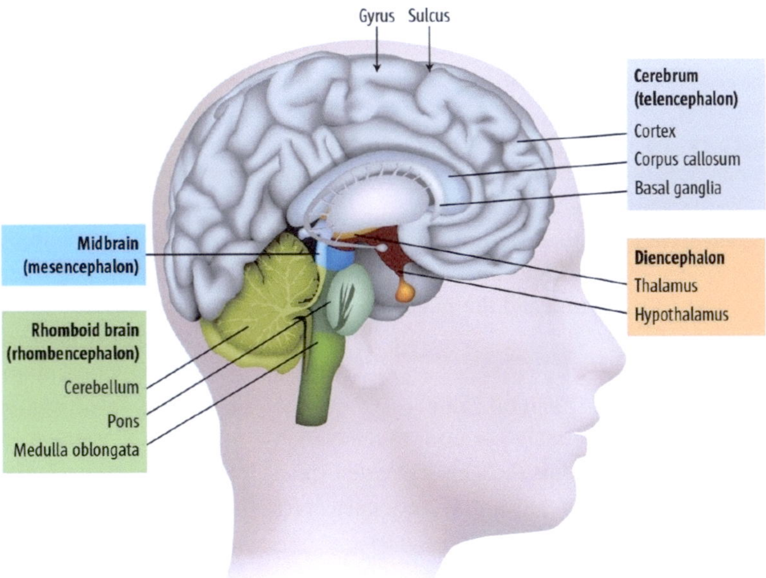

Fig. 2.15 Parts of the brain. © ARKANA Forum GmbH 2022. All Rights Reserved

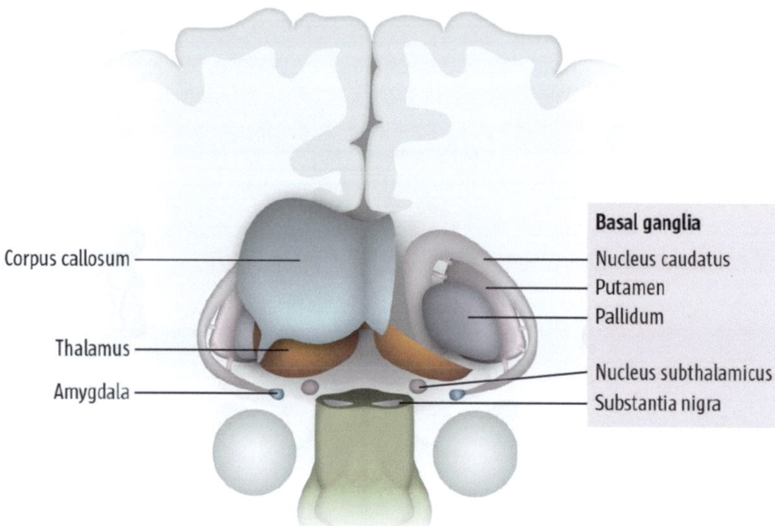

Fig. 2.16 Coronal section through the brain at the level of the basal ganglia. © ARKANA Forum GmbH 2022. All Rights Reserved

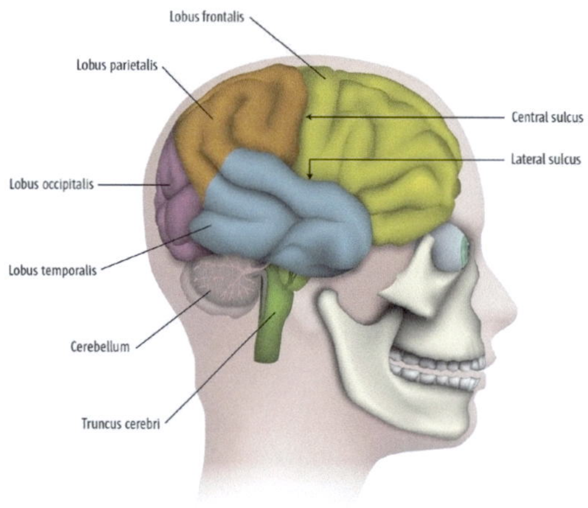

Fig. 2.17 The lobes (lobi) of the cerebrum. © ARKANA Forum GmbH 2022. All Rights Reserved

Lobus Frontalis (Frontal Lobe)

The frontal lobe includes the primary motor cortex (precentral gyrus) and the motor speech area (Broca's area).

Lobus Parietalis (Parietal Lobe)

It is located immediately posterior to the precentral gyrus and contains the sensory cortex (postcentral gyrus). The precentral and postcentral gyri are separated by the central sulcus.

Lobus Occipitalis (Occipital Lobe)

The occipital lobe contains the visual cortex.

Lobus Temporalis (Temporal Lobe)

It includes the sensory language area (Wernicke's area), which is responsible for language comprehension, the primary auditory cortical fields (Heschl's transverse gyri), and the hippocampal formation, which is relevant for memory functions.

Both the motor and sensory cortex are assigned to specific parts of the body in the periphery (**somatotopic organization**). This "functional map" is called **homunculus** ("little man") (Fig. 2.19). Knowledge of this somatotopic organization of the motor and sensory cortex is of particular importance for the neurosurgeon and the monitoring team.

What is particularly remarkable regarding the **somatotopic organization** is that the size of the cortical area does not correlate with the size of the peripheral body part it represents. Rather, the size of the cortical area in the homunculus, i.e., the number of neurons, depends on the tasks assigned to it. In terms of the motor system, this means that the number of neurons in the motor cortex depends on the precision of the corresponding body part required for movement. For

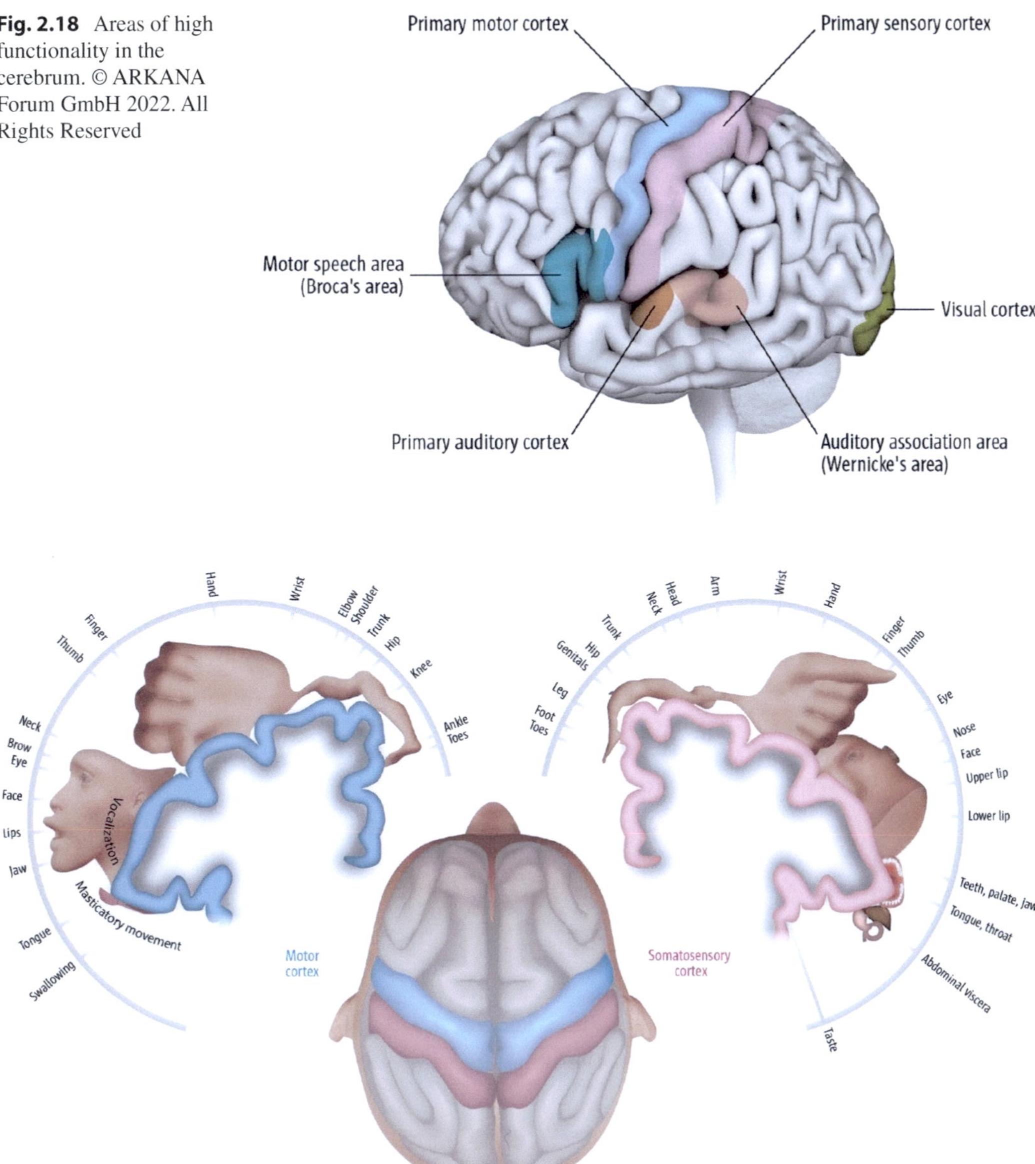

Fig. 2.18 Areas of high functionality in the cerebrum. © ARKANA Forum GmbH 2022. All Rights Reserved

Fig. 2.19 Motor homunculus (left), somatosensory homunculus (right). © ARKANA Forum GmbH 2022. All Rights Reserved

example, large cortical areas are available for muscles that are responsible for speech formation or facial expressions. They are thus represented oversized in the homunculus. In the sensory cortex, the necessary number of neurons depends on the density of the sensory receptors in the different body regions (e.g., the skin, the internal organs, or the muscles and joints). Particularly sensitive body regions such as the lips, tongue, and soles of the feet are therefore prominent in the sensory cortex of the homunculus. This somatotopic representation is not only found in the cortex but is also maintained throughout the pyramidal tract.

The **cerebellum** is located in the posterior fossa and is separated from the cerebrum by a thick layer of the dura mater, the tentorium cerebelli. Like the cerebrum, the cerebellum contains gray matter on its outside and white matter at its inside. The cerebellum is composed of the two cerebellar hemispheres and the cerebellar vermis (vermis cerebelli). It is connected to the brainstem by the superior, middle, and inferior cerebellar peduncles. The convolutions of the cerebellum are much smaller than in the cerebrum and are called folia. The cerebellum represents the most important center for the coordination of movement and fine motor skills.

The **diencephalon** lies immediately below the cerebrum. It encloses the third ventricle on both sides and is composed of the thalamus, epithalamus with epiphysis, subthalamus, metathalamus, and hypothalamus. Caudally, the diencephalon merges into the midbrain. The largest portion of the diencephalon (about 4/5) is made up by the thalamus, which serves as a switching and filtering station of ascending signals from the spinal cord, brainstem, and cerebellum before they ascend further into the cortex to become conscious. The thalamus is therefore also referred to as the "gateway to consciousness." It contains numerous nuclear areas and both afferent (ascending) and efferent (descending) connections. The diencephalon additionally contains centers for olfactory, visual, and auditory functions, as well as centers for surface and depth perception and the emotional processing of sensory information.

The **brainstem** consists of the midbrain (mesencephalon), the pons, and the medulla oblongata. It can be understood as a large signal highway on which all ascending and descending pathways run. In the corresponding nuclear areas, these signals are partially switched. In addition, the brainstem contains an essential regulatory center for vital body functions such as respiration, cardiac activity, and circulation, as well as the nuclei of cranial nerves III–XII, furthermore, a nuclear area which macroscopically appears dark due to its high content of iron and melanin, called substantia nigra. The loss of nerve cells in the substantia nigra leads to Parkinson's disease.

The **cranial nerves** (Fig. 2.20) are numbered from I to XII according to the order of their exit from the CNS. The first two cranial nerves—the olfactory nerve and the optic nerve—arise from the cerebrum and are not nerves in the true sense. Both show structural characteristics of the central nervous system and represent therefore overlaying parts of the telencephalon. Cranial nerves III to XII arise from the brainstem (Fig. 2.21).

I. *N. olfactorius* (**Olfactory Nerve**)

It transmits olfactory sensations to the processing centers of the telencephalon (corpus amygdaloideum, gyrus parahippocampalis, etc.).

II. *N. opticus* (**Optic Nerve**)

Signals received by the eyes are transmitted through the optic nerve. The fibers receiving impulses from the nasal half of the visual fields of both eyes cross to the opposite side in the so-called optic chiasm (chiasma opticum). Further, the signals are transmitted via the tractus opticus to the visual cortex.

III. *N. oculomotorius* (**Oculomotor Nerve**)

Cranial nerves III, IV, and VI are involved in eye movements. The oculomotor nerve supplies both the internal and four of the six external eye muscles (M. rectus medialis, M. rectus superior, M. rectus inferior, M. obliquus inferior) and the eyelid lifter (M. levator palpebrae). The internal muscles are responsible for pupil reactions and adjusting (accommodating) the eye to different object distances. The external eye muscles move the eyeball.

IV. *N. trochlearis* (**Trochlear Nerve**)

Like the oculomotor nerve, this is a motor eye nerve. It innervates the superior oblique muscle (M. obliquus superior) which lowers the eye and rolls it inward.

V. *N. trigeminus* (**Trigeminal Nerve**)

The trigeminal nerve is a mixed nerve with sensory and motor fibers. The sensory fibers form its main part and transmit sensory stimuli from the face. The sensory portion of the trigeminal nerve is divided into three branches: The ophthalmic nerve

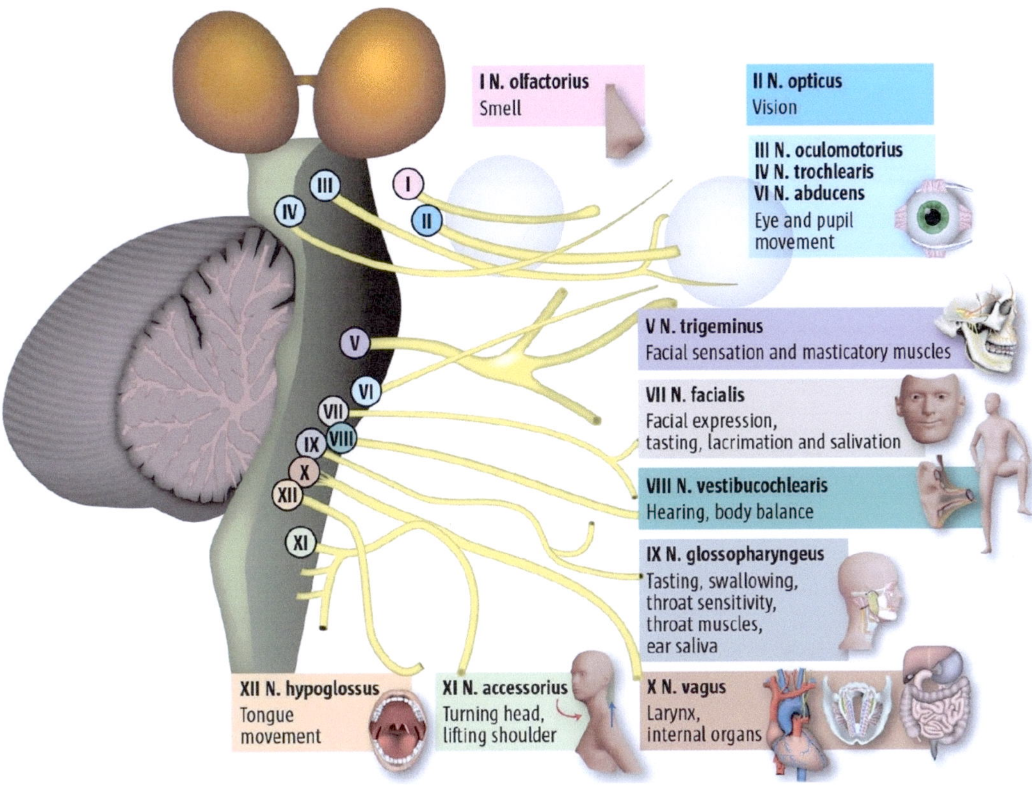

Fig. 2.20 Illustration of the twelve cranial nerves and their functions. © ARKANA Forum GmbH 2022. All Rights Reserved

supplies the area above the eye, the maxillary nerve concerns the midface, and the mandibular nerve covers the mandible. The motor fibers innervate the masticatory muscles.

VI. *N. abducens* (**Abducens Nerve**)

Besides the oculomotor nerve, this is the only cranial nerve that leaves the brainstem at its frontal aspect. The abducens nerve controls the lateral rectus muscle (M. rectus lateralis) and is responsible for the outward movement of the eye.

VII. *N. facialis* (**Facial Nerve**)

Its main function is to innervate the facial muscles and the stapes muscle (M. stapedius) in the middle ear. A small portion of the nerve (N. intermedius) contains taste fibers of the anterior two-thirds of the tongue.

VIII. *N. vestibulocochlearis* (**Vestibulocochlear Nerve**)

It is responsible for the transmission of acoustic signals and for body balance.

IX. *N. glossopharyngeus* (**Glossopharyngeal Nerve**)

It supplies the pharyngeal muscles and is thus an important nerve for swallowing (deglutition). In addition, the glossopharyngeal nerve transmits the signals for the taste of the posterior third of the tongue.

X. *N. vagus* (**Vagus Nerve**)

As the main parasympathetic nerve, it regulates functions of the internal organs during the resting phases of the body. One branch of the vagus nerve, the recurrent nerve (N. laryngeus recurrens) is responsible for the movement of the vocal cords.

XI. *N. accessorius* (**Accessory Nerve**)

It originates for the most part from the spinal cord, runs parallel to the spinal cord into the skull, and leaves the skull again via foramina at its base. Together

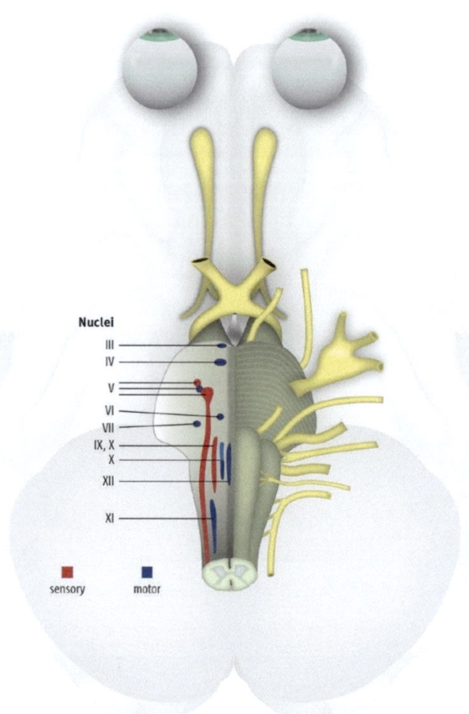

Fig. 2.21 Location of the cranial nerve nuclei and exit sites of the cranial nerves from the brain. © ARKANA Forum GmbH 2022. All Rights Reserved

with cranial nerves IX and X, it is involved in swallowing. Motorically, it supplies the sternocleidomastoid and trapezius muscles (M. sternocleidomastoideus and M. trapezius).

XII. *N. hypoglossus* **(Hypoglossal Nerve)**

It controls the movement of the tongue.

2.2.3.2 Blood Supply and Venous Drainage of the Brain

Blood supply to the brain is accomplished by two paired arteries supplying the right and left hemispheres, respectively: the internal carotid and vertebral arteries (Ae. carotides internae and Ae. vertebrales). The branches of the internal carotid artery are mainly responsible for supplying structures in the anterior and middle cranial fossae and smaller portions of the posterior cranial fossa. The branches of the vertebral artery supply the most parts of the posterior fossa and some portions of the mesial temporal lobe. Both circuits connect at the brain base to form a vascular ring, called circle of Willis (circulus arteriosus Willisii). Thus, in the event of occlusion of one vessel, the affected part of the brain can be supplied to a certain extent by the other circuit (Fig. 2.22).

The **venous blood** enters the large sinuses via deep and superficial cerebral veins and returns to the heart mainly via the internal jugular veins. Since the sinuses consist of duplications of the dura mater, the configuration of their walls is different from that of other venous vessels in the body (Fig. 2.23).

2.2.3.3 Spinal Cord

The spinal cord (Medulla spinalis) transmits signals from and to the processing centers in the brain. Similar to the brain, it is surrounded by bone, the spinal column, and the three-layered spinal meninges (meninges medullae spinalis). The outer aspect of the spinal cord consists of white matter which surrounds the gray matter lying inside.

The bilateral **spinal nerves** attach to the spinal cord by anterior and posterior roots, respectively. The posterior roots transmit afferent signals to the spinal cord. From here, the stimuli are sent to processing centers in the brain. The anterior roots conduct efferent signals to the periphery. Both motor and sensory pathways follow a precisely defined topography within the spinal cord (Fig. 2.24).

The lower end of the spinal cord, the **conus medullaris**, is located at the level of the third lumbar vertebra at birth and migrates upward as part of longitudinal growth. In adults, it is located at the level of the thoracolumbar junction (T12/L1). From there, the nerve fibers form the **cauda equina** before they leave the spine as spinal nerves in the lower vertebral segments. At all levels, the spinal nerves exit the spinal column through intervertebral foramina (foramina intervertebralia). Table 2.1 presents the assignment of the spinal nerves to the corresponding segments of the spinal column. Figure 2.25 illustrates the segmental exits of the spinal nerves from the spinal cord and the spinal column.

Fig. 2.22 Brain territories supplied by the large vessels. © ARKANA Forum GmbH 2022. All Rights Reserved

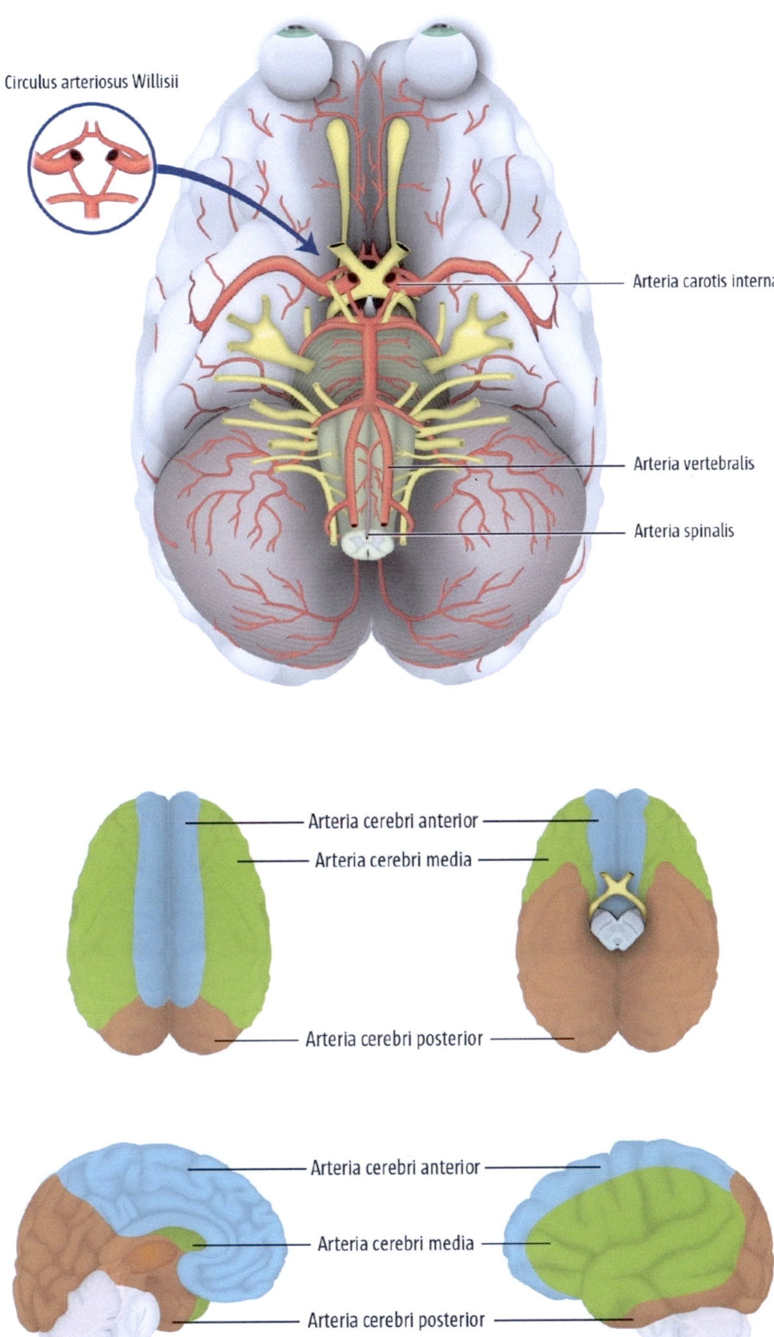

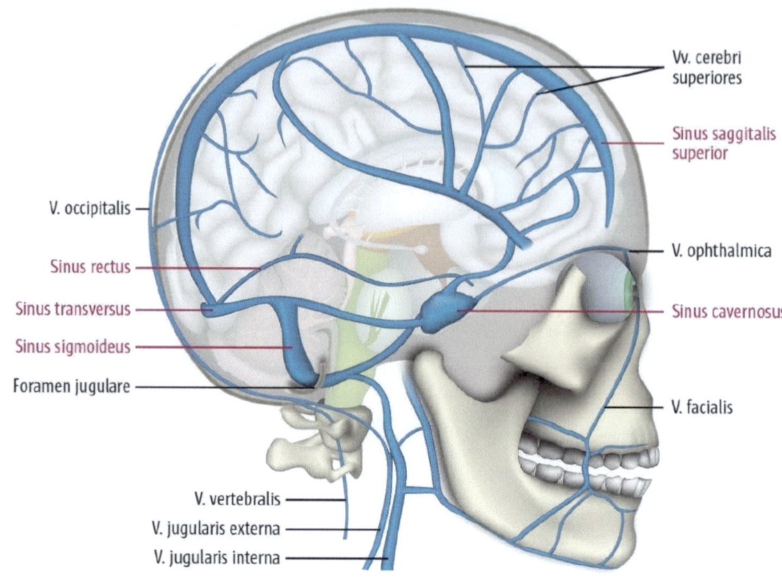

Fig. 2.23 Venous drainage of the brain. © ARKANA Forum GmbH 2022. All Rights Reserved

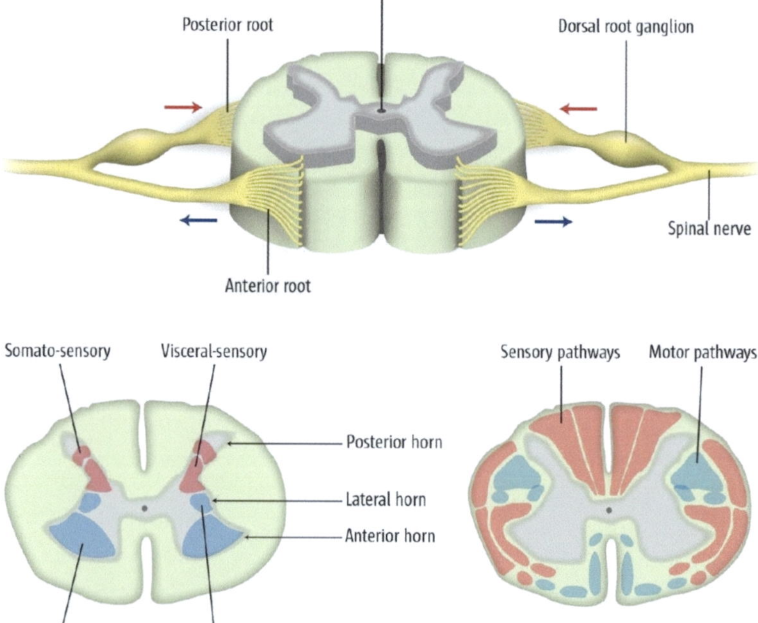

Fig. 2.24 Structure of the spinal cord. © ARKANA Forum GmbH 2022. All Rights Reserved

2.2.3.4 Blood Supply and Venous Drainage of the Spinal Cord

Arterial blood supply to the anterior part of the spinal cord is provided by the anterior spinal artery (A. spinalis anterior), which arises directly from the aorta. The dorsal part of the spinal cord is supplied by segmental vessels, the posterolateral spinal arteries (Ae. spinales posterolaterales) (Fig. 2.26). The spinal arteries form multiple anastomoses among each other.

Venous drainage of the spinal cord occurs through an epidural venous network which drains

Table 2.1 Spinal nerves and spinal segments

Spinal cord	Spinal column
8 pairs of cervical nerves (C1–C8)	7 cervical vertebrae (C1–C7)
12 pairs of thoracic nerves (T1–T12)	12 thoracic vertebrae (T1–T12)
5 pairs of lumbar nerves (L1–L5)	5 lumbar vertebrae (L1–L5)
5 pairs of sacral nerves (S1–S5)	5 sacral vertebrae (fused into the sacrum during development)

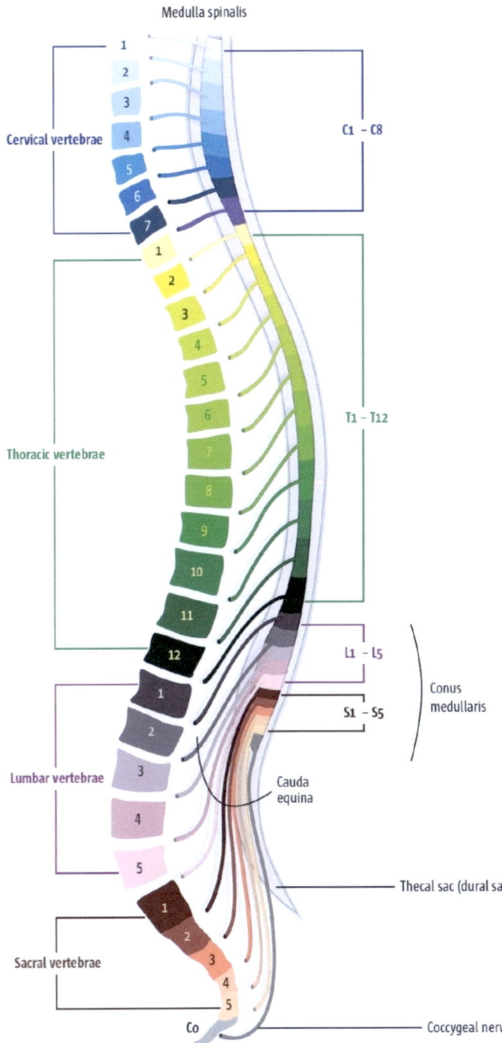

Fig. 2.25 Segmental exits of the spinal nerves from the spinal cord and the spinal column. © ARKANA Forum GmbH 2022. All Rights Reserved

into the epidural venous plexus, the anterior and posterior spinal veins (V. spinalis anterior, V. spinalis posterior), and from there into the large body veins (Fig. 2.27).

2.2.4 Peripheral Nervous System

The nerves leaving the spinal cord form the PNS. Microscopically, they consist mainly of the axons of the nerve cells, each surrounded by a myelin sheath. In the PNS, the myelin sheaths are formed by Schwann cells. It is supposed that the different composition of myelin in the central and peripheral nervous systems is partly responsible for the fact that the PNS, unlike the CNS, remains capable of regeneration after injury. The individual nerve fibers are grouped together by connective tissue to form nerve bundles, which in turn join to a peripheral nerve.

Of the **31 pairs of spinal nerves**, the 12 pairs of thoracic nerves (T1–T12) run to their target structures as individual nerves. The remaining nerves of the cervical, lumbar, and sacral spine intermingle shortly after leaving the spinal column to form a **plexus**, namely the cervical plexus, the brachial plexus (Fig. 2.28), the lumbar plexus, and the sacral plexus. The latter two are often summarized to the lumbosacral plexus (Fig. 2.29; Table 2.2). The formation of the plexus results in a multisegmental innervation of individual muscles. At the same time, some of the spinal nerves also innervate several muscles.

The **skin** is innervated via the individual spinal cord segments. The skin fields assigned to the respective spinal cord segments are called **dermatomes** (Fig. 2.30).

2.2.5 Somatic/Voluntary Nervous System

The somatic nervous system, also called voluntary nervous system, consists of parts of the CNS and PNS. It is responsible for the conscious per-

Fig. 2.26 Arterial blood supply of the spinal cord. © ARKANA Forum GmbH 2022. All Rights Reserved

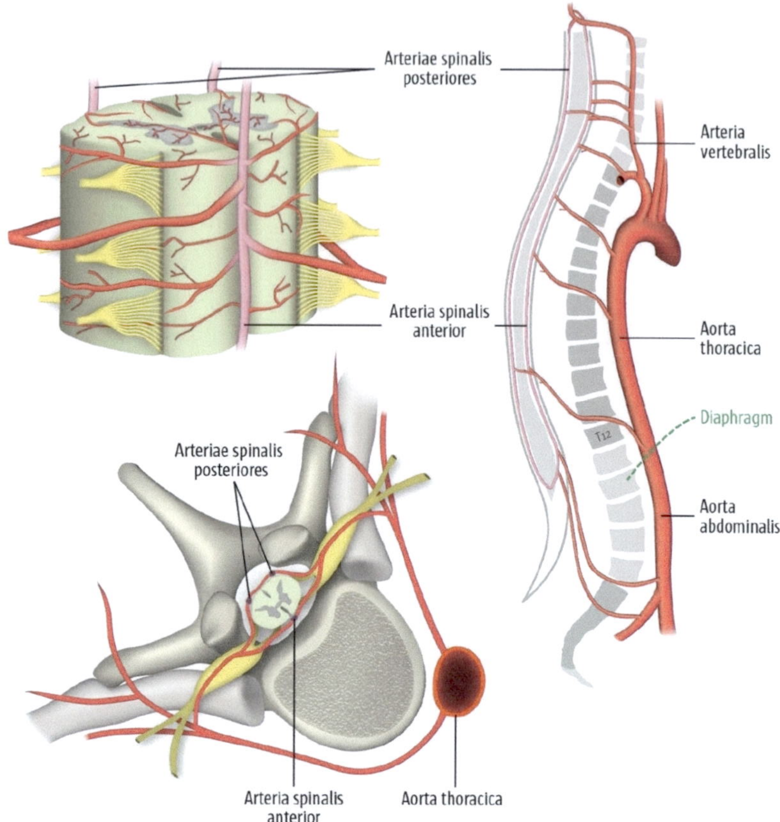

Fig. 2.27 Venous drainage of the spinal cord. © ARKANA Forum GmbH 2022. All Rights Reserved

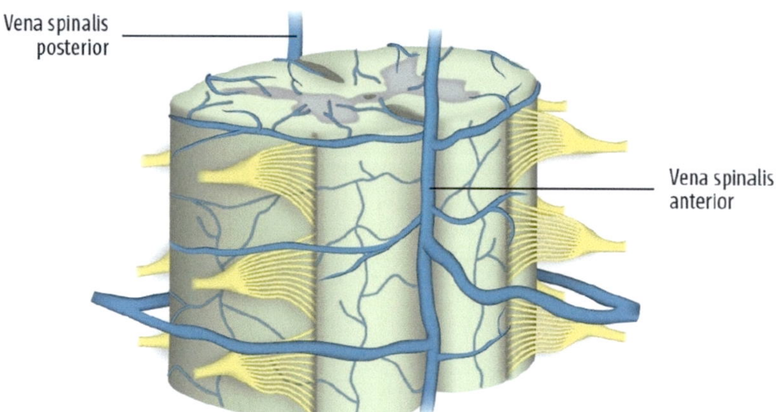

ception of external stimuli and for voluntary actions (e.g., via the muscles). Two systems are to be distinguished: the motor and the sensory system.

2.2.5.1 The Motor System

The motor impulses for voluntary movements are largely generated in the precentral gyrus. The most important motor pathway of the CNS is the

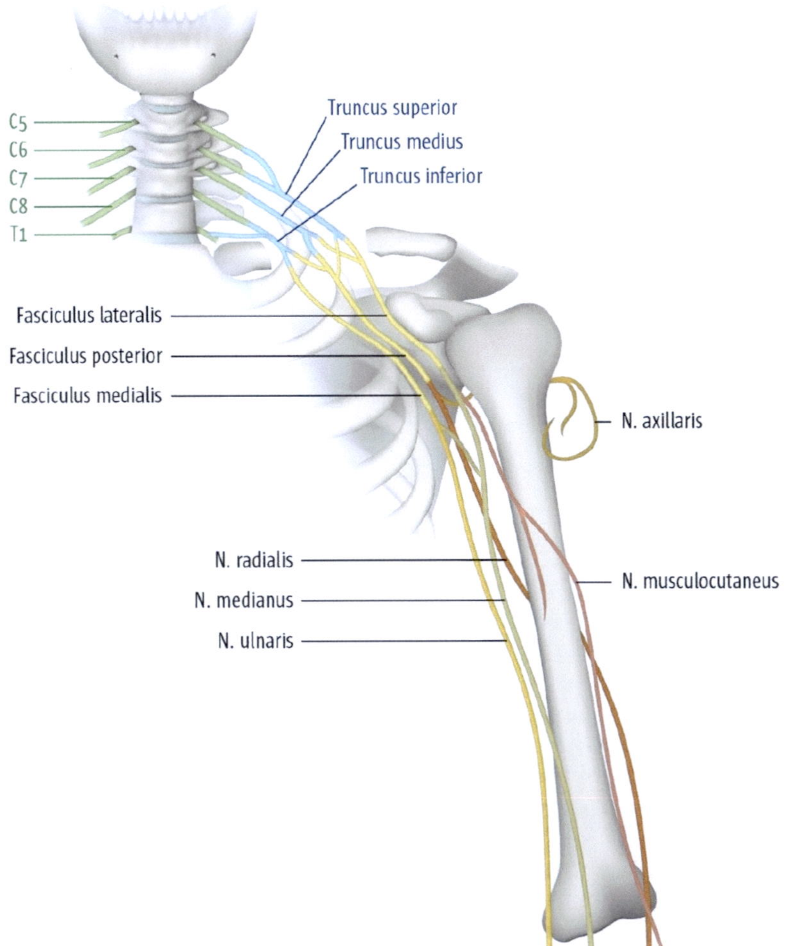

Fig. 2.28 The brachial plexus. © ARKANA Forum GmbH 2022. All Rights Reserved

corticospinal tract, also known as the **pyramidal tract**. Starting from the **first motoneuron**, the impulses are transmitted to the anterior horn of the spinal cord. The pyramidal tract crosses to the opposite side at the level of the medulla oblongata. At the anterior horn, switching to the **second motoneuron** (α-motoneuron) takes place. The signals leave the CNS through the anterior roots of the spinal nerves and reach the motor end plate via the peripheral nerves. This is where the stimulus is transmitted to the muscles (Fig. 2.31).

To enable an extremely rapid response, afferent stimuli can be switched directly to the motor system via peripheral circuits without reaching the brain. These are **reflexes** that are processed in the spinal cord and produce an immediate response. Reflexes occur unconsciously and cannot be influenced. A distinction is made between monosynaptic and polysynaptic reflexes.

The simplest **monosynaptic reflex** is the stretch reflex, or more accurately muscle stretch reflex (Fig. 2.32). **Polysynaptic reflexes** serve for protection and escape. For example, if a hot surface is touched with the hand, not only a single muscle is activated, but the whole arm is

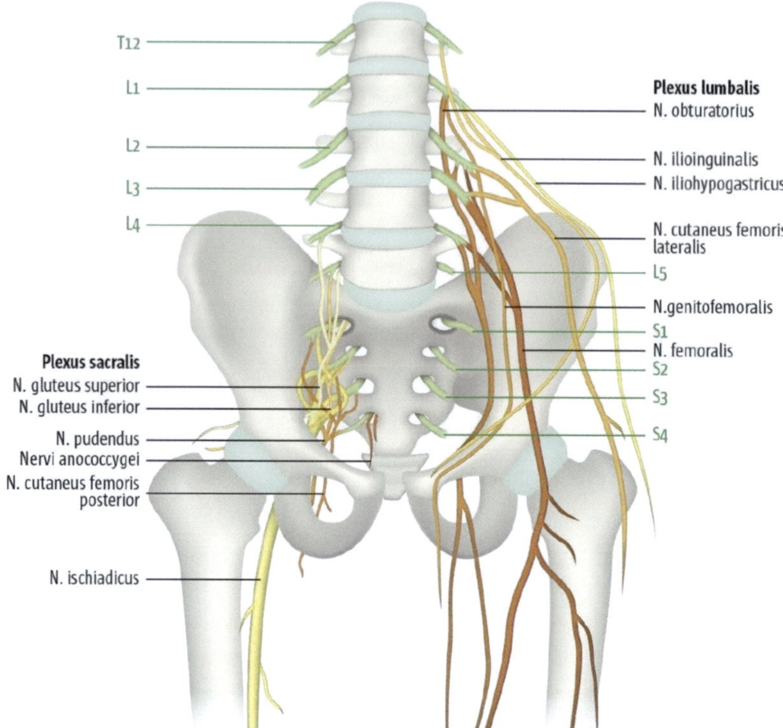

Fig. 2.29 The lumbosacral plexus. © ARKANA Forum GmbH 2022. All Rights Reserved

Table 2.2 Plexus and associated spinal nerves

Plexus	Spinal nerves
Cervical plexus	C1–C4
Brachial plexus	C5–T1 with proportions of C 4
Lumbar plexus	L1–L3 with proportions of L 4
Sacral plexus	L5–S5 with proportions of L 4

immediately withdrawn. Other examples of polysynaptic reflexes are the sucking reflex in newborns, the corneal reflex, and the bulbocavernosus reflex.

2.2.5.2 The Sensory System

The sensory system is responsible for perception and processing of both stimuli from the environment and from inside the body. One of the most important sensory pathways is the **dorsal column-medial lemniscus pathway** or **posterior column-medial lemniscus pathway** in the spinal cord. Through this pathway, information on tactile discrimination and proprioception from the periphery reaches the CNS. The **spinotha-** **lamic tract** consisting of two adjacent **anterior and lateral pathways** carries information about pain, temperature, pressure, and crude touch.

Signal processing in the sensory system is as follows: Receptors, e.g., in the skin, register information and pass it on to afferent nerve fibers. The cell bodies of the afferent nerve fibers are located in the dorsal root ganglia immediately before they continue to reach the spinal cord. From here, signals on tactile discrimination and proprioception enter the CNS without switching (**first neuron**) and ascend in the dorsal column of the spinal cord on the same side. Switching to the **second neuron** and crossing to the contralateral side occurs at the level of the brainstem. Information about pain, temperature, pressure, and crude touch switch to the second neuron and cross to the contralateral side directly at the level of entry into the spinal cord, and signals ascend in the opposite anterolateral pathways. Another switch of all sensory information to the **third neuron** occurs in the thalamus before reaching the cortical centers in the postcentral gyrus (Fig. 2.33).

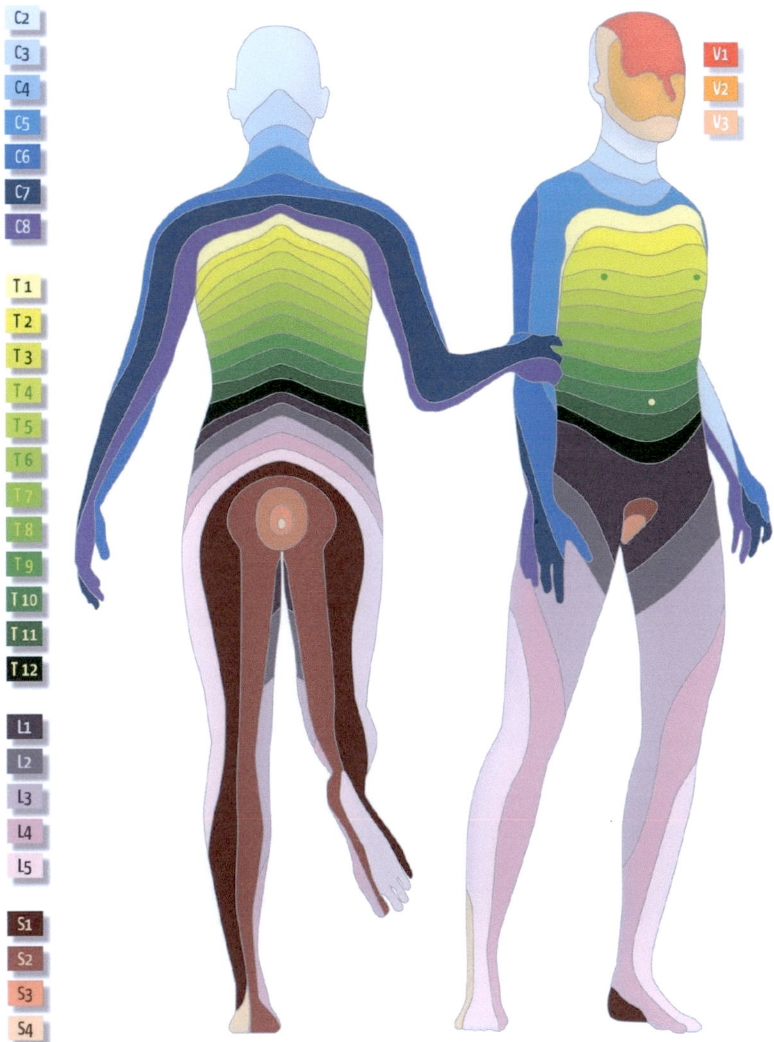

Fig. 2.30 Spinal cord segments and dermatomes. © ARKANA Forum GmbH 2022. All Rights Reserved

2.2.6 Vegetative/Autonomic Nervous System

The vegetative or autonomic nervous system works involuntarily (autonomously) and regulates vital functions such as breathing, circulation, digestion, and water balance. The efferent parts of the autonomic system are divided into sympathetic and parasympathetic fibers. While the neurons of the **sympathetic** system originate from the thoracolumbar spinal cord, part of the first neurons of the **parasympathetic** system arise from the nuclei of cranial nerves III, VII, IX, and X and another part from the sacral cauda equina. The sympathetic fibers join to the **sympathetic trunk** (truncus sympathicus) which runs parallel to the spinal cord (Fig. 2.34).

2.2.6.1 The Sympathetic System

The sympathetic system innervates smooth muscles of vessels, pupils, viscera, bladder, hair follicles, and various glands, as well as heart muscles. Its activation **prepares the body for escape**. That is, functions necessary for rapid energy gain, improved blood supply, and increase

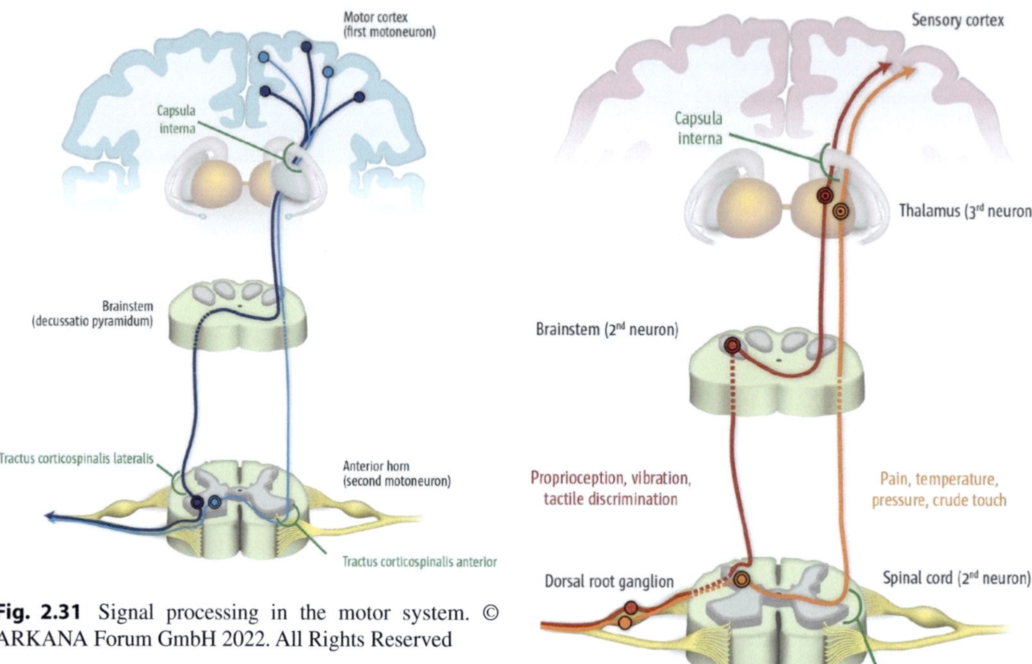

Fig. 2.31 Signal processing in the motor system. © ARKANA Forum GmbH 2022. All Rights Reserved

Fig. 2.33 Signal processing in the sensory system. © ARKANA Forum GmbH 2022. All Rights Reserved

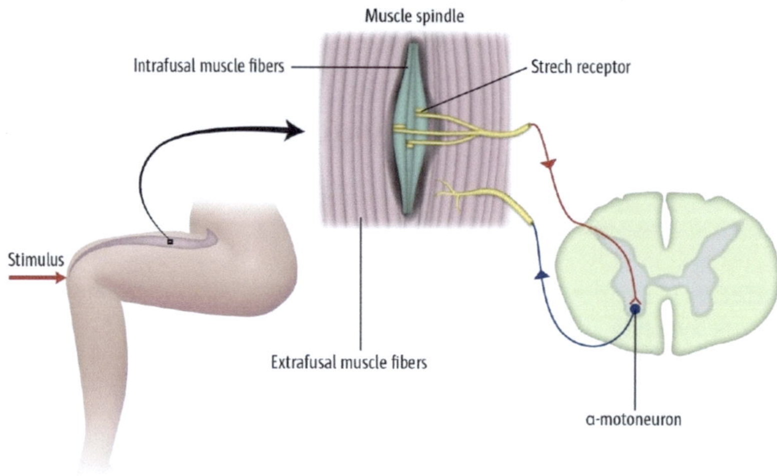

Fig. 2.32 Schematic illustration of a monosynaptic muscle stretch reflex (patellar tendon reflex). The stretching of the intrafusal muscle fibers of the quadriceps femoris muscle by the stimulus is registered by muscle spindles. An action potential is transmitted to the posterior horn of the spinal cord. Here, the signal switches to the α-motoneuron of the same muscle. This results in a contraction of the extrafusal muscle fibers. © ARKANA Forum GmbH 2022. All Rights Reserved

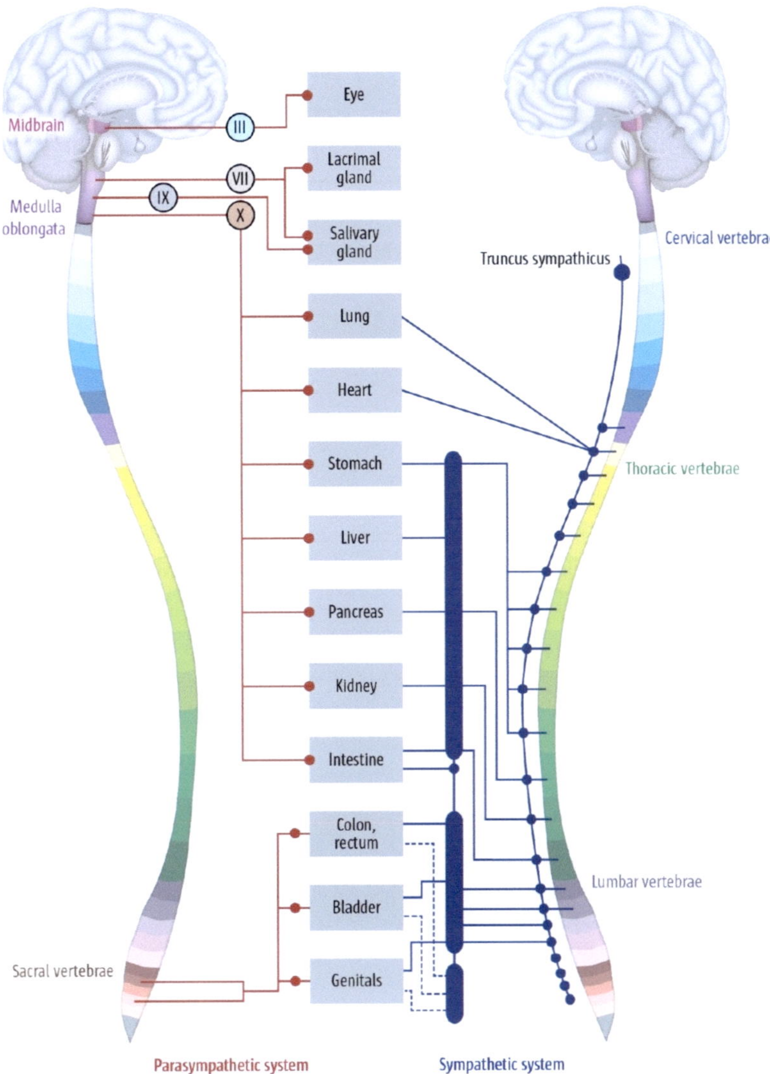

Fig. 2.34 Overview of the vegetative/autonomic nervous system. © ARKANA Forum GmbH 2022. All Rights Reserved

of the ability to perceive the environment are activated. Constriction of the vascular walls increases blood pressure. At the same time, the smooth muscles of the viscera (e.g., bladder, intestines, etc.) are inhibited. Reduction in the activity of the sympathetic system expands the vessel walls again.

2.2.6.2 The Parasympathetic System

The parasympathetic nervous system controls in particular the **activity of the internal organs**. It inhibits the cardiac action, lowers blood pressure, and increases the activity of the intestines and glands. In the sacral area, it causes the bladder

and intestines to empty and regulates sexual function. The heart, lungs, and intestines down to the last third of the transverse colon are supplied by the parasympathetic fibers running in the vagus nerve. The rectum, urinary bladder, and genital organs are innervated by the sacral parasympathetic fibers.

2.3   The Musculoskeletal System

The musculoskeletal system, also known as the locomotor system, provides stability and movement of the body and protects vital organs. It comprises two main components: The passive and the active system.

The **passive musculoskeletal system** or supporting apparatus consists of the skeleton with its various components such as bones, cartilage, joints, intervertebral discs, and ligaments (Fig. 2.35).

The **active musculoskeletal system** comprises skeletal muscles, which can move individual parts of the skeleton against each other or fix them in a specific position. In addition to the muscles, it also includes fasciae, tendons, tendon sheaths, and synovial bursae of the joints (Figs. 2.36 and 2.37).

The muscular system is controlled by the nervous system although some muscles such as the cardiac muscles can be completely autonomous. Movements can be voluntary or involuntary. For these reasons, there are three distinct **types of muscles** (Fig. 2.38).

Smooth muscles: Smooth muscles are controlled by the autonomic nervous system. They require low energy to maintain tension (tone) and form the muscle walls of the internal organs,

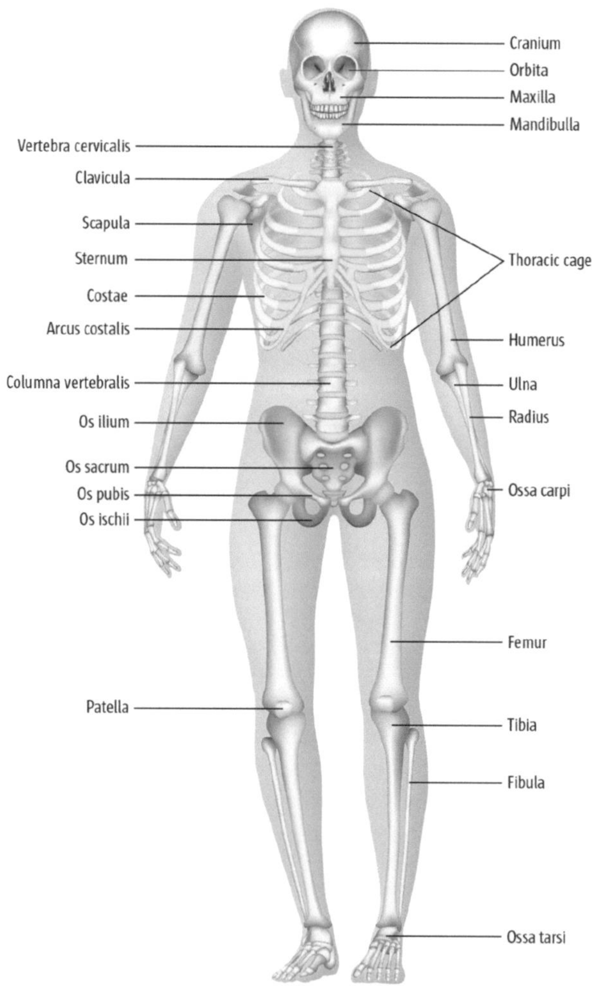

Fig. 2.35 Overview of the human skeleton in front view (passive musculoskeletal system). © ARKANA Forum GmbH 2022. All Rights Reserved

Fig. 2.36 Overview of the human muscular system in front view (active musculoskeletal system). © ARKANA Forum GmbH 2022. All Rights Reserved

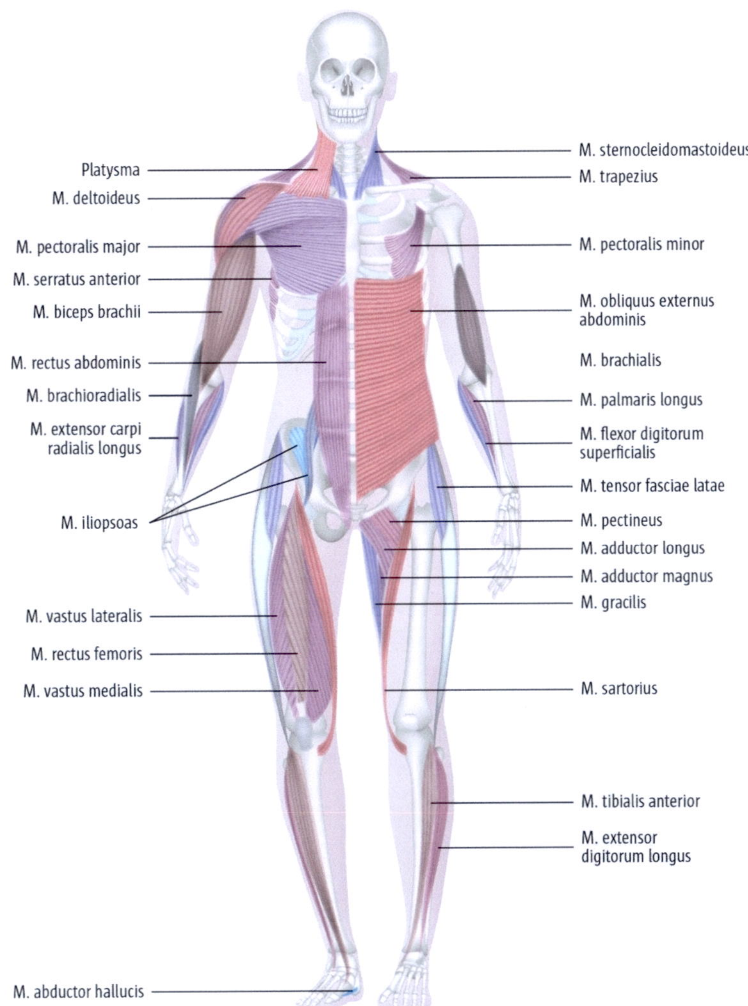

including the gastrointestinal tract, the urogenital tract, the bronchial system, and the vessels.

Skeletal muscles: Skeletal muscles owe their striated structure to different filaments, which facilitate a fast conversion of an impulse into a movement. They build up the muscles of the active musculoskeletal system, but are also found in the tongue, pharynx, larynx, and esophagus. The skeletal muscles are mainly controlled voluntarily by the somatic nervous system.

Cardiac muscles: Cardiac muscles represent a special type of striated muscles, which are controlled by the autonomic nervous system, but can also activate themselves, as they have their own conduction system, called the cardiac conduction system.

Fig. 2.37 Overview of the human muscular system in rear view (active musculoskeletal system). © ARKANA Forum GmbH 2022. All Rights Reserved

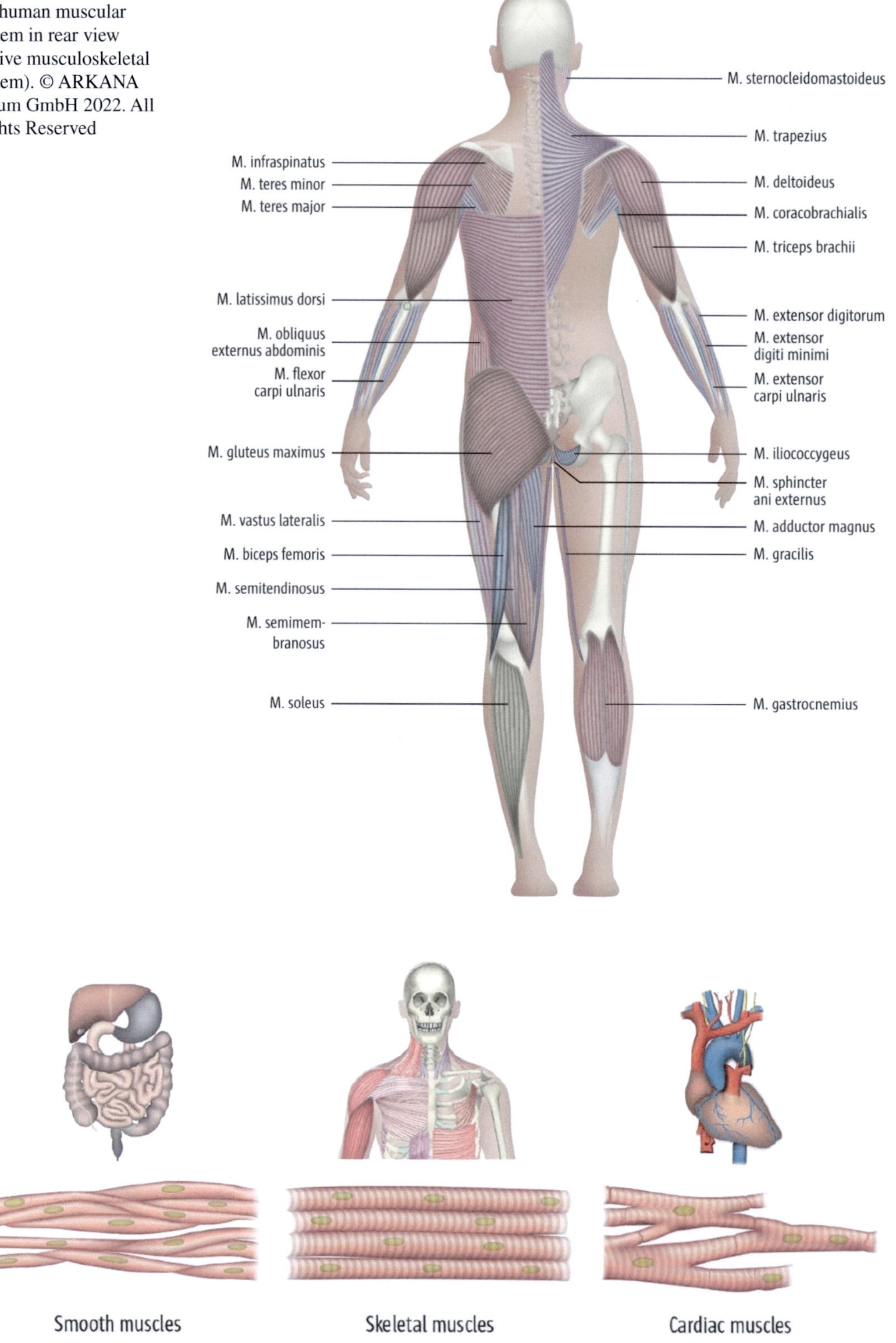

Fig. 2.38 Different types of muscles. © ARKANA Forum GmbH 2022. All Rights Reserved

2.4   Test Questions

1. Into which parts can the nervous system generally be divided and what functions do they each have?
2. Name the individual structures of a nerve cell (neuron) in the Fig. 2.39 (numbers 1–7) and describe the signal processing represented by the red arrows.
3. What are the functions of the glial cells surrounding the nerve cells?
4. What is a synapse and what is its function?
5. Describe the different phases of the action potential on the basis of the Fig. 2.40 and the role of sodium and potassium.
6. What does saltatory conduction mean and which structures in the axons are important in this process?
7. What is the motor end plate?
8. Name the different meninges and spaces lying in between using the illustration. What is meant by sinuses? (See Fig. 2.41).
9. What is the cerebrospinal fluid? Describe the circulation of the cerebrospinal fluid.
10. What is meant by gray and white matter? Where is it located in the brain and spinal cord, respectively?
11. Name the different parts of the brain on the basis of the illustration (See Fig. 2.42).
12. Name the different lobes of the cerebrum and the most important functional areas in the Fig. 2.43. Describe the basic functions of these areas.
13. In which part of the brain is the thalamus located and what is its function?
14. Which parts make up the brain stem, and what essential functions do they represent?
15. Use the Fig. 2.44 to name the 12 cranial nerves and the most important function of each.
16. Which arteries supply the brain with blood? What is meant by the circulus arteriosus Willisii?
17. Describe the structure of the spinal cord and the organization of the spinal nerves.
18. Which arteries supply the spinal cord with blood?
19. What is meant by the term dermatome?
20. What is meant by the terms brachial plexus and lumbosacral plexus?

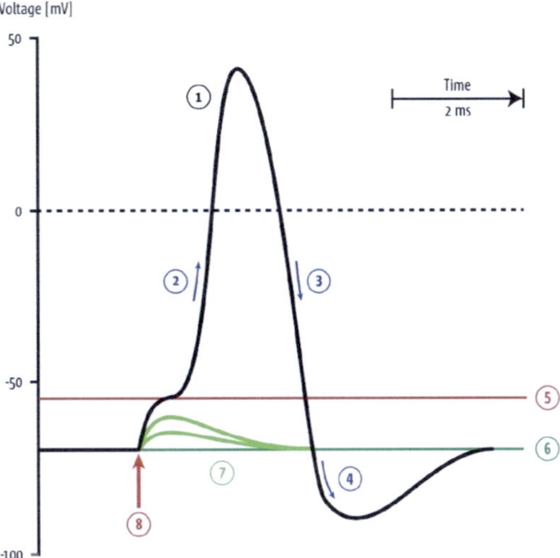

Fig. 2.40 Test question—Time course of an action potential. © ARKANA Forum GmbH 2022. All Rights Reserved

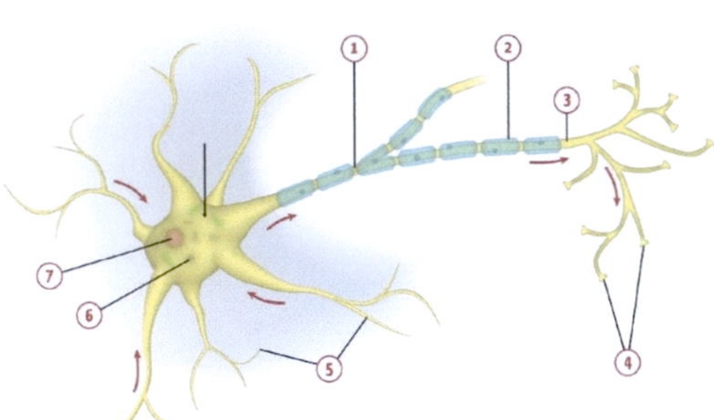

Fig. 2.39 Test question—Structure of a nerve cell (neuron). © ARKANA Forum GmbH 2022. All Rights Reserved

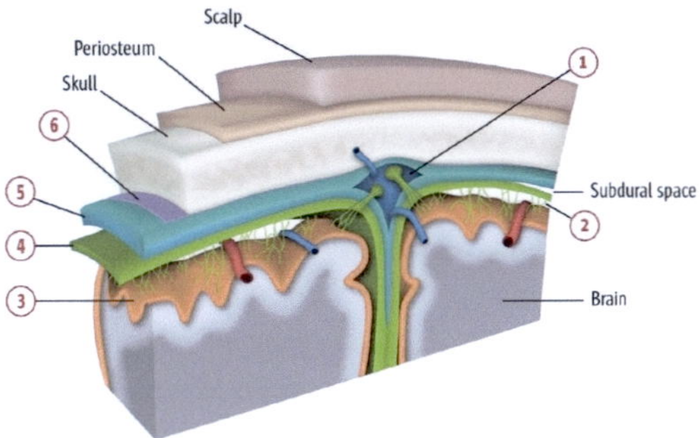

Fig. 2.41 Test question—Structure of the meninges. © ARKANA Forum GmbH 2022. All Rights Reserved

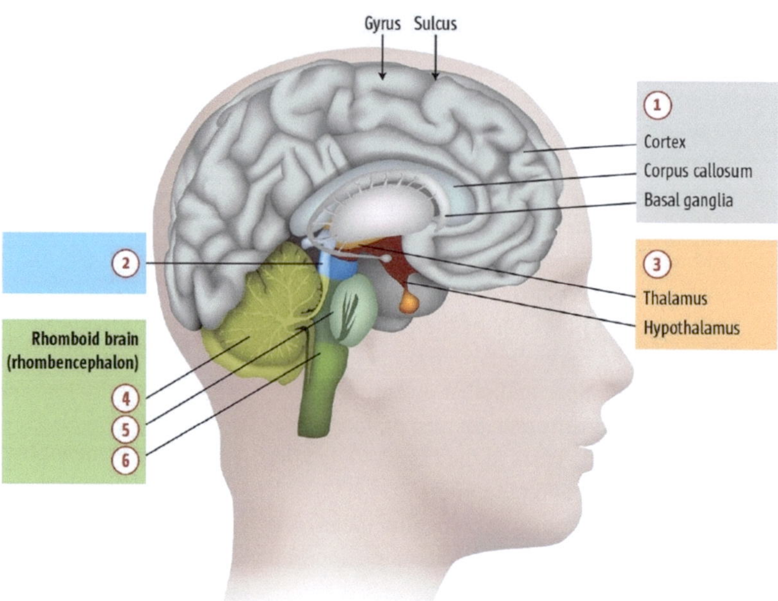

Fig. 2.42 Test question—Parts of the brain. © ARKANA Forum GmbH 2022. All Rights Reserved

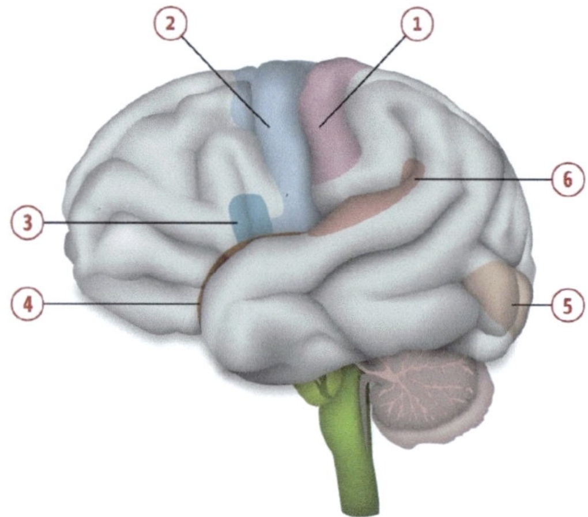

Fig. 2.43 Test question—Areas of high functionality in the cerebrum. © ARKANA Forum GmbH 2022. All Rights Reserved

21. Which two somatosensory systems do you know and what information is transmitted via each respective system?
22. Describe the signal course of a tactile discriminating sensory perception.
23. Describe the signal course of a motor impulse for a voluntary movement on the basis of the illustration. See Fig. 2.45.

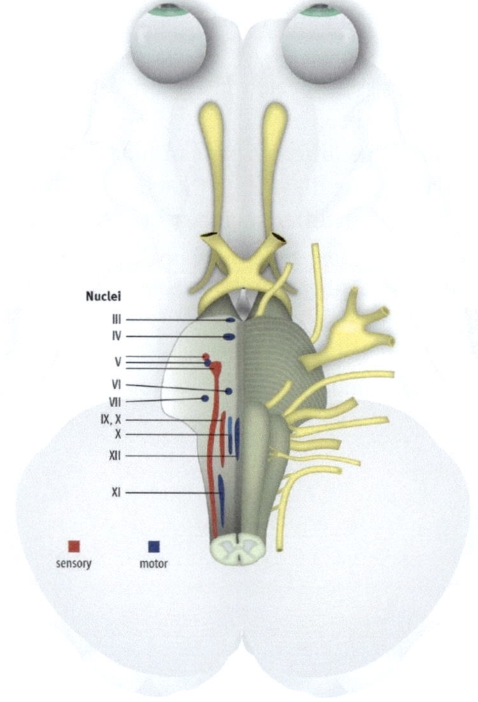

Fig. 2.44 Test question—Location of the cranial nerve nuclei and exit sites of the cranial nerves from the brain. © ARKANA Forum GmbH 2022. All Rights Reserved

24. Describe the signal course of a simple muscle stretch reflex on the basis of the Fig. 2.46.
25. What parts does the autonomic nervous system consist of and what functions do they each represent?
26. What types of muscles exist? Where do they occur, and what are their functions?

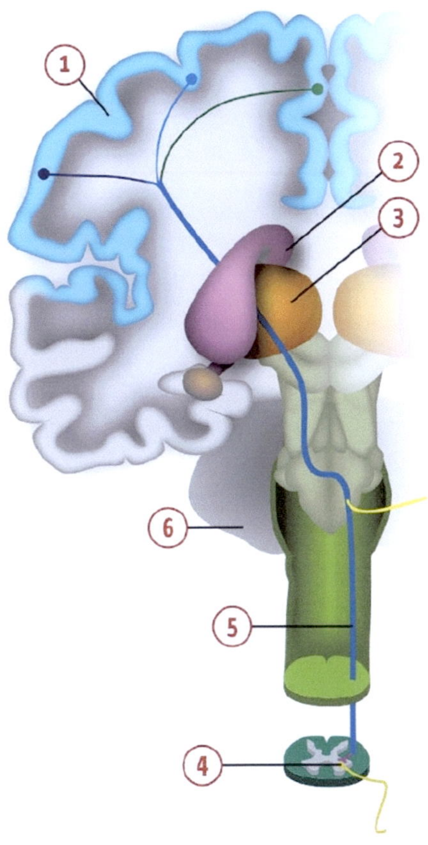

Fig. 2.45 Test question—Signal processing in the motor system. © ARKANA Forum GmbH 2022. All Rights Reserved

Fig. 2.46 Test question—Schematic illustration of a muscle stretch reflex (patellar tendon reflex). © ARKANA Forum GmbH 2022. All Rights Reserved

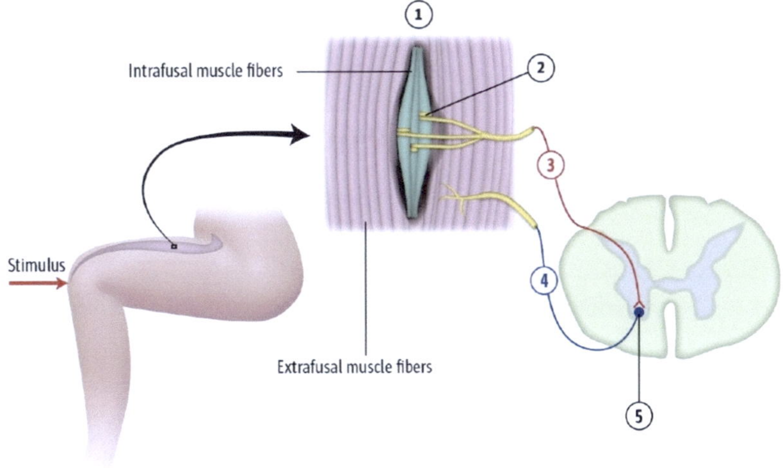

Technical Basics

3

Celine Wegner and David MacDonald

Contents

3.1 Physical Parameters

3.1.1 Electrical Current

Formula symbol: I
  Unit: Ampere (A)

Electrical current is the flow of charged particles though a conductor. Its intensity is the rate of flow. Electrons flow in the wires of a neurostimulator circuit, while ions normally flow through the body tissue between the stimulating electrodes.

3.1.2 Electrical Voltage

Formula symbol: V

C. Wegner (✉) · D. MacDonald
ARKANA Forum GmbH, Emmendingen, Germany
e-mail: c.wegner@arkana-forum.com

© The Author(s), under exclusive license to Springer Nature Switzerland AG 2024
J. Zentner et al. (eds.), *Intraoperative Neuromonitoring*,
https://doi.org/10.1007/978-3-031-46125-5_3

Unit: Volt (V)

Electrical voltage is the potential difference between two points in a circuit, such as between two neurostimulation electrodes. In the broadest sense, it can be understood as the force or "pressure" that moves the electrical current through the circuit.

3.1.3 Electrical Resistance

Formula symbol: R

Unit: Ohm (Ω)

Electrical resistance is the opposition to *direct current* (DC) flow through an electrical conductor.

3.1.4 Electrical Impedance

Formula symbol: Z

Unit: Ω

Impedance is like resistance but is the opposition to *alternating current* (AC) flow through an electrical conductor. Unlike resistance, impedance varies with the frequency of the AC.

3.1.5 Ohm's Law

Ohm's law defines the relationship between I, V, and R or Z and has two forms:

$I = V/R$ (DC circuit)

$I = V/Z$ (AC circuit)

Thus, current intensity is equal to the voltage divided by the resistance or impedance of the circuit.

3.1.6 Electrical Charge

Formula symbol: Q

Unit: Coulomb (C)

Atoms, constituents of all material, contain negatively charged electrons and positively charged protons. In the normal state, their numbers are equal, and the atom is electrically neutral. If an imbalance is created by external influences, a charge equalization takes place automatically, causing the flow of electric current. The electric charge indicates the electron excess or electron deficiency of an electrically charged material.

3.1.7 Electrical Energy

Formula symbol: E

Unit: Joule (J)

According to the law of conservation of energy, the total energy of a closed electrical system remains constant. Electrical energy is the amount of energy that is transferred by means of electric current. Electrical energy can be converted to heat energy.

The most important parameter for the definition of effective neurostimulation is the charge *transferred* by a pulse defined as the integral of current over the time or width of the pulse, known as pulse duration (D). It can be thought of as the amount of electricity delivered by the pulse. For a rectangular pulse, the transferred charge is simply the product of pulse amplitude and duration.

Calculation formula: $E = I^2 \times D \times R = V \times I \times D = V \times Q$

3.1.8 Electrical Current Density

Formula symbol: J

Unit: A/m^2

The electrical current density is the current per unit cross-sectional area of an electrical conductor. For neurostimulation, mainly current density at the electrode-tissue interface is considered, which depends on electrode surface area. The smaller the area, the higher the current density.

Calculation formula: $J = I/A$, where A is electrode surface area

3.2 Stimulation

3.2.1 Type of Pulses

At least two electrodes or poles are required to make stimulation current flow through tissue. During the stimulation pulse, electrons flow through the stimulator circuit toward and accumulate at one pole that becomes negatively charged, and electrons flow away from the other pole that becomes positively charged. By convention, the direction of current flow is defined as the direction of positive flow, which is opposite to electron flow. The negatively charged pole is the cathode, the positively charged pole the anode. Usually, the cathode is indicated by a black marking and the anode by a red marking. Under normal safe stimulation conditions, electrons do not flow into or out of tissue at the poles. Instead, there is a capacitive charge transfer at the electrode-tissue interface due to repulsion or attraction of negatively charged anions and positively charged cations in the tissue fluid electrolyte. Specifically, anions flow away from the cathode toward the anode, while cations flow away from the anode toward the cathode. This is normally the tissue current that stimulates neural targets.

The poles can be used in different configurations for stimulation. With **bipolar stimulation**, both poles are near the neural target and current flows focally between them (Fig. 3.1). This is often used for direct cortical stimulation during awake craniotomies. It is also used for stimulating focally along the course of axons in nerves or the spinal cord. In this case, the cathode is more active because anodal block may occur under the anode, so that action potentials more readily propagate away from the cathode. Consequently, this technique may be thought of as **bipolar cathodal stimulation**. With **monopolar stimulation**, one pole is near the neural target and the other is distant (Fig. 3.2). The current flow is less focal and at high intensity may spread to activate neurons away from the target, so particular attention must be paid to the threshold intensity. In

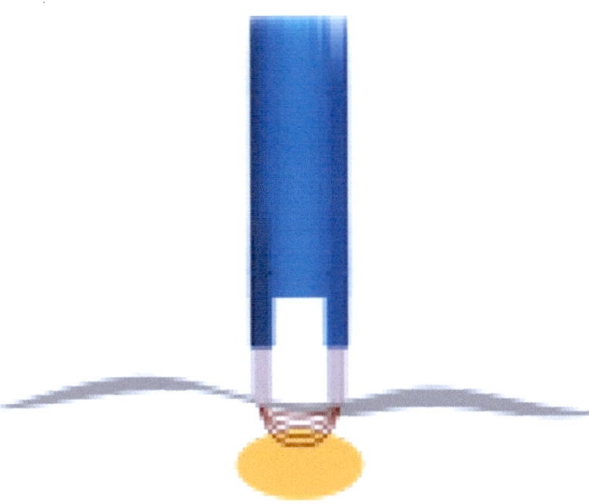

Fig. 3.1 Bipolar stimulation. © ARKANA Forum GmbH 2022. All Rights Reserved

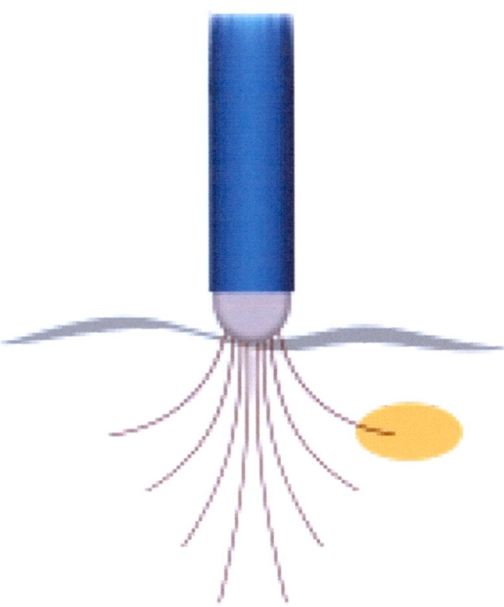

Fig. 3.2 Monopolar stimulation. © ARKANA Forum GmbH 2022. All Rights Reserved

monopolar cathodal stimulation, the cathode is near the target, and in **monopolar anodal stimulation**, the anode is near the target. These two different configurations are used for the stimulation of different target structures. For example, while monopolar cathodal stimulation is preferred for axon stimulation, monopolar anodal stimulation provides better results for activation of pyramidal cells of the cortex.

With monopolar stimulation, the penetration depth of the stimulation current is approximately proportional to the stimulation intensity. The rule of thumb for application of subcortical monopolar stimulation in the brain is a penetration depth of 1 mm at a set stimulation current of 1 mA using 0.5 ms pulse duration [1–3].

The functional principle of **depolarization** of a nerve by **bipolar cathodal stimulation** is shown in Fig. 3.3. Delivering of the negative charge causes an excess of positive charge to accumulate intracellularly under the cathode. This leads to depolarization, and the action potential propagates in both directions. Under the anode, on the other hand, hyperpolarization occurs due to accumulation of negative charge in the intracellular space, which prevents further propagation of the action potential in that direction. This is also known as anodal block. However, the anodal block can be overcome by higher stimulation intensities [4].

Stimulation pulses can have one or two phases (Fig. 3.4). **Monophasic stimulation** induces current in one direction. **Biphasic stimulation** induces current in one direction during the first phase and then the opposite direction in the second phase, essentially reversing the anode and cathode. This mode is important for safe language mapping and is sometimes used for transcranial motor evoked potential (MEP) spinal cord monitoring. **Alternating monophasic stimulation** provides a stimulation current alternately in each direction by switching the anode and cathode between successive trials. Thus, symmetric monitoring of homologous brain areas or nerves can be achieved from both poles.

The stimulation pulse is additionally characterized by the parameters described in Fig. 3.5.

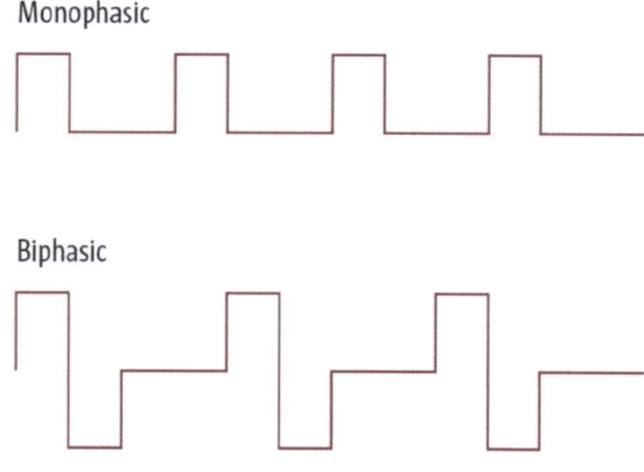

Fig. 3.4 Monophasic and biphasic stimulation pulses. © ARKANA Forum GmbH 2022. All Rights Reserved

Fig. 3.3 Depolarization of a nerve by cathodal stimulation. © ARKANA Forum GmbH 2022. All Rights Reserved

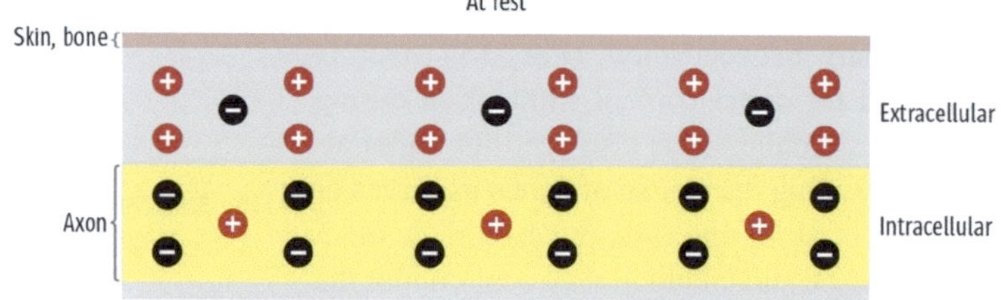

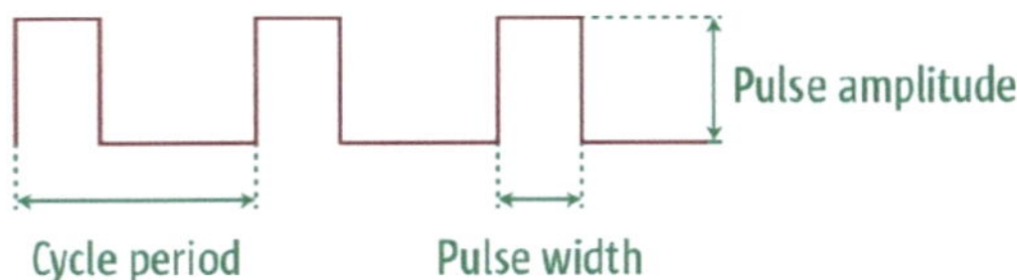

Fig. 3.5 Parameters of a stimulation pulse. © ARKANA Forum GmbH 2022. All Rights Reserved

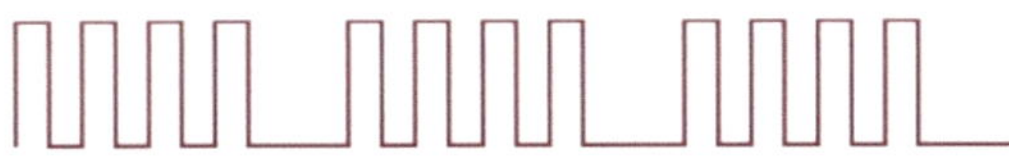

Fig. 3.6 Train stimulation. © ARKANA Forum GmbH 2022. All Rights Reserved

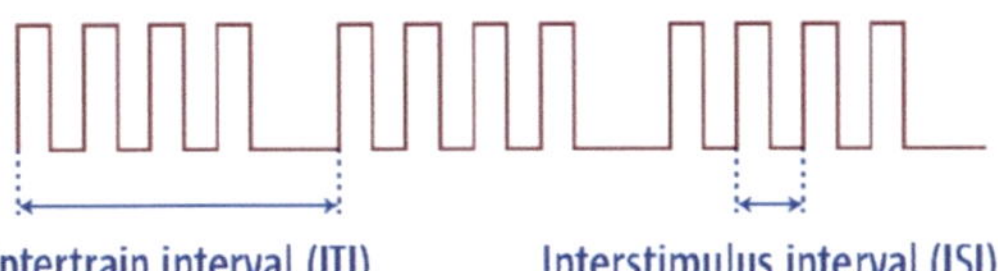

Fig. 3.7 Parameters of train stimulation. © ARKANA Forum GmbH 2022. All Rights Reserved

Train stimulation (Fig. 3.6) represents a way to overcome the inhibitory effects of anesthesia, e.g., during motor cortex stimulation. It constitutes the standard technique for eliciting intraoperative muscle MEPs. Parameters characterizing train stimulation are given in Fig. 3.7.

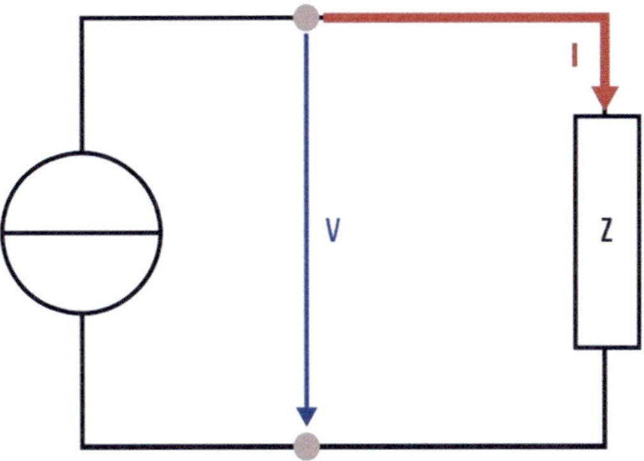

Fig. 3.8 Constant current stimulation. © ARKANA Forum GmbH 2022. All Rights Reserved

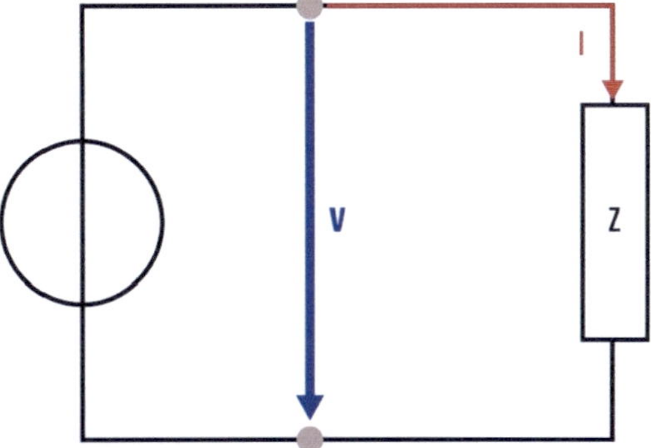

Fig. 3.9 Constant voltage stimulation. © ARKANA Forum GmbH 2022. All Rights Reserved

3.2.2 Frequency

The frequency indicates the rate of repetitions in periodic processes.

Formula symbol: f
Unit: Hertz (Hz)
Calculation formula: $f = $ repetitions/second

3.2.3 Stimulators

A distinction must be made between **constant current** and **constant voltage** stimulators, advantages and disadvantages of which are often the subject of controversial discussion. The principles of both stimulation modalities are shown in Figs. 3.8 and 3.9. Figure 3.10 gives an over-view of the main differences between both techniques.

With **constant current stimulation**, stimulation occurs at the selected current and is independent of impedance because the device automatically adjusts voltage to maintain the chosen current (Fig. 3.8).

The following formula applies:

Current $I = V/Z$

With **constant voltage stimulation**, activation always takes place with the set voltage, but the current depends on the impedance (Fig. 3.9).

The following formula applies:

Voltage $V = I \times Z$

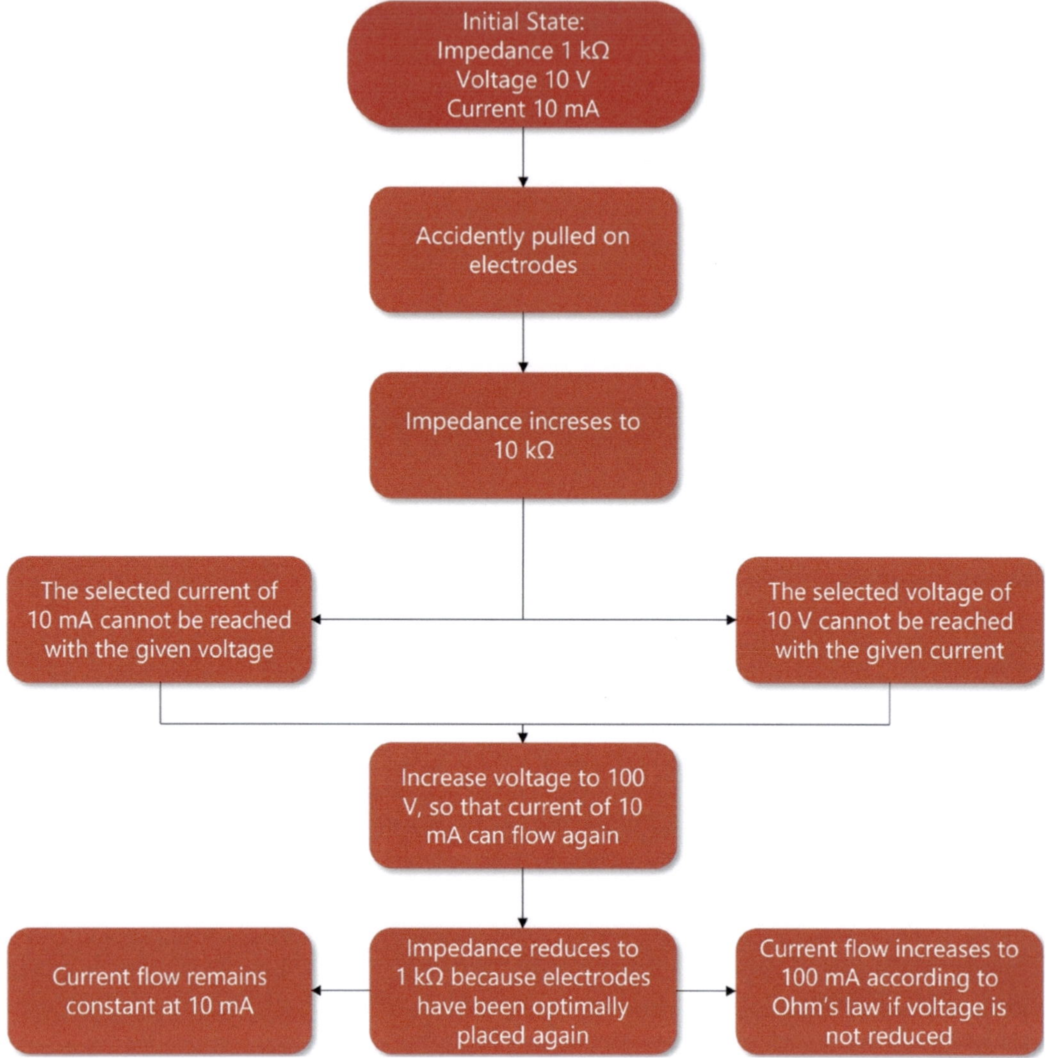

Fig. 3.10 Differences between a constant current and a constant voltage stimulator.© ARKANA Forum GmbH 2022. All Rights Reserved

3.3 Signal Acquisition

Various systems are available for the acquisition of electrophysiological signals, which differ depending on the manufacturer. However, the underlying measurement technique is based on the same principles.

3.3.1 Amplifier Technique

Differential amplifiers are used for the acquisition of bioelectric signals. They amplify the difference of the voltages between two inputs. The connection of these inputs to the tissue is established by the respective recording electrodes.

Interfering signals can also act on the recording electrodes from a greater distance, such as far-field potentials from distant bioelectric tissues, or extraneous electromagnetic fields. However, with proper technique the interference effects on the two recording electrodes and the associated inputs of the amplifier are almost the same, which reduces the difference of these interference effects to a minimum. This is known as common-mode rejection. The use of differential amplifiers leads to a typical biphasic signal when recording a nerve action potential (Fig. 3.11).

For registering the electromyogram (EMG) and MEPs, differential amplifiers are used to make bipolar recordings, both inputs of which come from a specific muscle group. Thus, a spe-cific differential bipolar signal on the monitor can be assigned to the respective monitored muscle (Fig. 3.12). Some headboxes are designed to operate only in this differential-bipolar mode, with each pair of inputs being assigned to one amplifier.

Recordings of somatosensory, auditory, and visual evoked potentials (SEPs, AEPs, VEPs) as well as the electroencephalogram (EEG) can be bipolar or referential. In referential recordings, for each negative input to various differential amplifiers, there is a positive input that serves as a common reference. Thus, in contrast to bipolar measurement of muscle groups, it is sufficient to use one measuring electrode for each measuring point, which is displayed against a common ref-erence (Fig. 3.13). The electrode that is close to the generator is the active electrode and is con-nected to the negative input, while the inactive or less active common reference is connected to the positive input. Some headboxes are designed to operate in referential mode, with several inputs for active electrodes and one input for the com-mon reference.

The output from the differential amplifier is filtered with a hardware **high-pass filter**. This means that low frequencies, i.e., slow oscillations of the signal such as baseline fluctuations, are already deleted in the amplifier. Usually, the cut-off frequency for this filter, which specifies which low frequencies are to be deleted from the signal, is adjustable. Short and fast potentials (e.g., nerve action potentials or AEPs) are mainly character-ized by high frequencies. In order to delete as many interfering lower frequencies as possible, the hardware filter should be set higher in such a case. With the EEG, however, the slow fluctua-tions, i.e., the low frequencies, are also important for the interpretation. The cutoff frequency of the high-pass filter should therefore be set low here.

For further processing, the signal is **digitized**. This means that the analog uninterrupted signal from each amplifier is sampled at an adjustable frequency. After this conversion, therefore, instead of a continuous signal, only discrete data

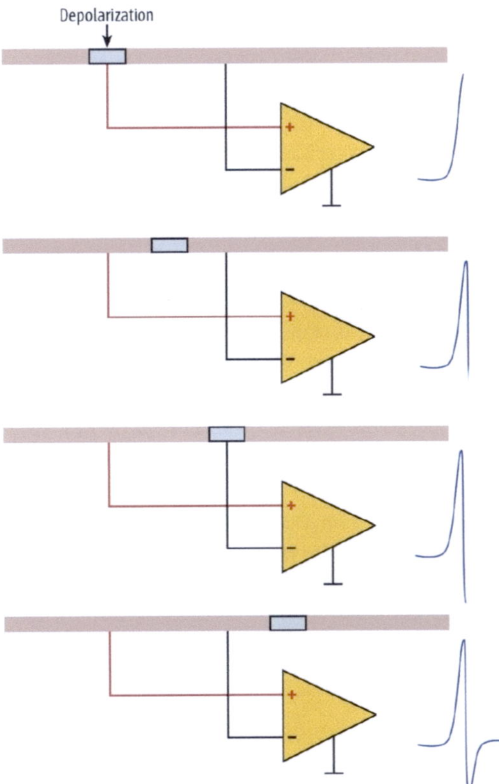

Fig. 3.11 Recording of a biphasic nerve action potential with a differential amplifier. © ARKANA Forum GmbH 2022. All Rights Reserved

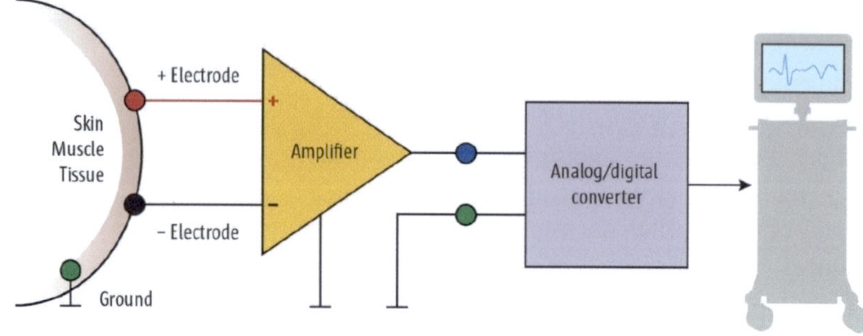

Fig. 3.12 Schematic illustration of the function of a differential amplifier for bipolar recordings from a muscle group. © ARKANA Forum GmbH 2022. All Rights Reserved

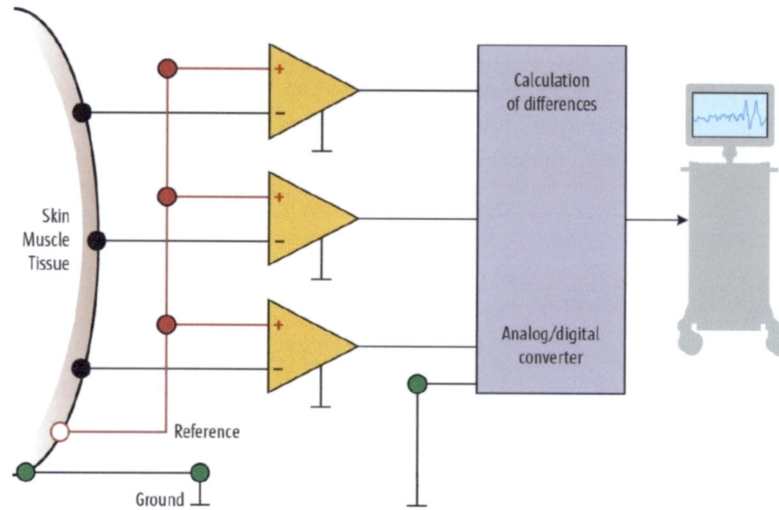

Fig. 3.13 Schematic illustration of the function of a differential amplifier for referential recordings. © ARKANA Forum GmbH 2022. All Rights Reserved

points are available with time resolution according to the set **sampling rate**. Important in this context is the resolution not only in the time axis but also in the amplitude. The number of available data points in the amplitude is fixed by the bit depth of the digital converter (usually 16 bits), but the expected dynamic **measuring range**, i.e., the range in which the amplitude of the signal usually falls, is adjustable. For example, EMG signals are in the 50 µV to several mV range, while evoked potential signals range from <1 to several µV. The better the measuring range is matched to the actual voltages recorded, the better the amplitude resolution. This adjustment is also called **amplification** or **gain** in some systems. The following applies here: the smaller the signal, the larger the selected amplification should be. Ideally, the settings on the hardware merely keep the amplifier in the operating range and protect it from saturation effects. Further sig-

nal processing is done by **software filters**, which ensure maximum flexibility.

> *The recommended settings in hardware and software for the respective monitoring modalities can be found in the operating instructions of the monitoring system or obtained from the manufacturer, and in published IONM guidelines or recommendations.*

3.3.2 Signal Processing

Further signal processing serves to display the signal as optimally as possible on the screen. It takes place after the digitization and before the visualization of the signal. A display adapted to the respective signal in the best possible way is achieved by the application of various **software filters**. The use of high-pass and low-pass filters serves to flexibly adapt the displayed frequency bandwidth to the main frequency components of the wanted signal. Unwanted interfering frequencies below or above the signal's bandwidth can be suppressed in this way. It should be noted that filters can distort the signal, for example, in amplitude and latency. They should therefore always be set as narrow as necessary to reject unwanted noise, but also wide enough to contain most of the signal's frequency content. Corresponding recommendations for these settings are given by the manufacturers and published IONM guidelines.

The **notch filter** represents a special type of filter that removes only a very limited frequency range of the signal. It is usually used for filtering the frequency of the line voltage (50 or 60 Hz, depending on the country).

Similar to the hardware, the **high-pass filter** acts in software. This means that this filter deletes low frequencies from the signal, but only after digitization and before display. The high-pass filter in the software is usually more flexible to adjust than the high-pass filter in the hardware.

A **low-pass filter** deletes high-frequency oscillations from the signal. This filter can suppress amplifier noise, for example. The lower the cutoff frequency of this filter is set, the smoother the signal becomes. Also, with this filter the setting depends on the expected signal. For fast signals like AEPs or MEPs, the cutoff frequency should be set relatively high (1500–3000 Hz). For slower signals such as SEPs or VEPs, the cutoff frequency can be set somewhat lower to suppress noise and improve the quality of the signal. Note that the maximum possible low-pass cutoff frequency is limited by the sampling rate of the digital-to-analog converter. Specifically, it must be less than half the sampling rate to avoid aliasing (Nyquist-Shannon sampling theorem). For example, if the sampling rate is 4000 Hz, then the maximum low-pass filter cutoff would be about 1500 Hz; if the sampling rate is 8000 Hz, then the cutoff can be increased to about 3000 Hz.

Not all disturbances can be eliminated by filtering. Another common method of signal processing is averaging. Averaging is useful when a time-locked signal present in every recording sweep is overwhelmed by random noise of similar or larger amplitude. The noise consists mainly of biologic EEG, EMG, or electrocardiographic signals as well as electromagnetic interference. By averaging a number of sweeps (N), the time-locked signal averages in although modified by some jitter, while random noise amplitude gradually declines by $\sqrt{N}$ but never reaches zero. Thus, averaged signals are estimates distorted by some degree of jitter and residual noise. Their trial-to-trial reproducibility determines their accuracy. The N required to accurately reproduce a signal depends on its signal-to-noise ratio.

3.3.3 Disturbance Variables

The signals recorded during neuromonitoring can be very small in amplitude. Due to the many electrical devices placed in the operating room, despite modern amplification technology and shielding measures, interference with the signal cannot be completely avoided, which can overlay the monitoring signals and make interpretation difficult. By meticulous **placement of cables, electrodes, and devices**, these interferences can be minimized in a first step. Only then the software settings should be changed as necessary.

An important disturbance variable in the operating room is the **line voltage**, at a frequency of **50 or 60 Hz** (Fig. 3.14). This interference is caused by all devices in the operating room that are supplied with electrical power. In a first step, interference by the line voltage can be minimized by placing cables of the recording electrodes as far away as possible from power cables and other electrical equipment (electric blankets, high-

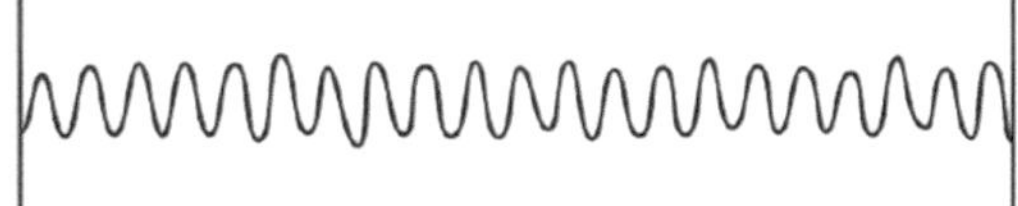

Fig. 3.14 Signal with strong interference due to the 50/60 Hz line voltage. © ARKANA Forum GmbH 2022. All Rights Reserved

frequency surgical equipment, microscope, etc.). In addition, ensuring low balanced recording electrode impedances below 2–5 kΩ reduces electromagnetic interference. Furthermore, tightly braiding or twisting together the cables of the recording electrodes is essential. This is because recording leads that are close together throughout their paths pick up electromagnetic interference with nearly the same amplitude, so that common-mode rejection cancels out the interference in the differential amplifiers. Interference can also be caused by surgical instruments, e.g., skull clamps, hooks, or holders. Cables of recording electrodes should therefore be placed at a distance from these instruments.

Additional noise can be caused by **dissection instruments** (electrosurgery, drills, ultrasound equipment). Electrosurgery in particular can cause large disturbances in the recorded signals, which cannot be avoided. Electrophysiological measurements can therefore only be made outside the respective surgical steps. The latest bipolar electrosurgery instruments use continuous impedance measurement to automatically activate the current upon tissue contact. This measurement can interfere with the signal recording even between applications of the electrosurgery instruments and can be seen as a periodically occurring curve in the biosignal. Furthermore, many devices now also use continuous impedance measurements to check for adequate tissue contact of electrodes (e.g., the neutral electrode of the electrosurgical device or the electrodes used to monitor the depth of anesthesia). These impedance measurements also occur as periodic disturbances in the monitoring signals.

3.4 Test Questions

1. What does Ohm's law describe?
2. Complete the following drawing with the names of the parameters of stimulation sequences (Figs. 3.15 and 3.16).
3. What is the difference between monopolar anodal and monopolar cathodal stimulation?

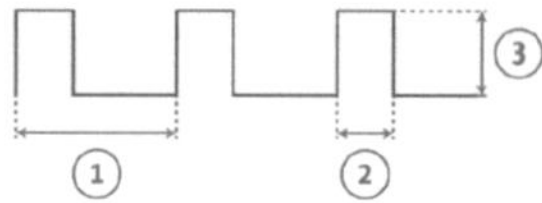

Fig. 3.15 Test question—Parameters of a stimulation pulse. © ARKANA Forum GmbH 2022. All Rights Reserved

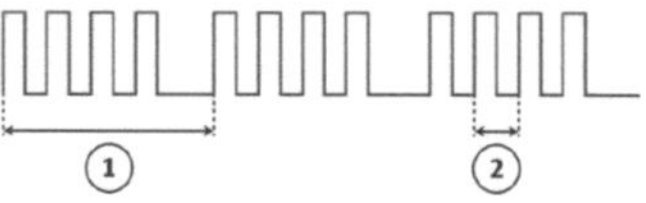

Fig. 3.16 Test question—Parameters of train stimulation. © ARKANA Forum GmbH 2022. All Rights Reserved

4. Describe the differences between a constant current stimulator and a constant voltage stimulator.
5. What is the difference between monopolar and bipolar stimulation? Which type of stimulation is used for what application?
6. What are the differences between bipolar and referential recordings and what purposes are they used for?
7. Complete the following text:

   The output from the differential amplifier is filtered with a hardware high-pass filter. This means that _________ frequencies, i.e., __________ oscillations of the signal such as baseline fluctuations, are already deleted in the amplifier. Usually, the cutoff frequency for this filter, which specifies which frequencies are to be deleted from the signal, is adjustable. Short and fast potentials (e.g., nerve action potentials or AEPs) are mainly characterized by __________ frequencies. In order to delete as many lower interfering frequencies as possible, the hardware filter should be set __________ in such a case. With the EEG, however, the slow fluctuations, i.e., the __________ frequencies, are also important for the interpretation. The cutoff frequency of the high-pass filter should therefore be set __________ here.
8. What types of software filters exist? Describe them briefly.
9. What possible disturbance variables do you know and how can the influence of these variables be minimized?

References

1. Kombos T, Süss O, Kern BC, Funk T, Hoell T, Kopetsch O, et al. Comparison between monopolar and bipolar electrical stimulation of the motor cortex. Acta Neurochir. 1999;141:1295–301.
2. Nossek E, Korn A, Shahar T, Kanner AA, Yaffe H, Marcovici D, et al. Intraoperative mapping and monitoring of the corticospinal tracts with neurophysiological assessment and 3-dimensional ultrasonography-based navigation. J Neurosurg. 2011;114(3):738–46.
3. Raabe A, Beck J, Schucht P, Seidel K. Continuous dynamic mapping of the corticospinal tract during surgery of motor eloquent brain tumors: evaluation of a new method: clinical article. J Neurosurg. 2014;120(5):1015–24.
4. Vogel RW. Understanding anodal and cathodal stimulation [internet]. The ASNM Monitor. 2017; https://www.asnm.org/blogpost/1635804/290597/Understanding-Anodal-and-Cathodal-Stimulation

Technical Accessories

4

Celine Wegner

Contents

There are disposable and reusable accessories. Disposable material is already sterile packaged and is disposed of after use. Reusable accessories used in the sterile field must be re-sterilized after use in the hospital's central sterile supply department. Non-sterile material must be disinfected after use according to the manufacturer's instructions.

C. Wegner (✉)
ARKANA Forum GmbH, Emmendingen, Germany
e-mail: c.wegner@arkana-forum.com

4.1 Stimulation and Recording Electrodes

4.1.1 Stimulation Probes

Stimulation probes are mainly used for localization and functional control of motor nerves and for mapping of the motor and sensory cortex. A very wide range of stimulation probes is available: monopolar, bipolar, and tripolar, each in different lengths and configurations (Figs. 4.1, 4.2, 4.3, 4.4, and 4.5).

Monopolar stimulation probes have a larger spread of the stimulation current than bipolar probes and are therefore often used to first get an overview in the surgical field and to estimate whether a nerve is involved or not, and approximately how far away it is, if at all [1, 2]. Therefore, monopolar stimulation probes are mainly applied

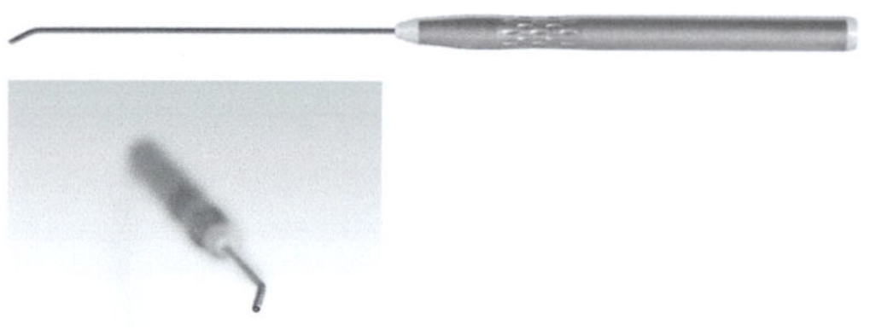

Fig. 4.1 Bipolar concentric stimulation probe. © ARKANA Forum GmbH 2022. All Rights Reserved

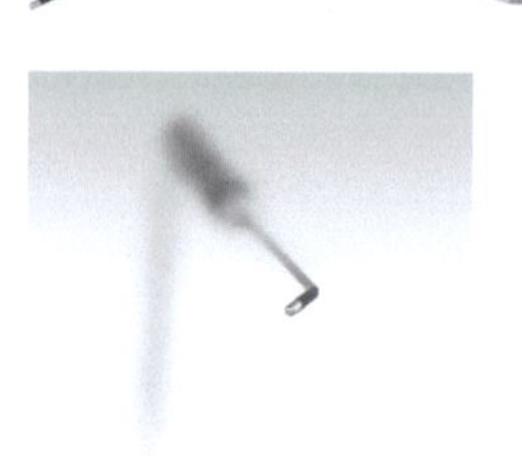

Fig. 4.5 Monopolar stimulation probe. © ARKANA Forum GmbH 2022. All Rights Reserved

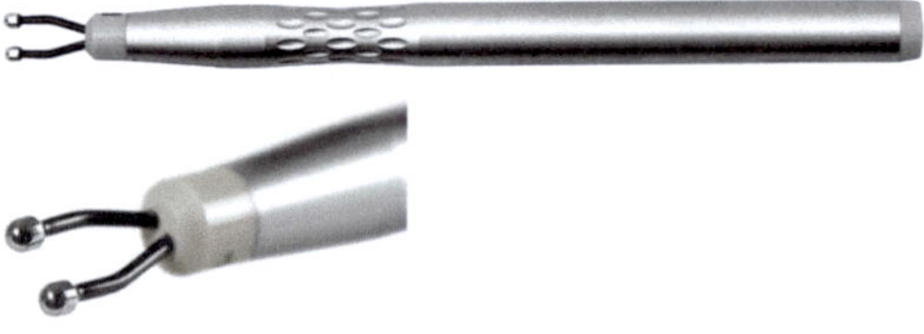

Fig. 4.2 Bipolar fork probe. © ARKANA Forum GmbH 2022. All Rights Reserved

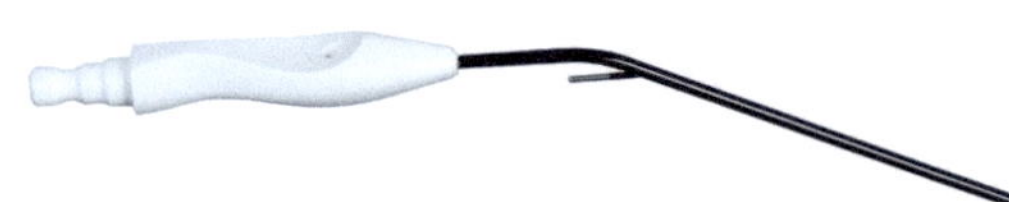

Fig. 4.6 Mapping suction probe. © ARKANA Forum GmbH 2022. All Rights Reserved

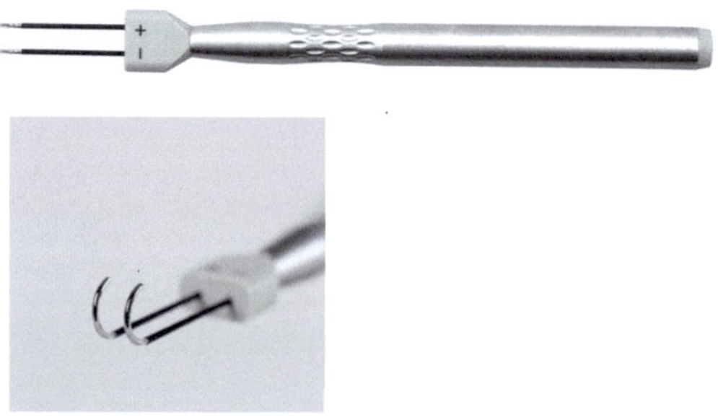

Fig. 4.3 Bipolar hook probe. © ARKANA Forum GmbH 2022. All Rights Reserved

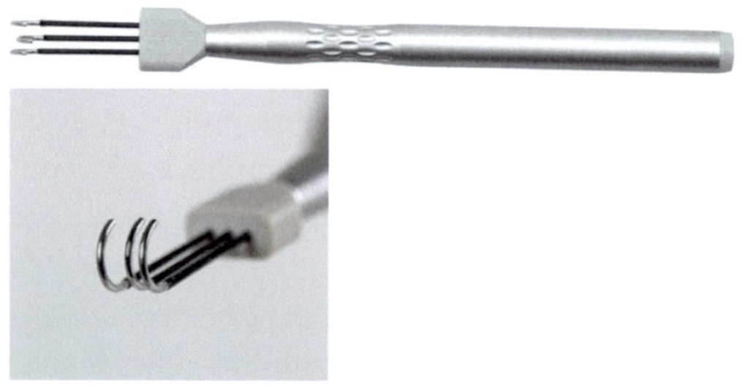

Fig. 4.4 Tripolar hook probe. © ARKANA Forum GmbH 2022. All Rights Reserved

in motor mapping, cranial nerve mapping, tethered cord surgery, and pedicle screw implantation.

Bipolar probes stimulate very selectively and are mainly used when a nerve is already visible, and it needs to be clarified which nerve it is, or when the nerve is to be functionally examined. Applications range from direct cortical stimulation, for example, for mapping the motor cortex or speech areas, and to triggering nerve action potentials. Bipolar concentric stimulation probes are used in particular for stimulation of peripheral nerves, cranial nerves, as well as at the brainstem.

Mapping suction probes (Fig. 4.6) represent a combination of conventional surgical suction devices and a monopolar stimulation probe. They enable the surgeon to suction and stimulate simultaneously during the procedure without having to change instruments. The mapping suction probe is insulated except for a small area at the tip of the probe. It has a connection for the stimulation cable near the handle. Otherwise, it is operated like a normal suction device.

4.1.2 Needle Electrodes

Needle electrodes can be used for both **stimulation** and **recording** of electrophysiological signals. For the registration of the electromyogram (EMG) as well as motor evoked potentials (MEPs), they penetrate directly into the belly of the muscle. Most needle electrodes used in clinical practice are made of stainless steel. However, if intraoperative magnetic resonance imaging (MRI) is planned, the use of platinum/iridium electrodes is advisable to reduce artifacts. Particularly in intraoperative MRI diagnostics, attention must be paid to the placement of needles and cables to avoid excessive heating or even burns [3]. Various commonly used needle electrodes are shown in Figs. 4.7, 4.8, and 4.9.

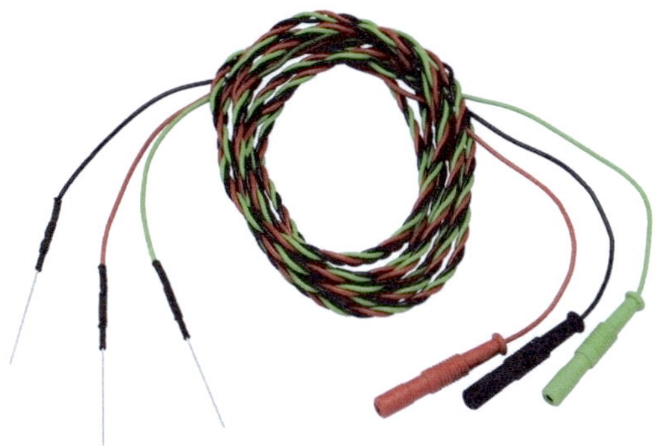

Fig. 4.9 Needle electrode, triple. © ARKANA Forum GmbH 2022. All Rights Reserved

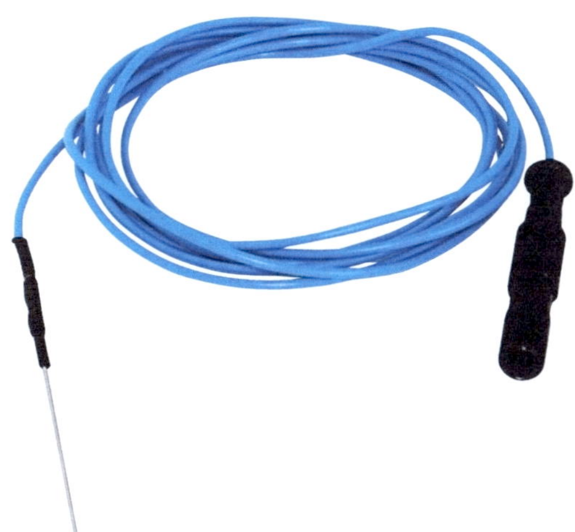

Fig. 4.7 Needle electrode, single. © ARKANA Forum GmbH 2022. All Rights Reserved

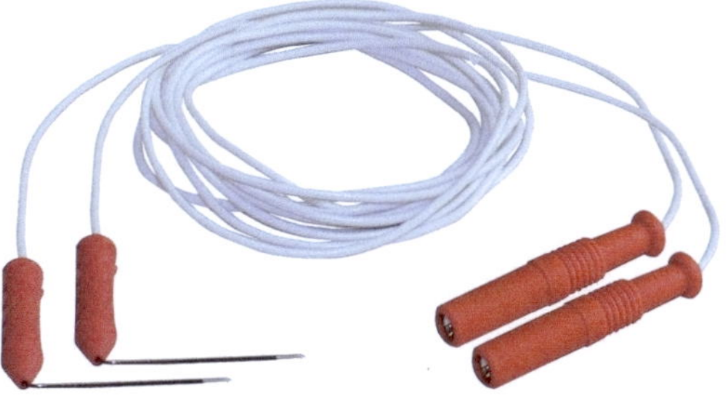

Fig. 4.10 Insulated needle electrodes. © ARKANA Forum GmbH 2022. All Rights Reserved

4.1.2.1 Insulated Needle Electrodes

In insulated needle electrodes, the electrode shaft is coated with an insulating material so that a signal can only be delivered or acquired at the tip (Fig. 4.10). These electrodes are particularly suitable for the stimulation of **deep-seated nerves** or for the recording from **deep-seated muscles**. They are used, for example, for selective recording from the masseter muscle in order to avoid the interference of signals from the mimic musculature.

4.1.2.2 Corkscrew Electrodes

The corkscrew shape of the needle allows the electrodes to be placed exactly at the desired position (Fig. 4.11). They are particularly suitable for application at the **scalp** and can be used for both **stimulation** and **recording**. Corkscrew electrodes are made of stainless steel. For placement, the electrodes are turned clockwise into the skin. They do not require any additional fixation. The electrodes are removed by turning them counterclockwise.

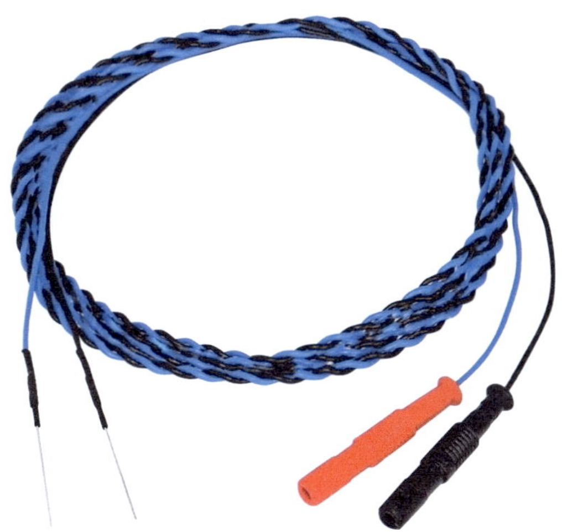

Fig. 4.8 Needle electrode, double. © ARKANA Forum GmbH 2022. All Rights Reserved

4.1.2.3 Double Needle Electrodes

Double needle electrodes are a special type of subdermal needle electrodes used to record **EMG** signals from the **face**, **mouth**, **throat,** and **neck** areas (Fig. 4.12). The advantage of double needles is especially that their placement takes less time, since only one electrode has to be inserted instead of the otherwise usual two electrodes and since the inter-electrode distance is always constant. Double needle electrodes have therefore proved particularly useful for application in muscles that are difficult to access.

4.1.2.4 Hook Electrodes

Hook electrodes are another special type of subdermal needle electrodes. They are used for recording electrophysiological signals mainly from the **facial region**. Their curved shape enables secure fixation in the tissue (Fig. 4.13).

4.1.2.5 Bipolar Needle Electrodes

In bipolar needle electrodes, both contacts necessary for recording are integrated in one needle. One pole is represented by the needle tip, the second pole by the needle shaft (Fig. 4.14). Due to the local proximity of the two contacts, this electrode facilitates a very **focused recording**.

4.1.2.6 Hookwire Electrodes

Hookwire electrodes are mainly used for recording electrophysiological signals from the **facial area** as well as the **mouth** and **throat**. They consist of a very thin stainless steel or silver wire that has been twisted individually or in pairs into a cannula for application. When the cannula is inserted, the wire hooks in the tissue like a small harpoon (Figs. 4.15 and 4.16). The cannula can then be retracted over the wire. After placement, the wires must be fixed very carefully. The cannulas attached to the wires

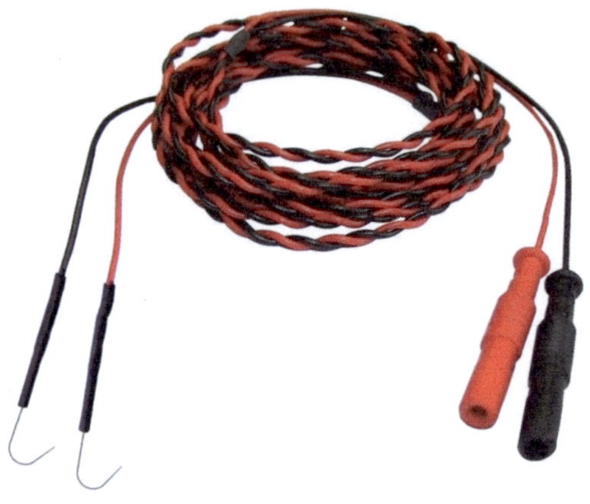

Fig. 4.13 Hook electrodes. © ARKANA Forum GmbH 2022. All Rights Reserved

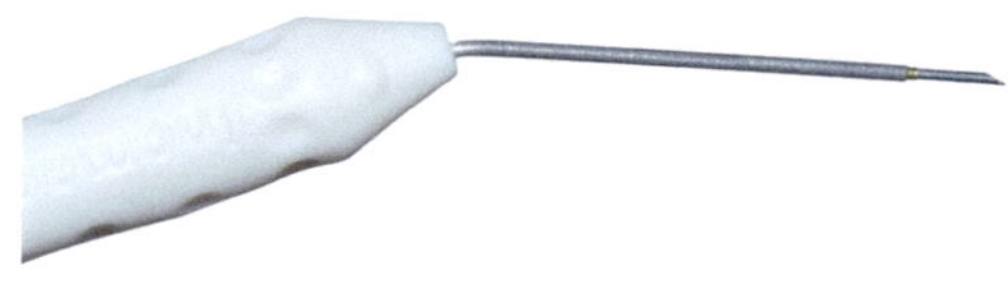

Fig. 4.14 Bipolar needle electrode. © ARKANA Forum GmbH 2022. All Rights Reserved

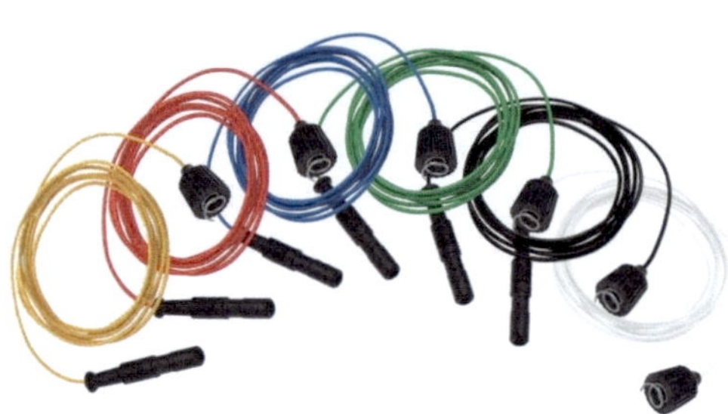

Fig. 4.11 Corkscrew electrodes. © ARKANA Forum GmbH 2022. All Rights Reserved

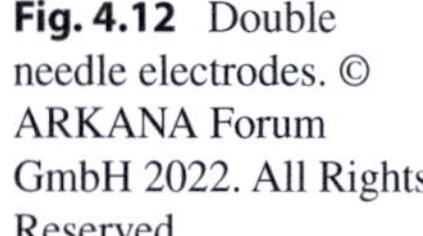

Fig. 4.12 Double needle electrodes. © ARKANA Forum GmbH 2022. All Rights Reserved

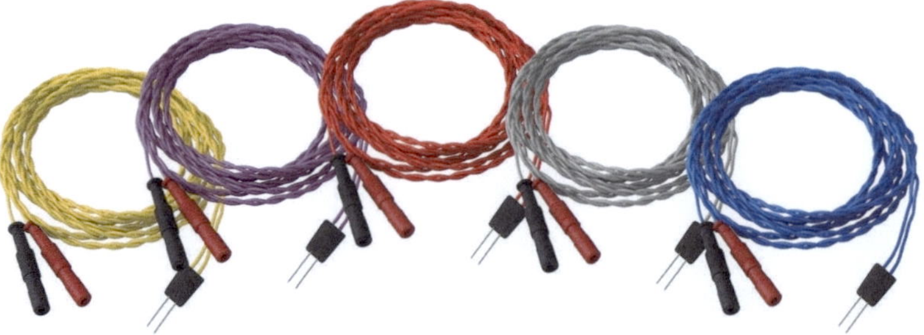

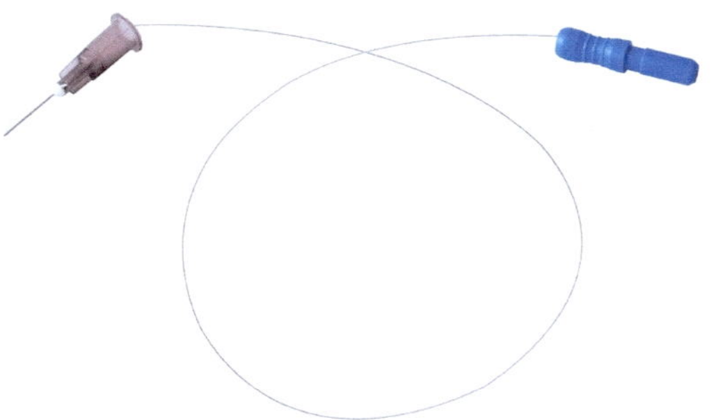

Fig. 4.15 Hookwire electrode, single. © ARKANA Forum GmbH 2022. All Rights Reserved

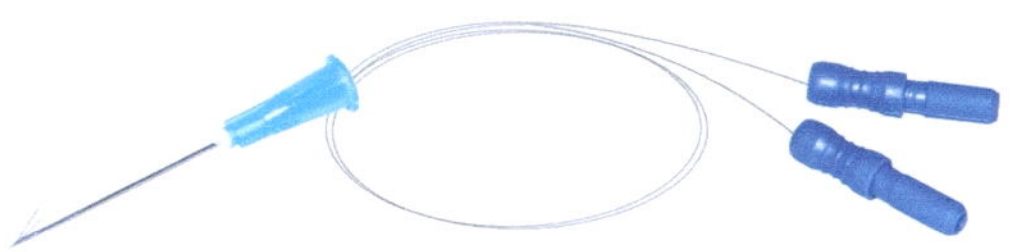

Fig. 4.16 Hookwire electrode, pair. © ARKANA Forum GmbH 2022. All Rights Reserved

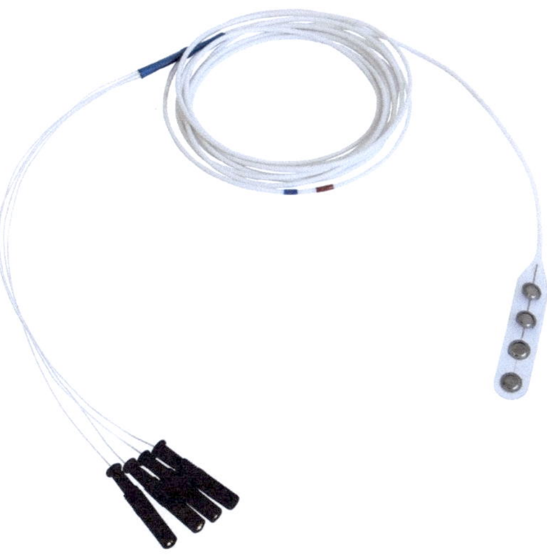

Fig. 4.17 Strip electrode, 1 × 4 contacts. © ARKANA Forum GmbH 2022. All Rights Reserved

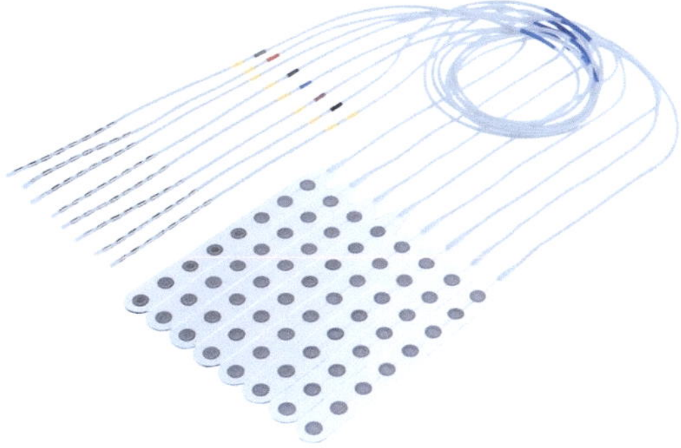

Fig. 4.18 Grid electrode, 8 × 8 contacts. © ARKANA Forum GmbH 2022. All Rights Reserved

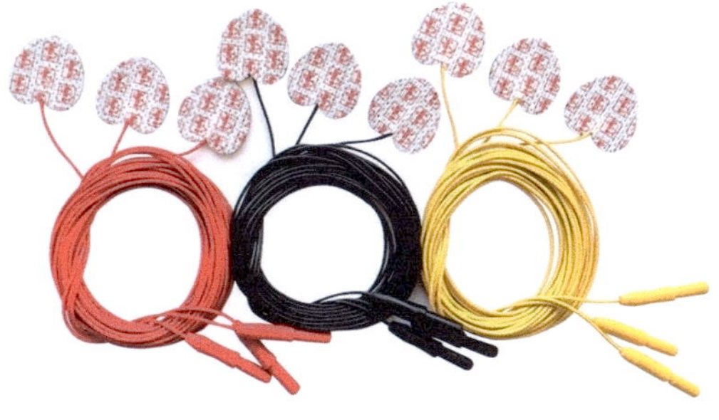

Fig. 4.19 Heart-shaped adhesive electrodes. © ARKANA Forum GmbH 2022. All Rights Reserved

must be positioned in such a way that the wires are not pulled out of the tissue by the weight of the cannulas.

4.1.3 Surface Electrodes

4.1.3.1 Strip and Grid Electrodes

Strip and grid electrodes can be used for both direct **cortical stimulation** and **recording** of electrophysiological signals, including the cortical **SEP phase reversal**. They consist of a silicone sheet in which discs made of platinum or stainless steel are embedded. The electrode assortment ranges from a single strip with 4 electrode contacts to configurations with 8 by 8 contacts (Figs. 4.17 and 4.18). When placing the electrode on the cortex, it is important to ensure that the cortex surface is not dry; otherwise the electrical contact may be insufficient. In case of doubt, the cortex surface should first be irrigated with sterile saline solution.

4.1.3.2 Adhesive Electrodes

Adhesive electrodes can be used for both **stimulation** and **recording** of electrophysiological signals. They are available in various sizes (Fig. 4.19). The adhesive surface is typically silver/silver chloride (Ag/AgCl). The skin must be prepared with gentle epidermal abrasion to reduce impedance before attaching the elec-

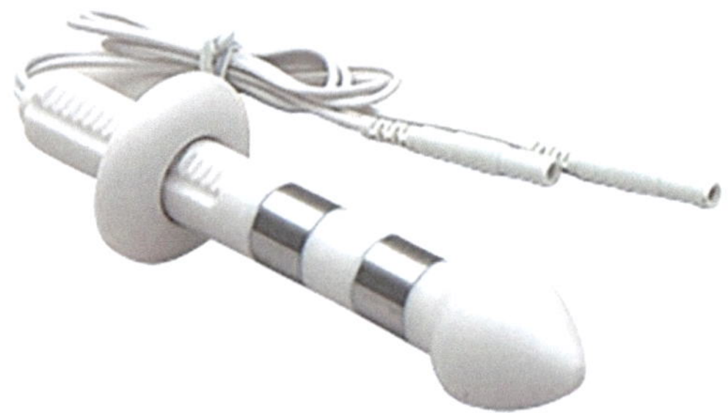

Fig. 4.20 Rectal electrode. © ARKANA Forum GmbH 2022. All Rights Reserved

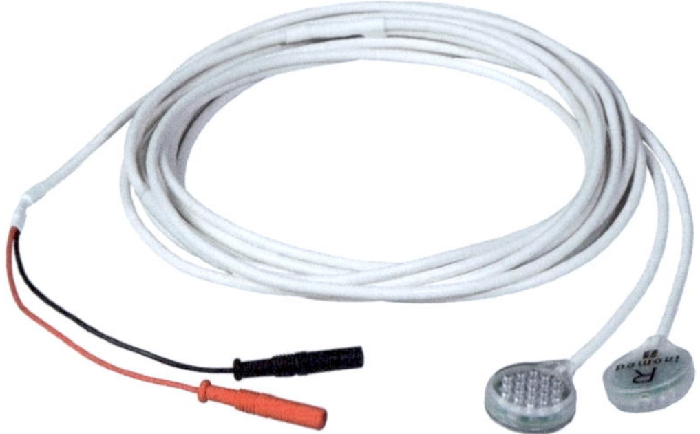

Fig. 4.21 Flash VEP eyelid discs. © ARKANA Forum GmbH 2022. All Rights Reserved

trodes. It should be noted that the adhesive properties may decrease during the course of surgery, causing impedances to increase. Adhesive electrodes are non-invasive and are therefore frequently used in children.

4.1.3.3 Rectal Electrodes

Rectal electrodes are used for the non-invasive recording of **EMG** signals from the **sphincter ani muscle**. They consist of a plastic body to which two stainless steel electrode contacts are attached (Fig. 4.20).

When placing the rectal electrode, it is important to ensure that no lubricant gel is used which could insulate the electrode contacts. To facilitate insertion, the electrode can be moistened with saline solution.

4.2   Special Accessories

4.2.1   Visual Evoked Potentials (VEPs)

Flash eyelid discs are used for triggering intraoperative VEPs. The flashes are applied via light emitting diode (LED) discs. An LED disc contains a large number of LEDs for homogeneous illumination of the eye (Fig. 4.21). The disc is placed on the closed eyelid and adhesively bonded there.

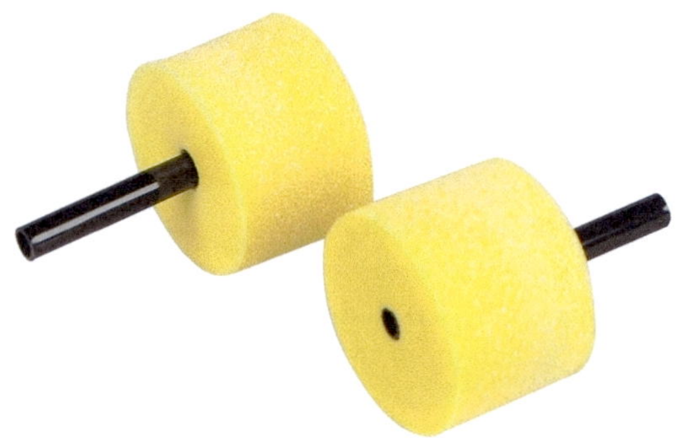

Fig. 4.22 Earplugs for AEP sound generator. © ARKANA Forum GmbH 2022. All Rights Reserved

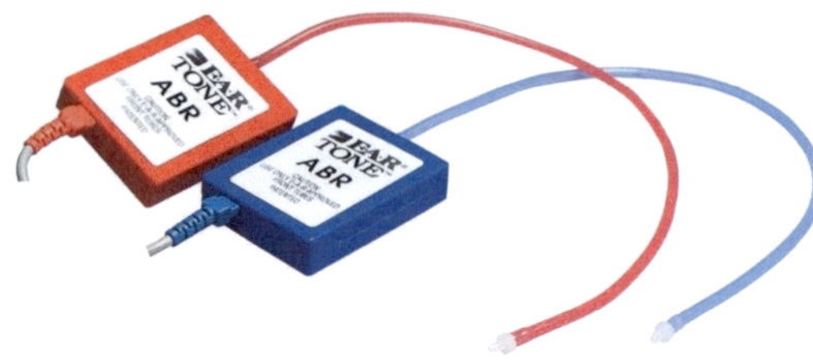

Fig. 4.23 AEP sound generators. © ARKANA Forum GmbH 2022. All Rights Reserved

4.2.2   Auditory Evoked Potentials (AEPs)

Earplugs (Fig. 4.22) and **sound generators** (Fig. 4.23) are used for eliciting AEPs. The soft foam rubber earplugs surround a rigid sound-conducting black tube. They are placed in the external auditory canal and connected via silicone tubes to the sound generators, which provide the acoustic stimulation pulses.

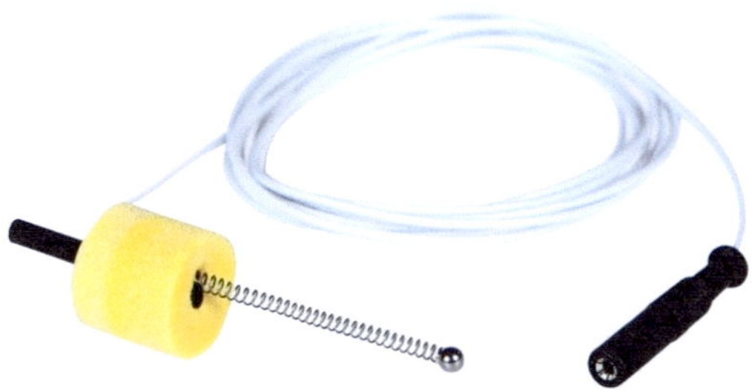

Fig. 4.24 Tympanic electrode. © ARKANA Forum GmbH 2022. All Rights Reserved

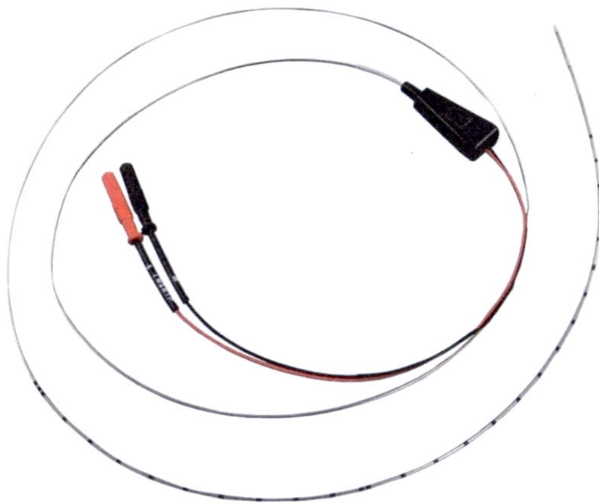

Fig. 4.26 Two-pole spinal epidural electrode. © ARKANA Forum GmbH 2022. All Rights Reserved

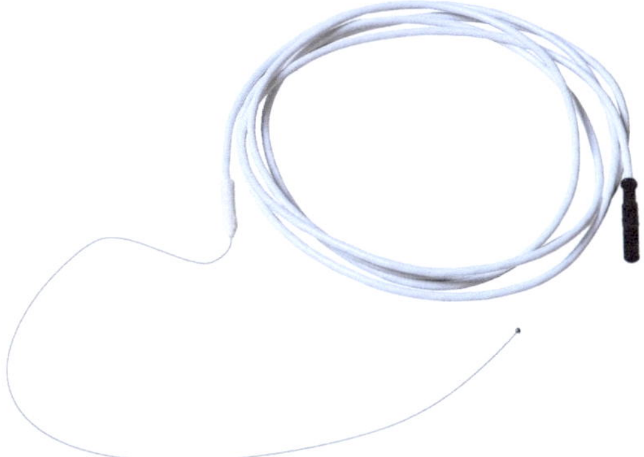

Fig. 4.25 Ball electrode. © ARKANA Forum GmbH 2022. All Rights Reserved

Tympanic electrodes facilitate simultaneous non-invasive stimulation and recording of AEPs. The AEP sound generator is connected to the short black tube. The ball at the end of the spring registers the electrophysiological signals (Fig. 4.24). The quality of AEP signals obtained with tympanic electrodes is usually better than when recorded over the mastoid because the ball electrode is closer to the origin site of the stimulus response.

Ball electrodes are mainly used for the recording of nerve action potentials (NAPs) from the cochlear nerve or wave I as well as the early components of the AEP. The ball and its wire are made of stainless steel (Fig. 4.25).

4.2.3 Spinal Recordings

Spinal epidural electrodes can be used for both stimulation and recording of electrophysiological signals. They are mainly used to register **D-waves** but can also be used to acquire spinal **SEPs** after stimulation of the tibial nerve or for spinal activation of cortical SEPs. The electrode is specially designed for use in the epidural space of the spinal cord. It consists of a silicone or polyamide tube with two or three stainless steel electrode contacts attached to its distal end (Fig. 4.26).

4.2.4 Monitoring of the Vagus Nerve

Continuous IntraOperative NeuroMonitoring (**CIONM**) **electrodes** are used intraoperatively for continuous stimulation of the vagus nerve. The electrodes consist of a silicone body with embedded electrode contacts (Fig. 4.27). After dissection of the vagus nerve, the electrode is looped around the nerve. It can be removed at the end of the operation by gently pulling on the electrode cable.

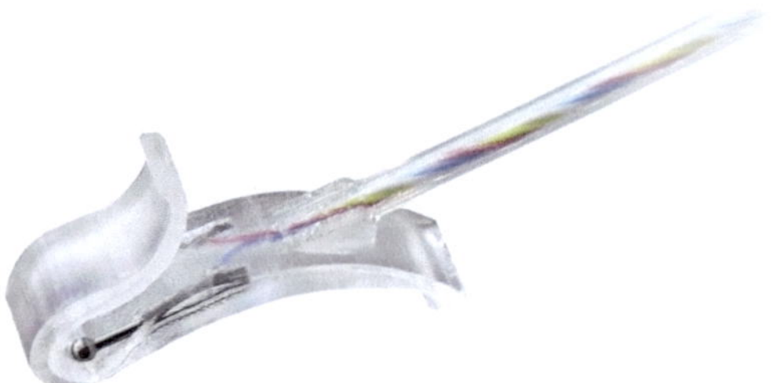

Fig. 4.27 CIONM electrode for stimulation of the vagus nerve. © ARKANA Forum GmbH 2022. All Rights Reserved

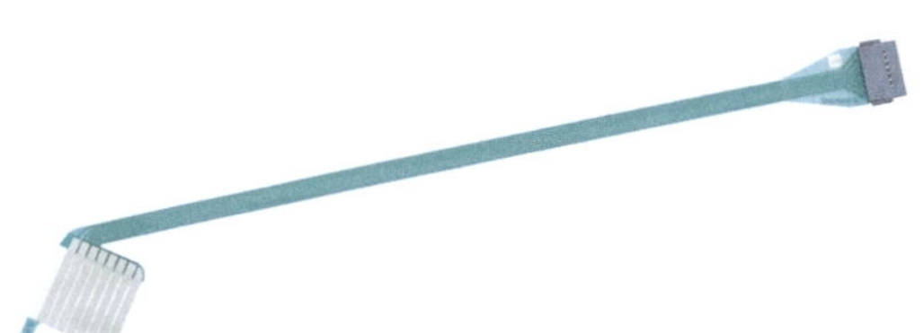

Fig. 4.28 Adhesive electrodes for ventilation tube attachment. © ARKANA Forum GmbH 2022. All Rights Reserved

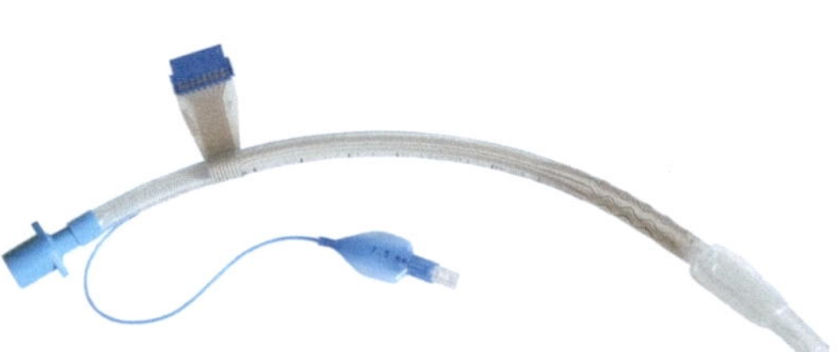

Fig. 4.29 Ventilation tube with integrated electrodes. © ARKANA Forum GmbH 2022. All Rights Reserved

Tube electrodes are used for the non-invasive recording of electrophysiological signals from the vocalis muscle, which is innervated by the laryngeal recurrent branch of the vagus nerve. Adhesive electrodes can be attached to any endotracheal ventilation tube (Fig. 4.28). Alternatively, a ventilation tube with an integrated electrode may be used (Fig. 4.29).

4.2.5 Diagnostics

Cup electrodes are mainly used for recording of electrophysiological signals from the scalp. They are made of gold- or silver-plated metal

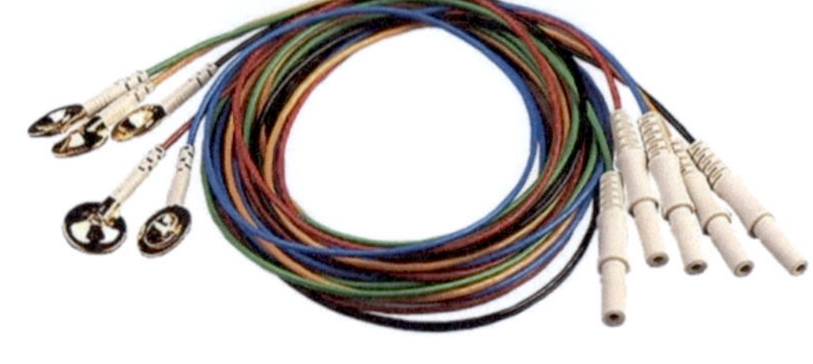

Fig. 4.30 Cup electrodes. © ARKANA Forum GmbH 2022. All Rights Reserved

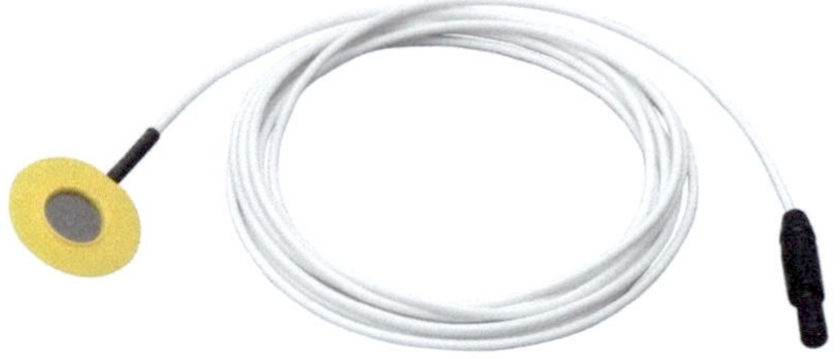

Fig. 4.31 Disc electrode. © ARKANA Forum GmbH 2022. All Rights Reserved

(Fig. 4.30). Before application, the scalp recording sites must be thoroughly degreased and prepared with gentle epidermal abrasion, otherwise the impedance will be too high. The cups are then filled with adhesive gel and bonded to the scalp. Cup electrodes are non-invasive and therefore the first choice for children.

Disc electrodes, similar to cup electrodes, are mainly used for recording of electrophysiological signals from the scalp. They consist of a plastic disc in which a silver-chlorinated metal disc is inserted (Fig. 4.31). Before placing the electrode, the scalp recording site must be thoroughly degreased and prepared with gentle epidermal abrasion to reduce impedance. Some adhesive gel is applied to the metal disk. After the electrode has been fixed, an adhesive ring is placed on the outer rim of the disc to prevent dislocation of the electrode. The adhesive rings must be changed after each application.

Bridge electrodes are used to record EEG signals from the scalp. They are in the form of a stamp with a small plate of silver/silver chloride attached to its end. A piece of felt is pulled over this stamp before the electrode is placed and fixed with small rubber rings (Fig. 4.32). The

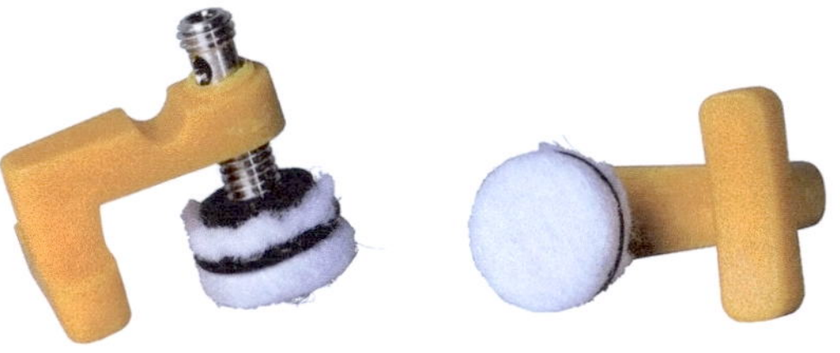

Fig. 4.32 Bridge electrodes. © ARKANA Forum GmbH 2022. All Rights Reserved

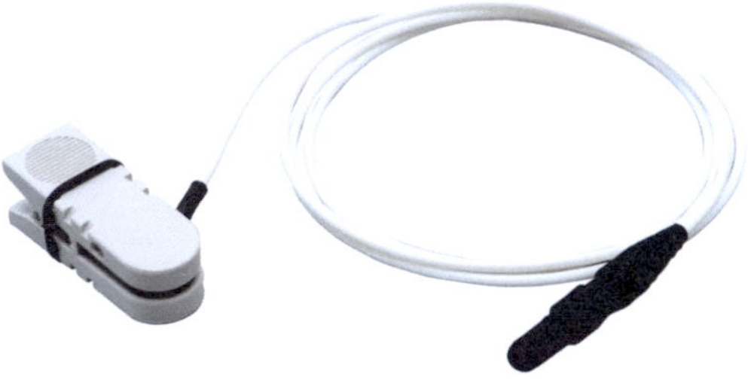

Fig. 4.34 Ear electrode. © ARKANA Forum GmbH 2022. All Rights Reserved

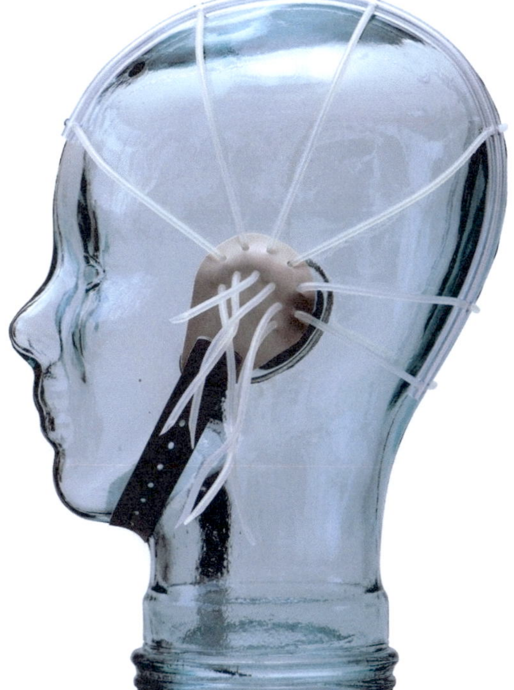

Fig. 4.33 Tube hood. © ARKANA Forum GmbH 2022. All Rights Reserved

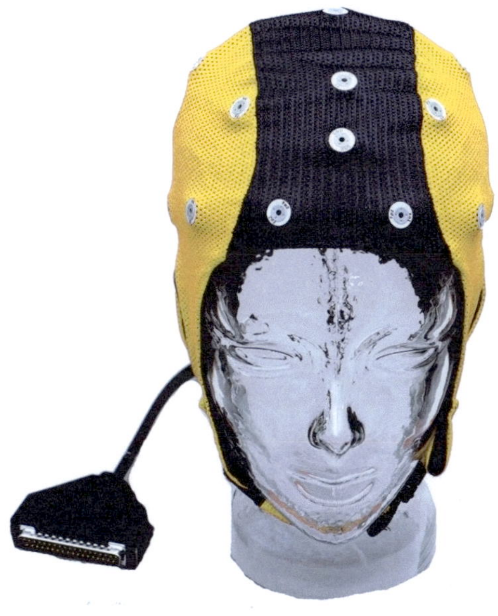

Fig. 4.35 EEG hood. © ARKANA Forum GmbH 2022. All Rights Reserved

electrodes are then immersed in saline solution to ensure good contact with the scalp. Bridge electrodes are used in combination with **tube hoods**, which are available in different sizes and fix the electrodes in selected position (Fig. 4.33). Before applying the electrodes, care should be taken to ensure that the felts are not dripping wet, as saline running down the head may cause electrode bridging. The felts must be changed after each application. As an alternative for soaked felts, good tissue contact can also be achieved by applying adhesive gel to the electrodes.

Ear electrodes are used for the non-invasive recording of electrophysiological signals from the ear. They consist of a plastic clip in which silver/silver chloride electrode discs are embedded on both sides (Fig. 4.34). The clip can be attached to the earlobe without additional fixation.

EEG hoods are used to record EEG signals from the scalp. They are available in different sizes and are placed on the head like a cap. On the inside, silver-chlorinated metal contacts are inserted into the hood tissue, the number of which varies depending on the hood configuration (Fig. 4.35).

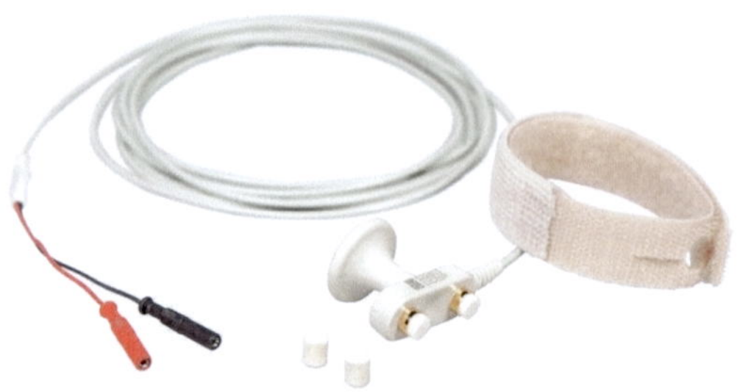

Fig. 4.36 Block electrode. © ARKANA Forum GmbH 2022. All Rights Reserved

Block electrodes are used in diagnostics, for example, for measuring nerve conduction velocity. They consist of a plastic molded part with two gold-plated sockets into which felt inserts soaked in saline solution or gold-plated inserts can be mounted (Fig. 4.36). A good fixation is important for application in order to avoid dislocation of the electrode.

References

1. Kombos T, Süss O, Kern BC, Funk T, Hoell T, Kopetsch O, et al. Comparison between monopolar and bipolar electrical stimulation of the motor cortex. Acta Neurochir. 1999;141:1295–301.
2. Szelényi A, Bello L, Duffau H, Fava E, Feigl GC, Galanda M, et al. Intraoperative electrical stimulation in awake craniotomy: methodological aspects of current practice. Neurosurg Focus. 2010;28(2):E7.
3. Sarnthein J, Lüchinger R, Piccirelli M, Regli L, Bozinov O. Prevalence of complications in intraoperative magnetic resonance imaging combined with neurophysiologic monitoring. World Neurosurg. 2016 Sep;93:168–74.

Modalities and Methods of Intraoperative Neuromonitoring

David MacDonald and Celine Wegner

Contents

D. MacDonald (✉) · C. Wegner
ARKANA Forum GmbH, Emmendingen, Germany

© The Author(s), under exclusive license to Springer Nature Switzerland AG 2024
J. Zentner et al. (eds.), *Intraoperative Neuromonitoring*,
https://doi.org/10.1007/978-3-031-46125-5_5

5.1 Electroencephalography (EEG)

The EEG represents the basis for the investigation of some evoked potentials (EPs). In addition, it enables the detection of **epilepsy typical potentials** during cortical stimulation. In epilepsy surgery, direct cortical EEG referred to as electrocorticography (ECoG) is used to optimize resection of the **epileptogenic area**. Moreover, the EEG allows the assessment of the **oxygen supply** to the brain during carotid endarterectomy and other cerebrovascular procedures. Finally, EEG recordings may be used to estimate the **depth of anesthesia**.

In this context, only a few basic features of the EEG will be discussed that are relevant for the understanding of IONM.

5.1.1 The 10–20 Electrode System

The basis for accurately placing the electrodes on the head is the 10–20 electrode system. For this purpose, the length of the **skull** is measured from the nasion (transition between the frontal bone and the nasal bone) to the inion (prominence of the occipital bone). The value of this distance corresponds to 100% and is divided into **10 and 20% sections** as follows: From the nasion, one first moves by 10%, then in four 20% steps and at the end again by 10% in the direction of the inion. Similarly, the distance between the two preauricular points (on both sides just in front of the tragus of the external auditory canal) is measured along the skull and divided according to the 10–20 rule in the same way as described for the longitudinal extent of the skull. Based on these coordinates, the electrodes are fixed to the scalp in several transverse rows. They are placed symmetrically at equal distances that are generally between 5 and 7 cm in adults, depending on head size.

The position of the electrodes is designated in relation to the topography of the brain (Fp for frontopolar, F for frontal, T for temporal, C for central, P for parietal, and O for occipital). They are further specified by odd and even numbers for left and right scalp sites, "z" for sagittal midline sites, and A for auricle sites on the left and right earlobe or mastoid (Figs. 5.1 and 5.2). The **percentage division** of the longitudinal and transverse extensions of the skull as described ensures that the desired brain areas are reliably covered even with different skull sizes. To achieve a higher resolution, additional rows of electrodes can be placed according to the 10–10 combinatorial nomenclature system, for example, the row CP midway between the rows C and P. The CP row is important for somatosensory evoked potential (SEP) monitoring. In adults, this row is about 3 cm behind the C row, depending on head size.

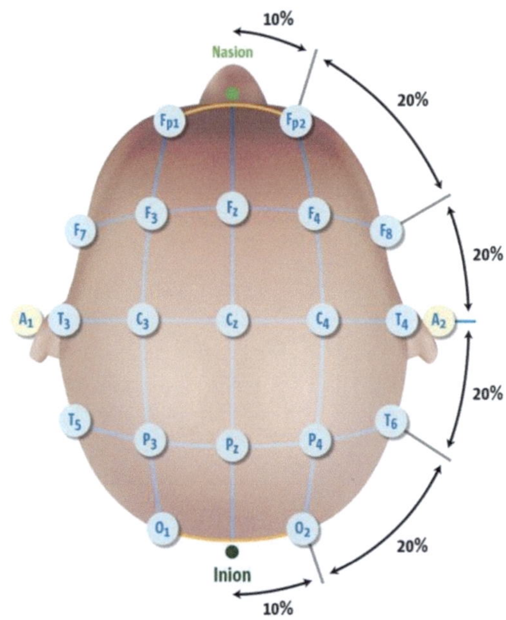

Fig. 5.1 The 10–20 electrode system from the top view. © ARKANA Forum GmbH 2022. All Rights Reserved

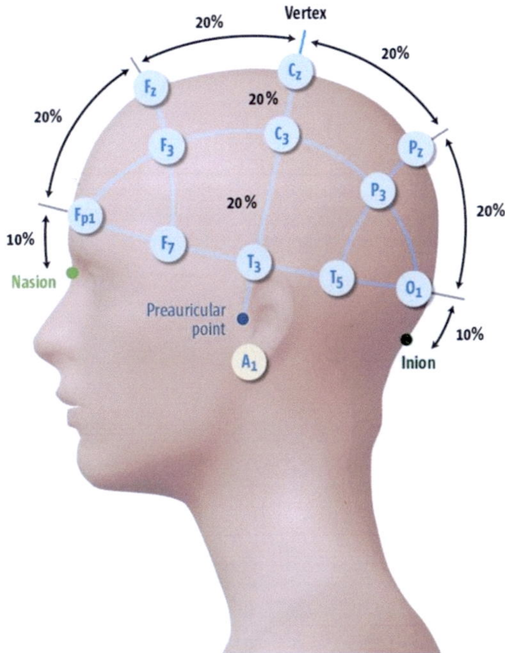

Fig. 5.2 The 10–20 electrode system from the side view. © ARKANA Forum GmbH 2022. All Rights Reserved

A modification of 10–20 nomenclature changes T3/4 to T7/8 and T5/6 to P7/8. However, here we will use the more widely-known original labels for these sites that are infrequently used for IONM.

5.1.2 Cortical Sources

The EEG is generated by the activity of **pyramidal cells**, which make up about 80% of the neurons of the cerebral cortex. Pyramidal cells show a typical morphology: From the cell body (soma), a single long dendrite ascends to higher layers of the cortex, where it branches (dendrite tree). At the soma, additional dendrites branch laterally and caudally. This is also where the axon originates, which runs to other cortical or subcortical areas. The pyramidal cells are arranged in vertical columns that extend from the surface to the depth of the brain.

Soma and dendrite tree form **two electrical compartments**. They receive excitatory and inhibitory input from subcortical sources.

Activation by **excitatory input** leads to a change in the resting membrane potential and to negativity of the activated area relative to the outside of the non-activated portions of the neuron. Thus, differences in charge occur between the apical area (negative) and the soma (positive). In the case of **inhibitory input**, this process takes place with reversed polarity.

Since the pyramidal cells are electrically coupled by gap junctions, their activity is synchronized over several square centimeters of the cortex. This creates **electrical dipoles**, the sum potential of which can be recorded from the scalp (Fig. 5.3).

5.1.3 Intraoperative EEG Recordings and Analysis

Diagnostic EEG recordings employ full-scalp montages of 16 or more channels, and sometimes this approach is used for monitoring carotid endarterectomy. Intraoperative ECoG during epilepsy surgery may also involve multiple channels. However, most intraoperative EEG recordings are limited to a few **channels**, mainly between **2 and 8**. The electrodes are connected to the EEG device. In the digital EEG devices commonly used today, the individual electrodes are recorded simultaneously against a common reference. These referential inputs can be displayed as recorded, or through digital subtraction and averaging displayed in any desired bipolar, common average, or source derivation montage. A montage is the arrangement or sequence of multichannel displays. The recording is done as a free-running EEG with a display time base of 10–60 s, depending on the intended application.

The **EEG is evaluated** by the experienced examiner mainly through viewing the waveforms. However, the frequency, amplitude, and phase of the EEG signals can also be digitally processed for quantitative analysis. An additional electrocardiogram (ECG) channel is recorded to identify electrocardiographic artifacts.

The **normal EEG** describes a basic activity comprising diverse frequency ranges, which differ between various brain areas as well as depend-

Fig. 5.3 Structure of a pyramidal cell and generation of a dipole by an excitatory input. © ARKANA Forum GmbH 2022. All Rights Reserved

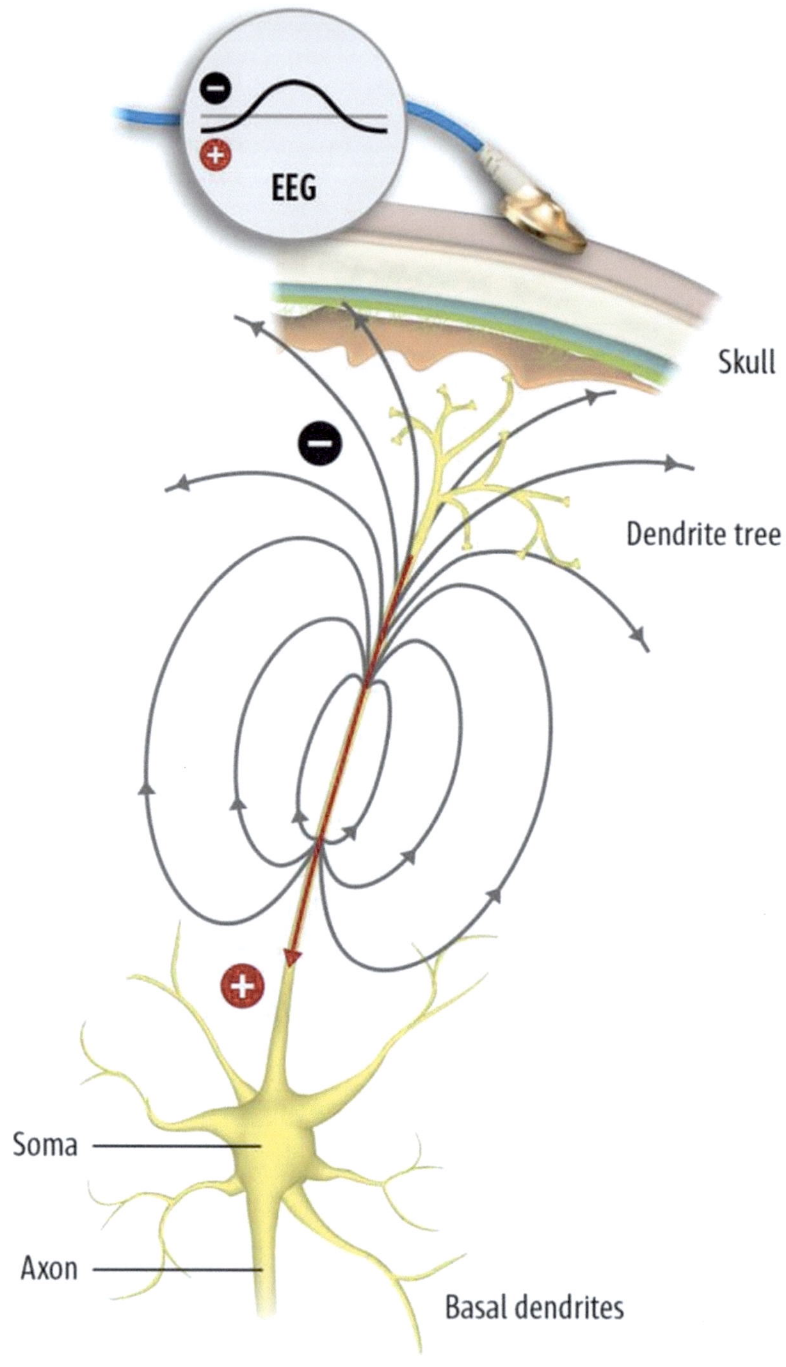

ing on the state of wakefulness. Figure 5.4 shows a normal EEG. The typical frequency ranges are listed in Table 5.1.

Atypical EEG patterns may be observed as **normal variants**, which do not have any pathological significance. They often occur only during

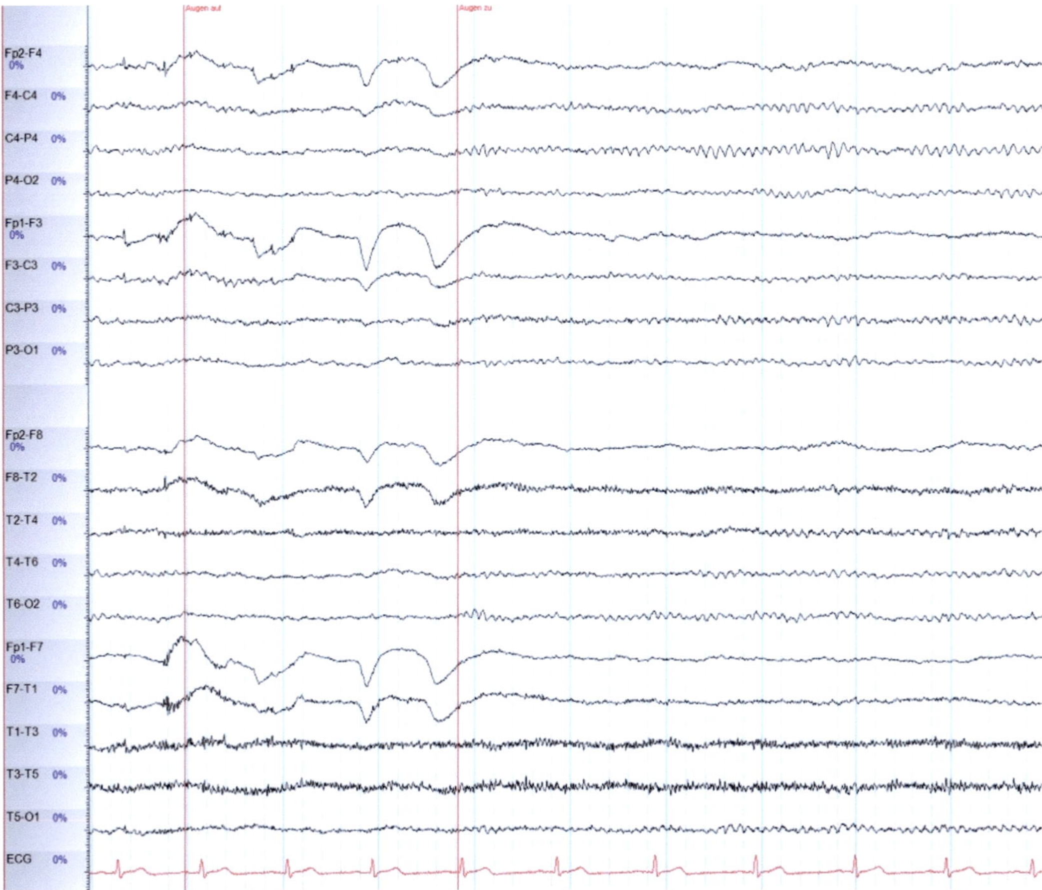

Fig. 5.4 Normal awake EEG. © ARKANA Forum GmbH 2022. All Rights Reserved

Table 5.1 Frequency ranges in the normal EEG

Designation	Frequency range in Hz	
	From	To
Alpha	8	13
Beta	>13	30
Theta	4	<8
Delta	0.5	<4

a limited period of time. Two examples are the fast and slow occipital alpha rhythm variants. In these variants, the frequency of the occipital rhythm is in the beta range (around 16 Hz) or in the theta range (around 4 Hz). Furthermore, the usual occipital alpha rhythm of about 8 Hz may be intermixed with the respective frequencies.

Pathological EEG patterns in the context of IONM include in particular epileptiform abnormalities such as spikes, sharp waves, polyspikes, and spike-and-wave complexes. Such patterns are frequently observed during intraoperative ECoG definition of resection borders in epilepsy surgery. Direct cortical stimulation may also occasionally be followed by epileptiform after-discharges that may indicate the risk of a stimulation-induced epileptic seizure (Fig. 5.5). During vascular interventions (e.g., carotid endarterectomy), EEG slowing in the delta range may be indicative of cerebral ischemia (reduced blood flow or impaired oxygen supply to the brain).

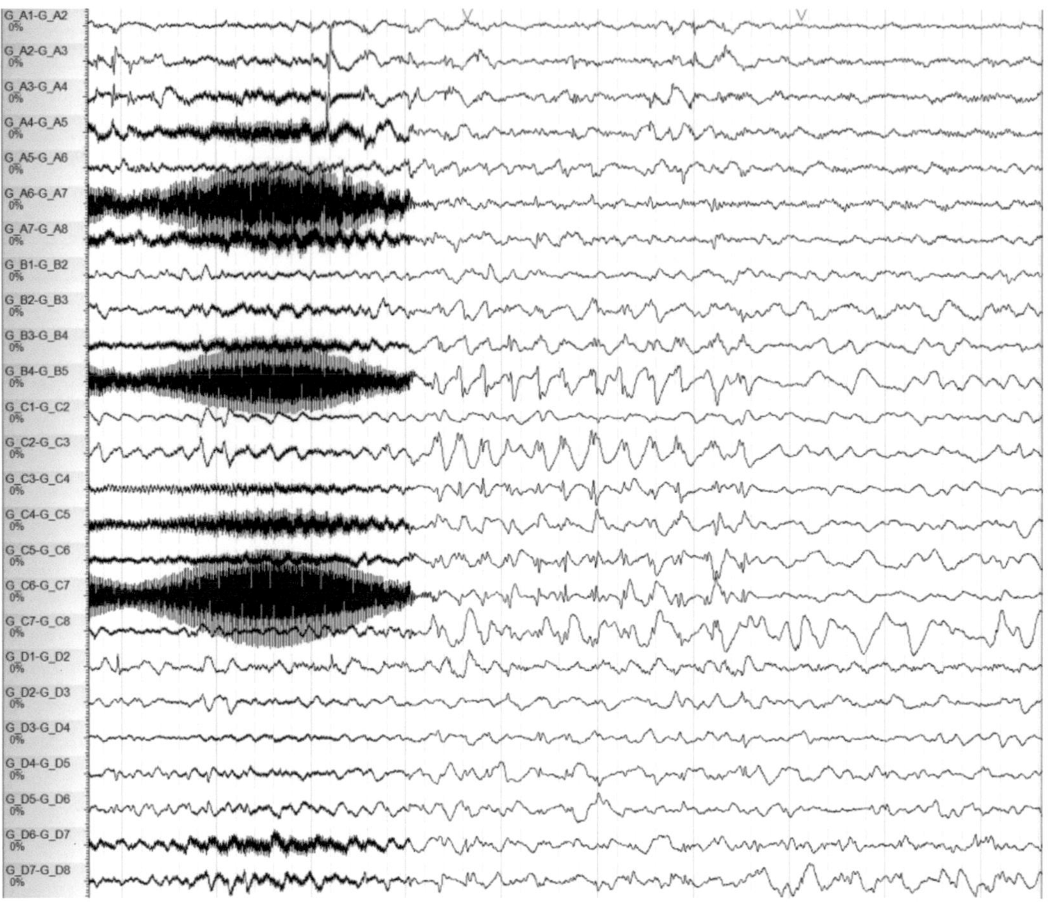

Fig. 5.5 A subdural grid ECoG showing 50 Hz direct cortical stimulation artifacts followed by stimulation-induced spike and spike-and-wave afterdischarges. © ARKANA Forum GmbH 2022. All Rights Reserved

5.2 Electromyography (EMG)

Electromyography measures the electrical activity of a muscle. For this, electrodes are placed in or over the muscle (intramuscular or surface electrodes) to record voltage changes from the muscle. On the one hand, the **spontaneous activity** of the muscle can be registered by continuous (free-running) EMG. On the other hand, the **compound muscle action potential (CMAP)** elicited by stimulation of a nerve can be assessed. During EMG monitoring, care must always be taken to ensure that muscle activity is not affected by the administration of muscle relaxants.

5.2.1 Continuous (Free-Running) EMG

Surgical manipulation of nerves and exposure to heat or cold can induce **spontaneous discharges** such as spikes, bursts, or trains. **Spikes** consist of bi- or triphasic waves with a single peak. **Bursts** represent sequential spikes with multiple peaks appearing within less than 200 ms. **Trains** are complexes of spikes or bursts with a longer duration in the range of seconds (Fig. 5.6). According to their characteristics and morphology, A-, B-, and C-trains are distinguished. A-trains are also known as neurotonic discharges.

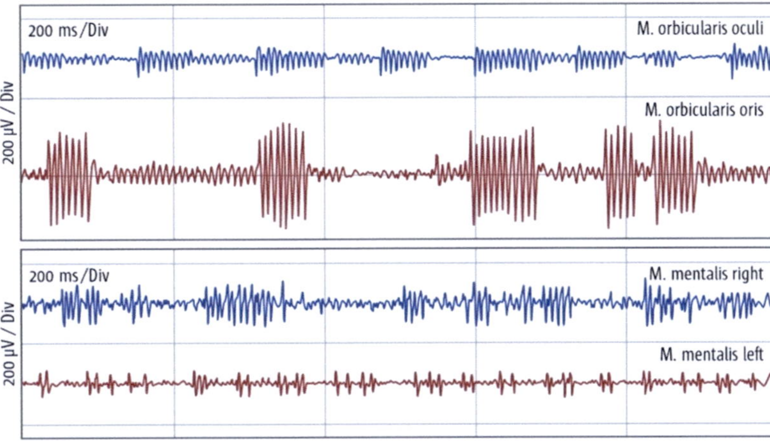

Fig. 5.6 Different trains of various amplitude, frequency and duration in facial EMG. © ARKANA Forum GmbH 2022. All Rights Reserved

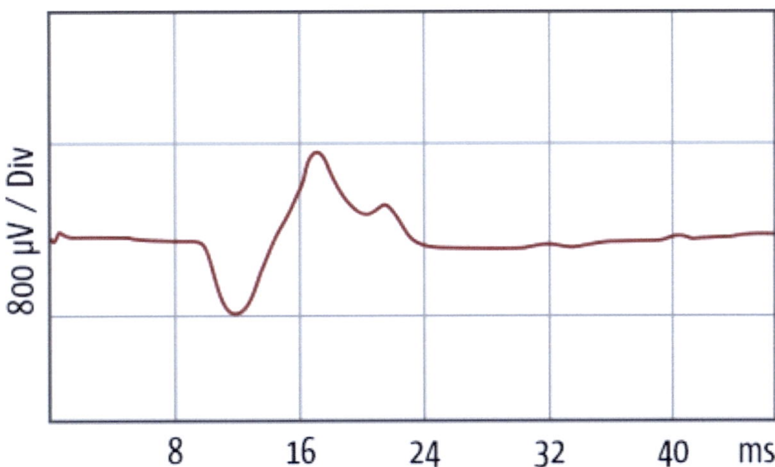

Fig. 5.7 CMAP of the M. vastus medialis. © ARKANA Forum GmbH 2022. All Rights Reserved

Continuous EMG is used to identify and monitor **motor nerves** or nerve branches intraoperatively. The EMG can be made audible via loudspeaker and provides the surgeon with continuous feedback on impending impairment of nervous structures.

Single spikes or bursts are usually not critical. In contrast, the surgeon should be informed about **persistent spikes and trains**, as these patterns of spontaneous activity often indicate postoperative deficits [1–4]. In particular, A-trains consisting of a low-amplitude and high-frequency sequence of spikes should be noted. For example, monitoring of the facial nerve has shown that these trains correlate with postoperative facial nerve paresis, with the degree of paresis depending on the total A-train time [5].

5.2.2 Compound Muscle Action Potential (CMAP)

Electrical stimulation of a peripheral motor nerve results in contraction of the innervated muscle, which can be assessed by recording a CMAP. This technique is known as triggered or stimulated EMG. Triggered CMAPs are used during dissection on **peripheral nerves**, in particular on **cranial nerves**. Usually, intraoperative registration of the CMAP is combined with continuous EMG. This provides the surgeon with the best possible feedback on any impending impairment of nerve structures, both continuously via audible EMG and selectively by stimulation-induced CMAPs. A typical CMAP is depicted in Fig. 5.7.

5.3   Electroneurography

Electroneurography is used to assess distal motor latency, motor and sensory nerve conduction velocities, and F-wave latency.

5.3.1   Motor Neurography

Stimulation is performed with a hand-held probe, hook electrodes, or surface electrodes. Common stimulation sites are median nerve, ulnar nerve, radial nerve, peroneal nerve, tibial nerve, and femoral nerve. **Recordings** are done directly from the nerve with hook electrodes or from the skin with surface electrodes. Figure 5.8 shows a typical potential.

The **F-wave** represents an indirect response resulting from antidromic excitation of the anterior horn cells under supramaximal peripheral stimulation.

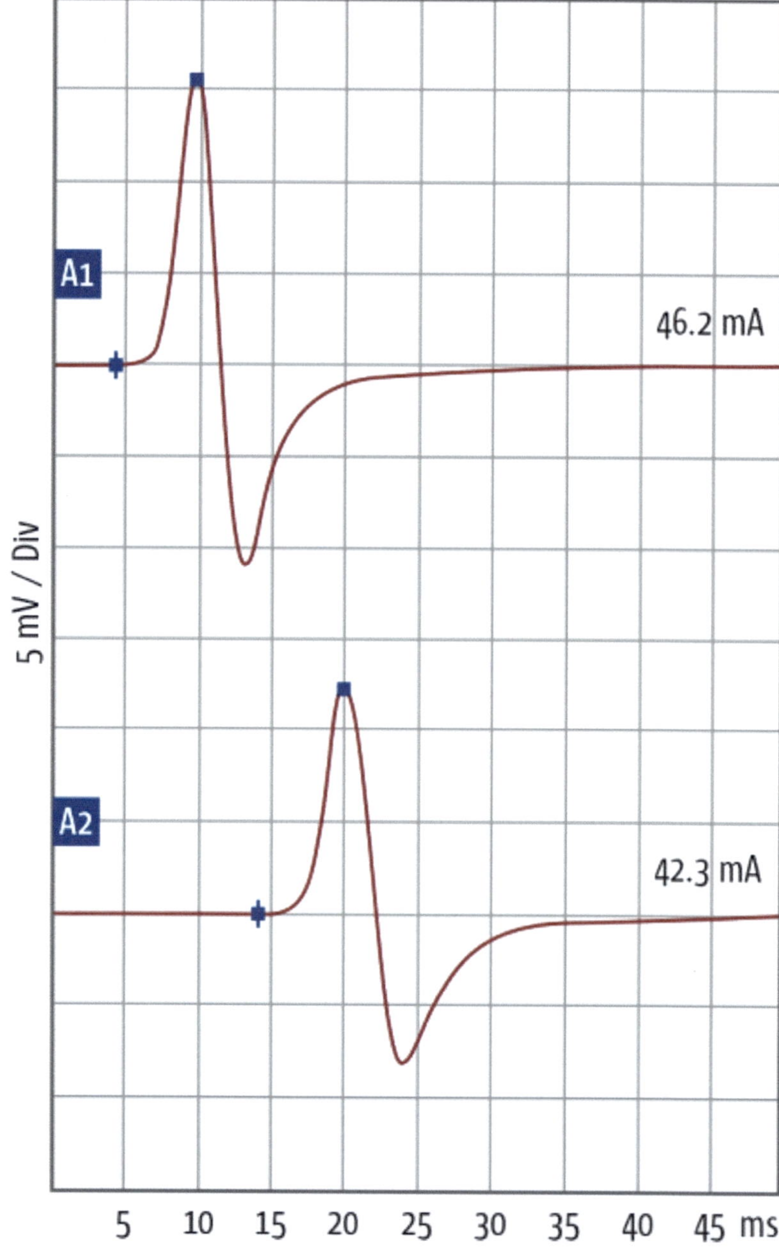

Fig. 5.8 Motor neurography of the tibial nerve recorded from the abductor hallucis muscle. Top: Potential after stimulation at the medial malleolus. Bottom: Response after stimulation at the popliteal fossa. © ARKANA Forum GmbH 2022. All Rights Reserved

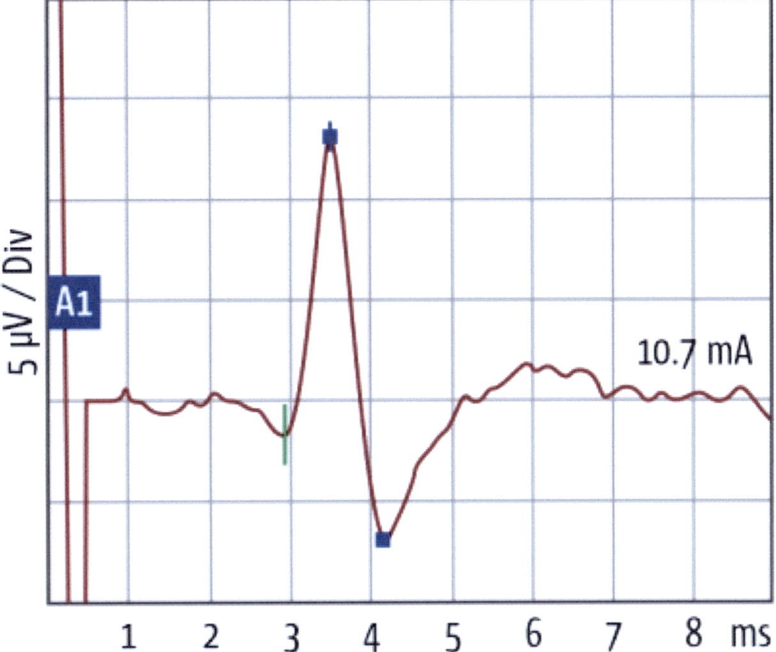

Fig. 5.9 Sensory neurography of the median nerve after stimulation of the index finger, recorded at the wrist. © ARKANA Forum GmbH 2022. All Rights Reserved

5.3.2 Sensory Neurography

Sensory neurography assesses nerve conduction velocity. The examination may be **orthodromic** (distal stimulation, proximal recording) or **antidromic** (proximal stimulation, distal recording). Frequently, hook electrodes are used for this application. With the three-pole hook electrode, propagation of the action potential in both directions can be generated by connecting the middle electrode as the anode. Figure 5.9 presents a typical potential.

5.4 Evoked Potentials (EPs)

Evoked potentials are elicited by a defined stimulus at a defined location. The **response is time-locked to the stimulus** and can be recorded as a typical wave from the various nervous structures or from the musculature. Individual waves of the signal obtained can be assigned to different **generators**. Important parameters for the evaluation of an evoked potential are onset or peak **latency** (delay between stimulus and response), **interpeak** latency (delay between the responses of two generators), and the **peak-to-peak amplitude** of a wave (Fig. 5.10).

> *It should be noted that the usual values given for the various modalities depend on the general conditions, in particular, body size, anesthesia, and temperature. The signals are always interpreted in side-by-side comparison and in relation to the individual baseline.*

Evoked potentials can provide important information about **afferent** and **efferent** pathways. Scalp or cortically recorded EPs are masked by spontaneous EEG or ECoG activity. Other sources of EP interference include EMG, ECG, and external electromagnetic fields. An important tool to obtain usable potentials is the **averaging** of multiple recording sweeps. The recurrent EP waveform present in every sweep gradually averages in although modified by jitter, while the amplitude of the uncorrelated random

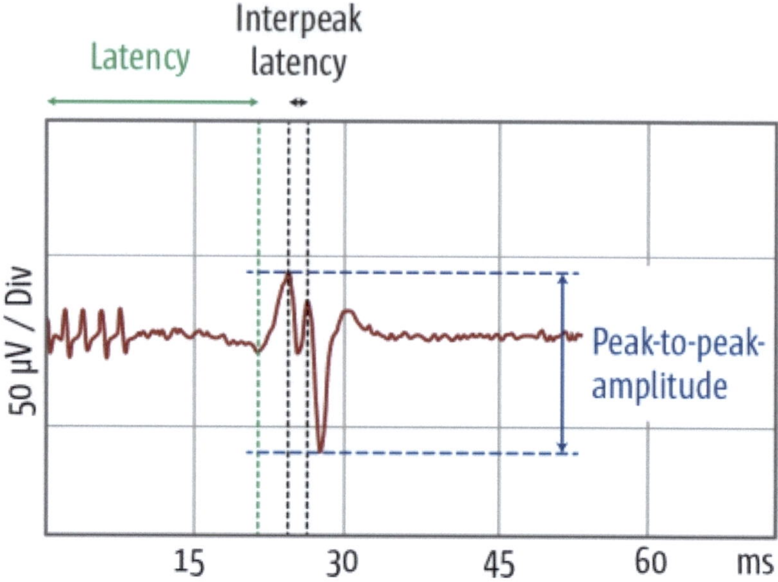

Fig. 5.10 Latency, interpeak latency and peak-to-peak amplitude of an evoked potential. © ARKANA Forum GmbH 2022. All Rights Reserved

interference gradually declines but never reaches zero. Thus, averaged EPs are estimates distorted by jitter and residual noise.

Depending on the site of stimulation and the monitored pathway, evoked potentials are either **somatosensory (SEPs), motor (MEPs), auditory (AEPs),** or **visual (VEPs)**. We can use SEPs and MEPs not only to monitor the ascending and descending pathways, respectively, but also to map sensory and motor areas in the brain (homunculus). This is referred to as **functional topographic mapping**.

> *The number of averaged sweeps needed to resolve an EP depends on the signal-to-noise ratio (SNR) that is related to ratio between the signal amplitude and the interference amplitude. To some extent, this varies with the distance of the generators from the recording electrodes. For example, averaging is not necessary for muscle MEPs since the recording electrodes are located directly at the generator, so the signal is large compared to interference. On the other hand, averaging 1000 or more sweeps may be needed for far-field recordings (e.g., brainstem AEPs, subcortical SEPs) to obtain a reproducible signal.*

> *A disturbance variable that plays a major role in the recording of evoked potentials is the line voltage frequency of either 50 or 60 Hz. In order to minimize the interference of this frequency during averaging, it is necessary to set the stimulation frequency to an odd divisor of 50 or 60 (e.g., 2.3 or 4.7 Hz). This will ensure that the oscillations occurring in the recording sweeps due to the disturbance appear with different delays after the stimulus and are thus minimized by averaging. Moreover, interferences can be reduced and the signal quality improved by tightly braiding or twisting the cables of the recording electrodes.*

> *By international agreement, potentials with a negative polarity are displayed as an upgoing "positive" deflection. However, the designation of the wave is based on its original polarity (N for negative, P for positive) and is completed by a consecutive number (e.g., N1, P1, N2, P2) or the mean latencies of the respective wave in awake normal control subjects (e.g., N20, P37).*

5.4.1 Somatosensory Evoked Potentials (SEPs)

We use SEPs to monitor dorsal column–medial lemniscus **ascending pathways** whenever they are at risk centrally or peripherally [6]. Stimulation is applied to a nerve of the arm or leg, and the monitored response is recorded from the scalp over sensory cortex. Control recordings from peripheral nerve or the spinal cord can be done distal to the surgical site.

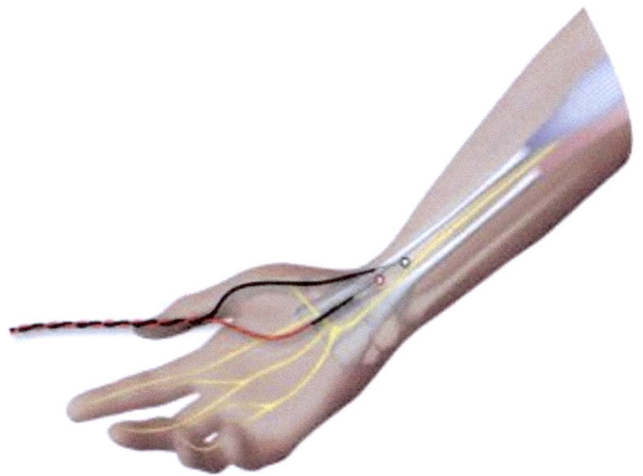

Fig. 5.11 Position of the electrodes for stimulation of the median nerve (red = anode; black = cathode). © ARKANA Forum GmbH 2022. All Rights Reserved

Traditionally, amplitude reduction of >50% or latency delay of >10% is considered critical. However, the warning criterion has recently been revised to visually obvious amplitude reduction from recent pre-change values that clearly exceed trial-to-trial variability, particularly if focal and abrupt. The surgeon should always be quickly informed of any negative trend unexplained by confounding factors. It is recommended not to wait until critical limits are reached. However, it is also important to avoid excessively frequent reports of minor deterioration that can interfere with surgery and jade surgeons to alerts, possibly leading to failure to intervene for truly pathological deterioration [6].

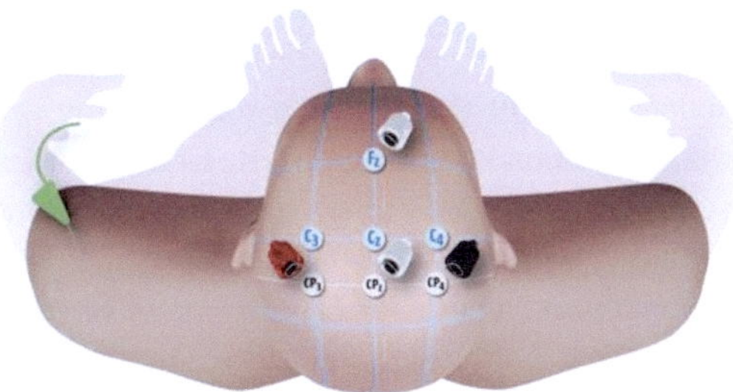

Fig. 5.12 Position of the electrodes for recording median nerve SEPs. © ARKANA Forum GmbH 2022. All Rights Reserved

Recording electrodes are placed according to the 10–20 system. Traditionally, points CP3 to Fz are used for recording right median nerve SEPs and CP4 to Fz for the registration of left median nerve SEPs (Fig. 5.12). However, recent recommendations advise CP3–CPz and CP4–CPz that usually have higher SNRs and therefore require less averaging. Sometimes CP3–CP4 and CP4–CP3 are best. Indeed, one can individually optimize the recording channels for each side [6].

5.4.1.1 Median Nerve SEPs

The examination of SEPs following stimulation of the median nerve is one of the most commonly used modalities of intraoperative neuromonitoring.

Stimulation is performed using a pair of electrodes placed at the wrist. The cathode is located 3 cm proximal to the wrist crease between the tendons of the palmaris longus and flexor carpi radialis muscles, and the anode is placed at the wrist crease along the course of the nerve (Fig. 5.11). Depolarization of the nerve occurs mainly at the cathode. At the anode, axons may be hyperpolarized. Thus, to prevent anodal block of the action potential by hyperpolarization, the cathode is always placed proximally [7].

When simultaneously recording EMG from the limb of SEP stimulation, observing the stimulation artifacts in the free-running EMG can verify correct setup, proper wiring, and adequate settings of the device.

The **action potential** triggered by stimulation initially runs along the median nerve. After entering the spinal cord in the area of the fifth cervical root to the first thoracic root, the potential rises in the dorsal column (fasciculus cuneatus) to the dorsal column nucleus (nucleus cuneatus) in the inferior medulla oblongata (**first neuron**). There, the **second neuron** begins, which crosses to the opposite side (decussates) in the lemniscus medialis and continues to ascend to the nucleus ventralis posterior of the thalamus. Here starts the **third neuron**, which finally reaches the primary sensory cortex in the postcentral gyrus.

The different **generators** can be recorded from the body surface. The **cubital fossa** potential recorded from a pair of electrodes medial to the biceps brachii tendon just above the cubital fossa crease and 3 cm proximal arises from the median nerve at the elbow. It requires minimal averaging due to very high SNR. **Erb's point** is located 2 cm above the mid-clavicle. Here, ascending sensory fibers in the brachial plexus are relatively superficial. The level of **cervical spine 5 or 7** indicates the transition from the peripheral to the central nervous system. At **cervical spine 2**, the signal can be recorded immediately before entering the brain. The Erb's point and cervical potentials may require substantial averaging due to low SNRs. A **subcortical** response of brainstem origin can be recorded via CP3 or CP4 ipsilateral to the stimulated nerve and referenced to the mastoid or contralateral Erb's point. However, it usually requires a lot of averaging due to very low SNR. In clinical practice, the **N20** potential from the **sensory cortex** contralateral to the stimulation side is the principal monitor. However, adding the cubital fossa potential provides valuable control for stimulus failure or distal limb conduction failure due to limb ischemia or pressure, without delaying surgical feedback. Additional recording sites may help evaluate other confounding factors such as brachial plexus conduction failure and anesthesia or vital parameters, but can slow surgical feedback (Fig. 5.13).

Rare patients have congenital nondecussation so that the second neuron does not cross to the other side but projects to the ipsilateral thalamus and sensory cortex. Accurately monitoring these patients requires reversed-lateralization scalp recording sites. Consequently, it is advisable to screen for this anomaly with an initial recording from CP3 and CP4 to the mastoid to determine which hemisphere generates the sensory cortex response.

A **typical potential** is shown in Fig. 5.14. Table 5.2 summarizes median nerve SEPs at different recording sites. Table 5.3 presents typical N20 peak latencies. Table 5.4 gives the parameters commonly used for stimulation and recording of median nerve SEPs.

The median nerve is particularly suitable for upper extremity SEPs because it has a large representation in the primary sensory cortex. Thus, a larger recording signal can be expected. However, for certain surgeries, for example, on peripheral nerves or the cervical spine, it may be necessary to monitor other or multiple sensory nerves, such as the **ulnar** and **radial nerves**. Nerves and associated spinal roots are listed in Table 5.5.

5.4.1.2 Tibial Nerve SEPs

Tibial nerve SEP recordings represent one of the standard techniques of intraoperative neuromonitoring.

Stimulation is achieved using a pair of electrodes placed at the ankle over the course of the tibial nerve. The cathode is located between the medial malleolus and the Achilles tendon, and the anode is placed 3 cm distal (Fig. 5.15).

In their simplest traditional form, **recordings** can be performed from the scalp according to the 10–20 system at CPz to Fz, independent of the side of stimulation (Fig. 5.16). This basic approach may be satisfactory for some patients, but is suboptimal due to low SNR. Advanced

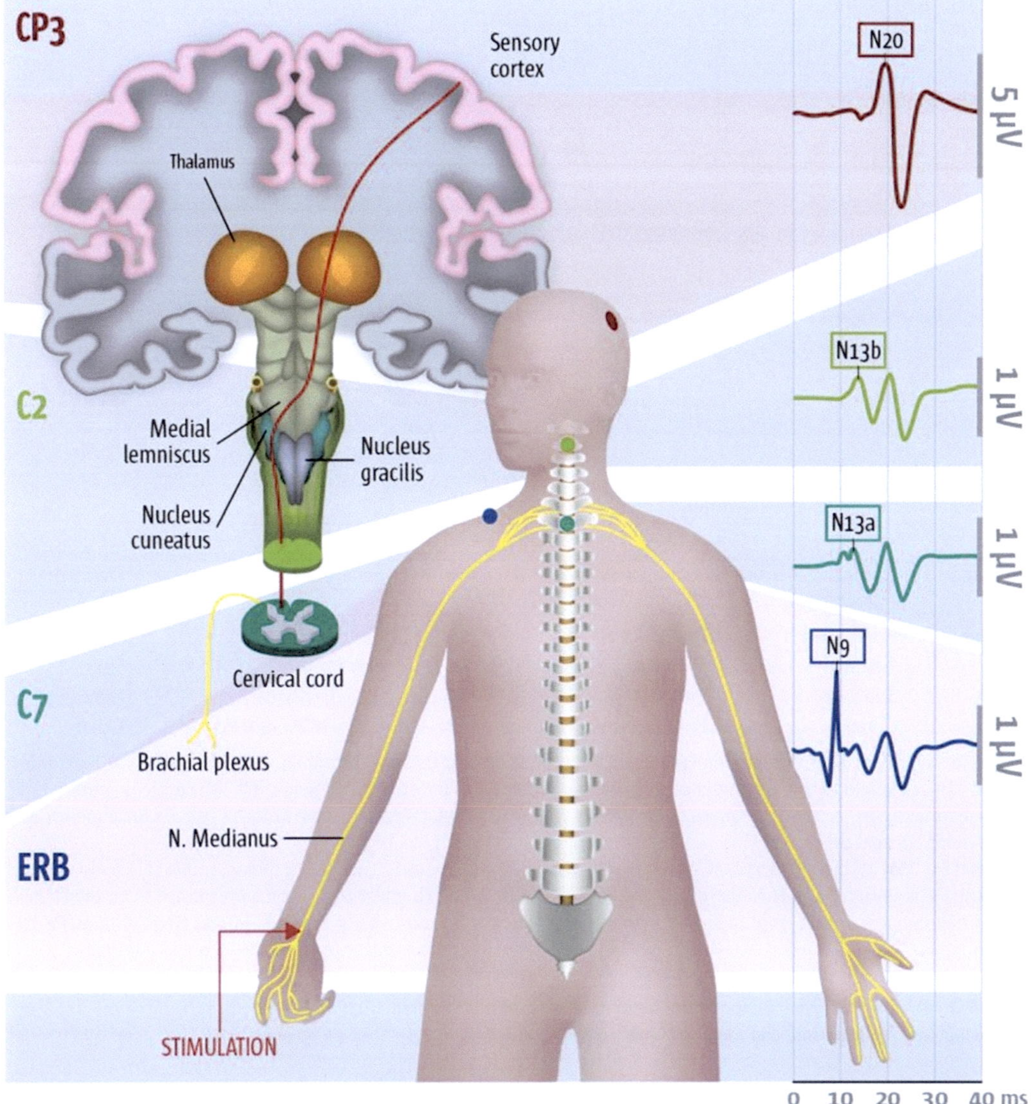

Fig. 5.13 Signal path of median nerve SEPs and their generators. © ARKANA Forum GmbH 2022. All Rights Reserved

neuromonitoring employs **SEP optimization** to ensure the best possible monitoring of all patients by maximizing the SNR [6]. This technique checks decussation by recording from CP3 and CP4 to the mastoid and compares all possibly optimal recording derivations. The best one for each side is then used for monitoring to provide the fastest possible surgical feedback.

The **action potential** triggered by the stimulation initially runs along the tibial nerve. At the lumbosacral junction (L5/S1), it enters the spinal canal, and at the level of the conus medullaris (T12/L1), it reaches the spinal cord via the posterior root. From there, the signal rises in the dorsal column (fasciculus gracilis) to the dorsal column nucleus (nucleus gracilis) in the inferior medulla

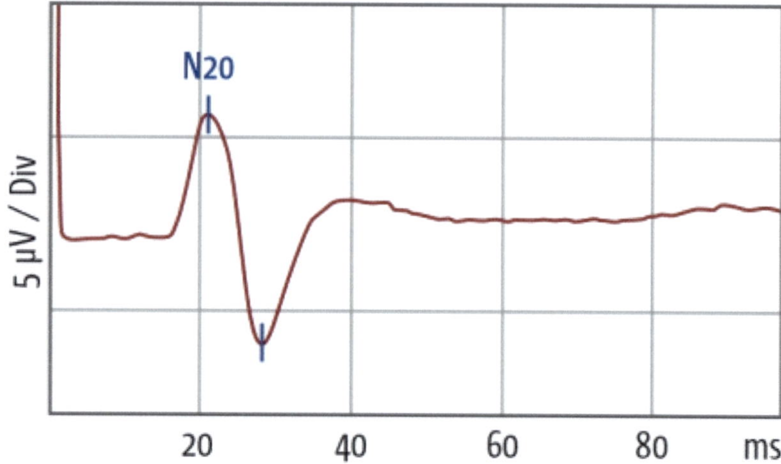

Fig. 5.14 Typical left median nerve SEP recorded with CP4–Fz. © ARKANA Forum GmbH 2022. All Rights Reserved

Table 5.2 Median nerve SEPs at different recording sites

		Monitoring derivations [6]		
Design.	Recording site	Traditional	Optimal (highest SNR)	Deflection
CF	Cubital fossa	–	CFd–CFp	Up
N9 or EP	Erb's point	EPi–EPc or EPi–Fz	EPi–M (optional)	Up
N13	Cervical	C5–EPc or C5–Fz	C5–M (optional)	Up
P14/N18	Subcortical	CPi–EPc	Omit, or fallback CPi–M[a]	Down/up
N20	Cortical	CPc–Fz or CPc–CPi	**CPc–CPz**[b], CPc–CPi, or CPc–Fz	Up

Design. designation, *SNR* signal-to-noise ratio, *CF* cubital fossa, *d* distal, *p* proximal, *EP* Erb's point, *M* mastoid, *CP* CP3 or CP4, *i* ipsilateral to the stimulated nerve, *c* contralateral to the stimulated nerve, *C5* 5th cervical spine
[a] The subcortical SEP is normally omitted due to very low SNR, but CPi–M may be a fallback spinal cord monitor in the case of poor cortical SEPs
[b] Optimal for 75% of median nerves. Consequently, one can routinely use it and check the other two if it seems possibly suboptimal, or initially compare the three and choose the best one (highest SNR) for monitoring. Note that CPc–Fz always has greatest signal amplitude, but also greatest EEG noise, so usually has suboptimal SNR. CPc–CPz has a smaller signal but lowest noise, so usually has highest SNR. Here, the *fastest reproducing* channel is optimal

Table 5.3 Typical N20 peak latency after median nerve stimulation. Note that the latency is depending on arm length. Anesthesia and hypothermia can increase peak SEP latencies

	Peak latency (ms)
Median nerve N20	17–21 ms

Table 5.4 Parameters for stimulation and recording of median nerve SEPs (recommended starting values are marked in bold)

Stimulation current	Supramaximal, usually 3–30 mA[a]
Stimulation frequency	2.1–5.1 Hz (select an odd divisor of 50 or 60 Hz)
Pulse form	Monophasic rectangular cathodal pulse
Pulse duration	200–500 µs (**200 µs**)
Low-pass filter	300 Hz (1000 Hz for peripheral recording)
High-pass filter	30 Hz (0.2 Hz for cubital fossa recording)
Time base	50–100 ms (**50 ms**)
Averaging	To medium–high reproducibility, usually 50–200 sweeps[b]

[a] The supramaximal stimulation intensity is that intensity which, when exceeded, does not elicit a higher amplitude of the response. At the beginning of measurements, the current intensity should be set as low as possible and adjusted step by step. One can quickly find supramaximal intensity by viewing single-sweep cubital fossa responses
[b] Valid interpretation requires SEP reproducibility. This means that consecutive recordings show nearly the same result, with <20–30% signal amplitude variation and approximate or nearly exact waveform superimposition. Less reproducible SEPs indicate a lot of residual noise and mandate caution

Table 5.5 Spinal roots of the typical nerves used for SEPs of the upper extremity

Nerve	Spinal roots
Median nerve	C5, C6, C7, C8
Radial nerve	C5, C6, C7, C8
Ulnar nerve	C7, C8, T1

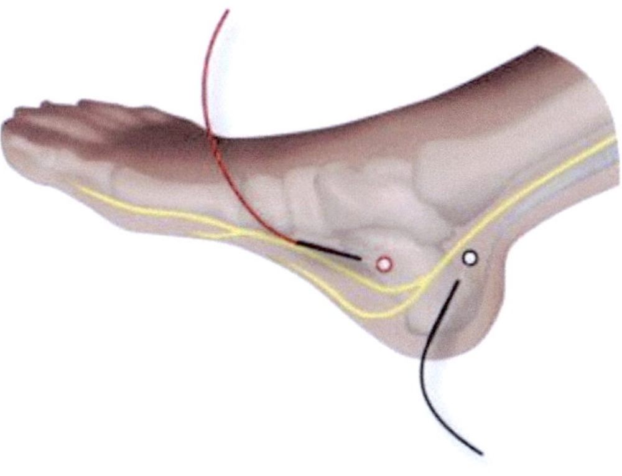

Fig. 5.15 Position of the electrodes for stimulation of the tibial nerve (red = anode; black = cathode). © ARKANA Forum GmbH 2022. All Rights Reserved

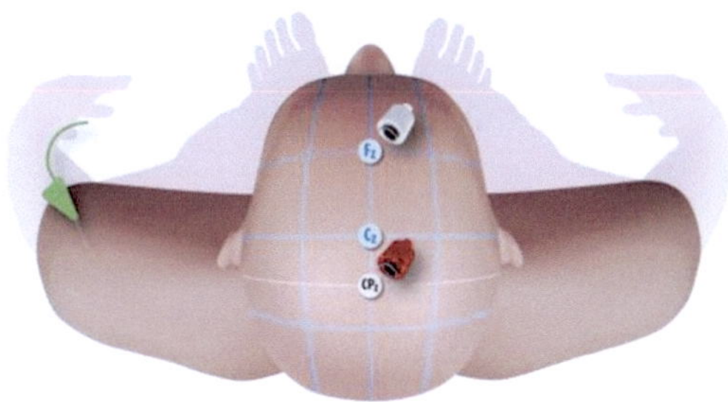

Fig. 5.16 Traditional position of the electrodes for recording tibial nerve SEPs. © ARKANA Forum GmbH 2022. All Rights Reserved

oblongata (**first neuron**). There, the **second neuron** begins, crossing (decussating) to the opposite side in the lemniscus medialis and continuing to ascend to the nucleus ventralis posterior of the thalamus. Here, the signal switches to the **third neuron**, which reaches the primary sensory cortex in the postcentral gyrus.

The **generators** in the central nervous system can be recorded at different sites from the skin surface. In clinical practice, the **sensory cortex P37** response is the principal monitor. However, adding the **popliteal fossa** potential provides valuable control for stimulus failure or distal limb conduction failure due to limb ischemia or pressure, without delaying surgical feedback. Additional thoracolumbar or subcortical recordings (Fig. 5.17) may help evaluate other confounding factors such as anesthesia or vital parameters, but can slow surgical feedback due to low SNR.

> *Although unilateral recording of the SEP is sufficient in principle, it is nevertheless recommended to record bilaterally to be able to interpret latency delays or amplitude reductions more quickly and reliably. If changes occur bilaterally, supratentorial surgical manipulation can most likely be excluded as the cause.*

A **typical potential** is shown in Fig. 5.18. Table 5.6 summarizes tibial nerve SEPs at different recording sites. Table 5.7 presents typical P37 peak latencies. Table 5.8 gives the parameters commonly used for stimulation and recording of tibial nerve SEPs.

Although the tibial nerve is preferred for stimulation due to its good accessibility, it may be advisable to use other nerves for triggering SEP of the lower extremities depending on the surgical requirements. If necessary, the **femoral nerve** and the **common fibular nerve** may be used. Nerves and associated spinal roots are listed in Table 5.9.

> *While one could monitor SEPs one limb at a time, stimulus interleaving with asynchronous parallel averaging or "shared stimulation" is highly advisable to speed surgical feedback. Left–right interleaving halves the acquisition time of median or tibial nerve SEPs by simultaneously recording both sides. Four-limb interleaving also halves acquisition time, but may not further accelerate monitoring because stimulus frequency must be reduced to accommodate the four staggered recording sweeps. Still, this technique enables concurrent four-limb recording and enhances SNR because cortical SEP signal amplitudes increase with slower stimuli.*

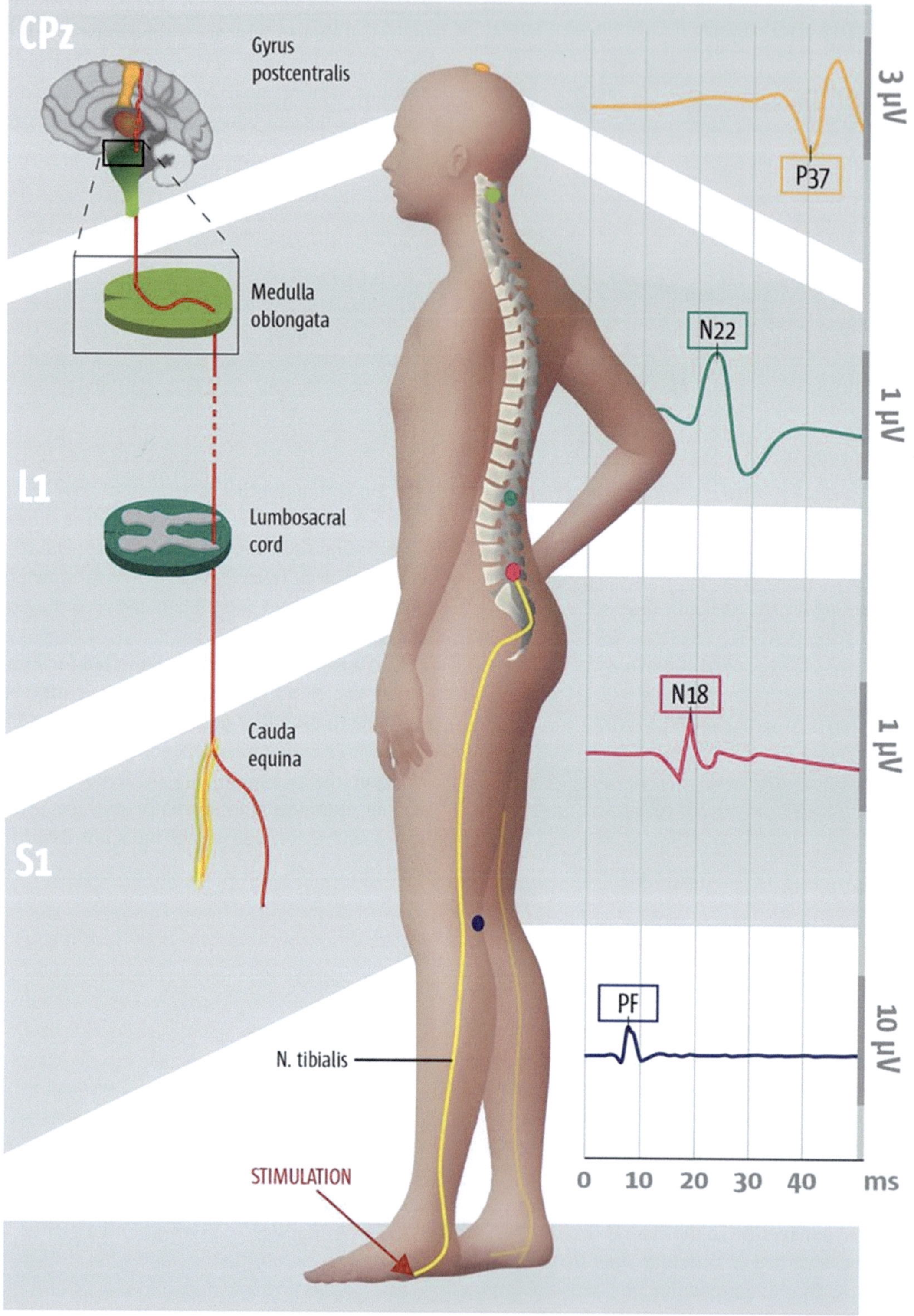

Fig. 5.17 Signal path and generators of tibial nerve SEPs. © ARKANA Forum GmbH 2022. All Rights Reserved

Fig. 5.18 Typical tibial nerve SEP recorded with CPz–Fz. © ARKANA Forum GmbH 2022. All Rights Reserved

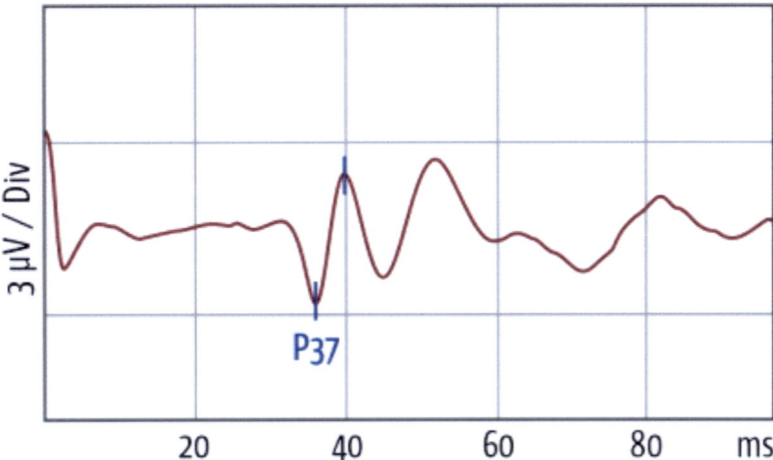

Table 5.6 Summary of tibial nerve SEPs at different recording sites

| | | Monitoring derivations [6] | | |
Design.	Recording site	Traditional	Optimal (highest SNR)	Deflection
N9 or PF	Popliteal fossa	PFd–PFp	PFd–PFp	Up
N22 or LP	Lumbar	T12–IC	Omit	Up
P31/N34	Subcortical	Fpz–C5	Omit, or fallback Fpz–M[a]	Down/up
P37	Cortical	CPz–Fz or CPz–Fpz	**CPz–CPc**[b], Cz–CPc, Pz–CPc, iCPi–CPc, CPi–CPc, or Cz–Pz	Down

Design. designation, *PF* popliteal fossa, *d* distal, *p* proximal, *T12* 12th thoracic spine, *IC* iliac crest, *C5* 5th cervical spine, *M* mastoid, *CP* CP3 or CP4, *iCP* CP1 or CP2, *postscript i and c* ipsilateral and contralateral to the stimulated nerve
[a] The subcortical SEP is normally omitted due to very low SNR, but Fpz–M may be a fallback spinal cord monitor in the case of poor cortical SEPs
[b] Optimal for 40% of tibial nerves and the best routine choice, but any of the six candidate channels may be optimal for an individual nerve. Consequently, the ideal approach is to initially compare them and choose the optimal one (highest SNR) for monitoring. Since all these channels have similar noise levels, the one with greatest signal amplitude is optimal

Table 5.7 Typical P37 peak latency after tibial nerve stimulation. Note that the latency is depending on height. Anesthesia and hypothermia can increase peak SEP latencies

	Peak latency (ms)
Tibial nerve P37	33–44

Table 5.8 Parameters for stimulation and recording of tibial nerve SEPs (recommended starting values are marked in bold)

Stimulation current	Supramaximal, usually 3–30 mA
Stimulation frequency	2.1–4.7 Hz (select an odd divisor of 50 or 60 Hz)
Pulse form	Monophasic rectangular cathodal pulse
Pulse duration	200–500 μs (**200 μs**)
Low-pass filter	300 Hz (1000 Hz for popliteal fossa recording)
High-pass filter	30 Hz (0.2 Hz for popliteal fossa recording)
Time base	100–200 ms (**100 ms**)
Averaging	To medium–high reproducibility, usually 50–300 sweeps

5.4.1.3 Trigeminal Nerve SEPs

Examination of SEPs after stimulation of the sensitive part of the trigeminal nerve is less common. It may be useful in surgical procedures on the brainstem or in the course of the trigeminal nerve.

Stimulation is performed using a pair of electrodes placed on the upper and lower lips (Fig. 5.19).

Recording is accomplished according to the 10–20 system at CP5 to Fz (right trigeminal nerve) or CP6 to Fz (left trigeminal nerve) (Fig. 5.20).

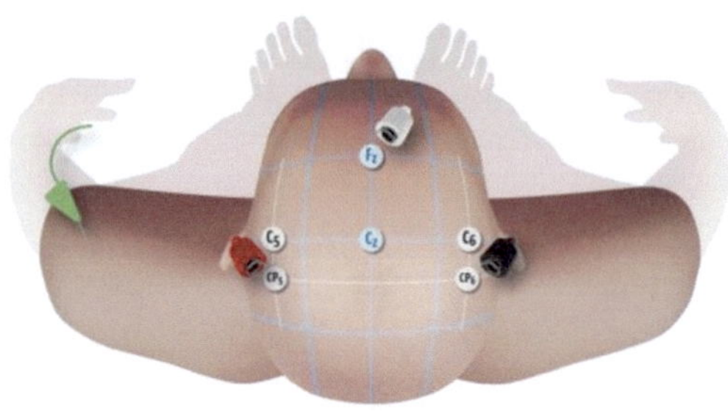

Fig. 5.20 Position of electrodes for recording trigeminal nerve SEPs. © ARKANA Forum GmbH 2022. All Rights Reserved

The **action potential** elicited by stimulation travels along the trigeminal nerve to its main sensory nucleus in the pons (**first neuron**). Subsequently, the signal switches to the contralateral side in the lemniscus trigeminalis, which is attached to the lemniscus medialis, and ascends to the nucleus ventralis posterior of the thalamus (**second neuron**). This is where the **third neuron** begins. It reaches the primary sensory cortex in the postcentral gyrus.

The **generators N13** and **P19** are available for recording. Due to the close spatial relationship between the stimulation and the recording site, the early potentials are often masked by the stimulation artifact. Reliably recordable is the down going positive peak at a latency of 19 ms (P19). The amplitude of the signal is measured from the preceding peak N13 to the peak P19.

Figure 5.21 shows the course of the three branches of the trigeminal nerve. A typical potential is depicted in Fig. 5.22. Mean latencies of trigeminal nerve SEPs are given in Table 5.10. Table 5.11 presents the parameters commonly used for stimulation and recording.

Table 5.9 Spinal roots of the typical nerves used for SEPs of the lower extremity

Nerve	Spinal roots
Femoral nerve	L1, L2, L3, L4
Common fibular nerve (Common peroneal nerve)	L4, L5, S1, S2
Tibial nerve	L4, L5, S1, S2, S3

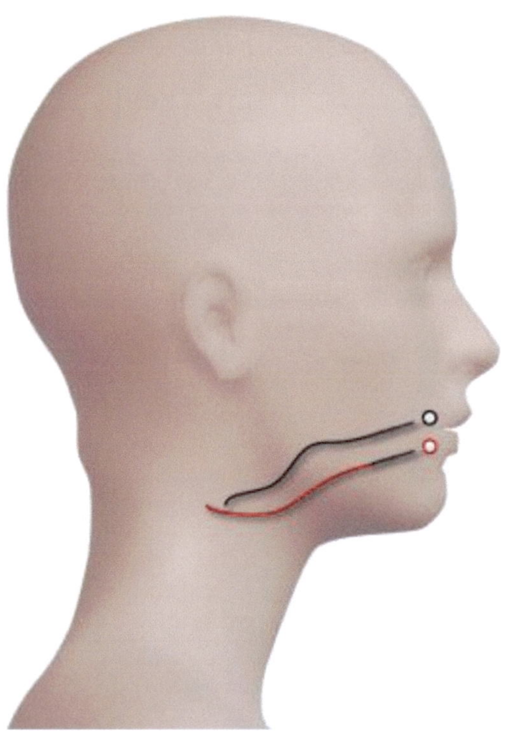

Fig. 5.19 Position of electrodes for stimulation of the trigeminal nerve (red = anode; black = cathode). © ARKANA Forum GmbH 2022. All Rights Reserved

The trigeminal nerve includes three main branches:

- *Branch 1: Ophthalmic nerve (eye branch)*
- *Branch 2: Maxillary nerve (upper jaw branch)*
- *Branch 3: Mandibular nerve (lower jaw branch)*

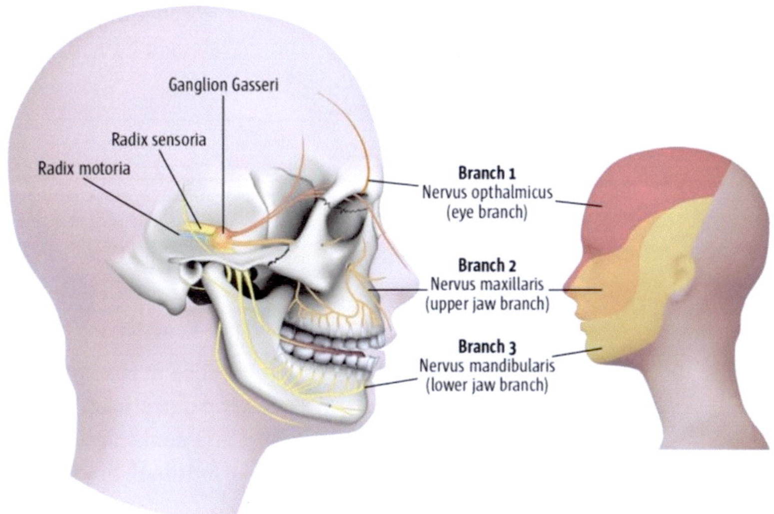

Fig. 5.21 Anatomical illustration of the three branches of the trigeminal nerve. © ARKANA Forum GmbH 2022. All Rights Reserved

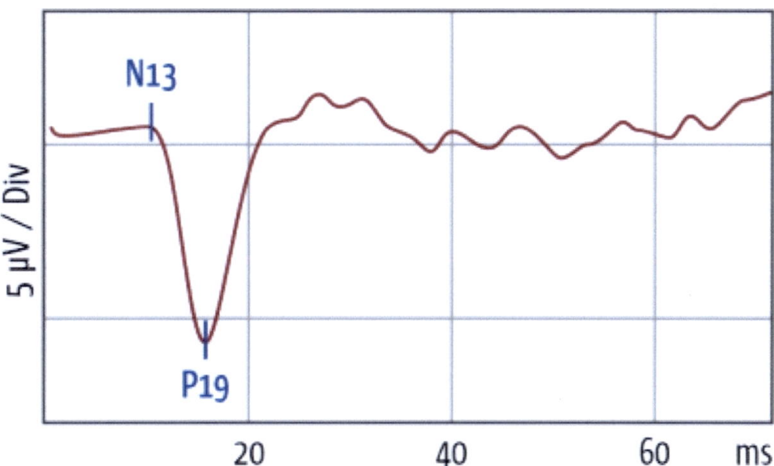

Fig. 5.22 Typical right trigeminal nerve SEP recorded with CP5–Fz. © ARKANA Forum GmbH 2022. All Rights Reserved

Table 5.10 Mean latencies of N13 and P19 and amplitude of P19 of trigeminal nerve SEPs under general anesthesia [8]. Note that these are mean values in patients undergoing surgery, so cannot represent normal values

	Mean latency (ms)	Amplitude (µV)
N13	12.4	–
P19	17.2	5.7

Table 5.11 Parameters for stimulation and recording of trigeminal nerve SEPs (recommended starting values are marked in bold)

Stimulation frequency	2.1–5.1 Hz (select an odd divisor of 50 or 60 Hz)
Pulse form	Monophasic or biphasic rectangular pulse
Pulse duration	200–300 µs (**200 µs**)
Low-pass filter	600 Hz
High-pass filter	20 Hz
Time base	60–100 ms
Averaging	To medium–high reproducibility, usually 50–200 sweeps

5.4.1.4 Pudendal Nerve SEPs

Monitoring of the sacral nerves can be accomplished by means of SEPs after stimulation of the sensory part of the pudendal nerve. This technique is used, for example, in selective dorsal rhizotomy or in the surgical treatment of the tethered cord syndrome.

Stimulation is performed via a pair of electrodes. In females, the cathode is placed near the clitoris and the anode between the outer and inner labia [9] (Fig. 5.23). In males, two cup electrodes are placed 2–3 cm apart on the dorsal penis. The cathode is located at the base of the penis (Fig. 5.24).

Recording is done according to the 10–20 system at CPz to Fz (Fig. 5.25).

> *For triggering pudendal SEPs, only surface electrodes are used in males. In females, stimulation is also viable via needle electrodes.*

The **action potential** runs along the sensory dorsalis clitoridis nerve in females and the dorsalis penis nerve in males, which each represent a terminal branch of the pudendal nerve. The pudendal nerve enters the spinal canal via the sacral plexus at the level of segments S1–S4 and the spinal cord through the posterior roots at the level of the conus medullaris (T12/L1). The signaling pathway is similar to the SEP after stimulation of the tibial nerve. The central conduction time of the pudendal nerve SEP is somewhat longer compared to other sensory nerves, which may be related to slower axons or possibly different pathways including more synapses [10].

Figure 5.26 depicts a typical potential. Similar to the SEP after stimulation of the tibial nerve, there is an initial positive wave followed by several negative–positive oscillations. Typical values for latencies are presented in Table 5.12. The parameters commonly used for stimulation and recording are summarized in Table 5.13.

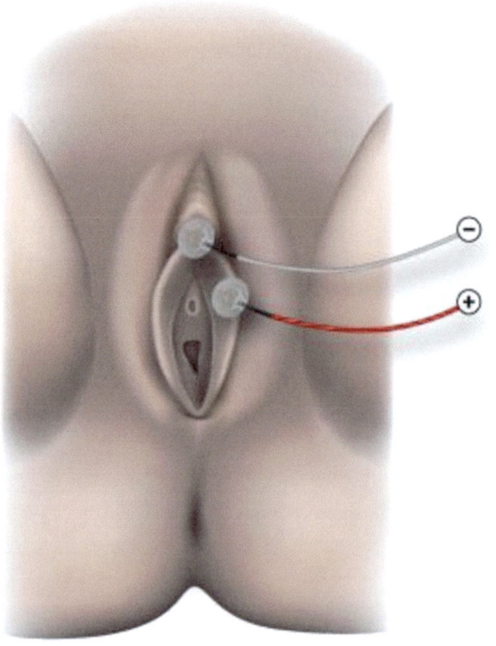

Fig. 5.23 Position of electrodes for stimulation of the pudendal nerve in females. © ARKANA Forum GmbH 2022. All Rights Reserved

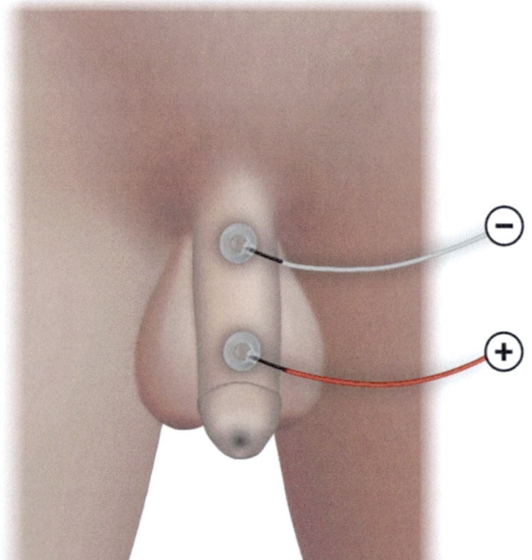

Fig. 5.24 Position of electrodes for stimulation of the pudendal nerve in males. © ARKANA Forum GmbH 2022. All Rights Reserved

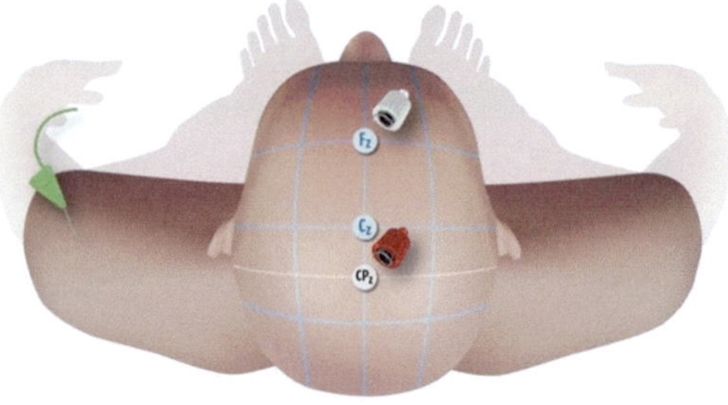

Fig. 5.25 Position of electrodes for recording pudendal nerve SEPs. © ARKANA Forum GmbH 2022. All Rights Reserved

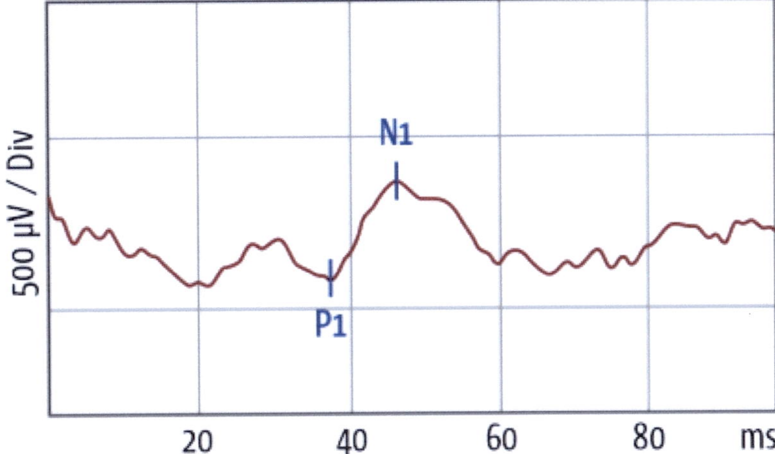

Fig. 5.26 SEP after stimulation of the pudendal nerve. © ARKANA Forum GmbH 2022. All Rights Reserved

Table 5.12 Typical intraoperative latencies of the pudendal nerve SEP. Latencies in females and males are similar [11]

	Latency (ms)
P1	35–40

Table 5.13 Parameters for stimulation and recording of the pudendal nerve SEP (recommended starting values are marked in bold)

Stimulation current	Supramaximal, usually 3–30 mA
Stimulation frequency	2.1–5.1 Hz (select an odd divisor of 50 or 60 Hz)
Pulse form	Monophasic rectangular cathodal pulse
Pulse duration	200–500 µs (**300 µs**)
Low-pass filter	800 Hz
High-pass filter	20 Hz
Time base	50–200 ms
Averaging	To medium–high reproducibility, usually 60–200 sweeps

5.4.2   Motor Evoked Potentials (MEPs)

Motor evoked potentials are used for intraoperative monitoring of the corticospinal **descending (efferent) pathways**.

Stimulation is performed with transcranial electric stimulation (through the skull) or directly on the motor cortex after craniotomy.

Recording of responses is usually accomplished from the associated target muscles. Thereby, distally located muscles are preferred due to their more extensive representation in the cortex [12]. Recording can also be done invasively from the different levels of the spinal cord.

5.4.2.1 Transcranial Stimulation and Recording

Stimulation is performed using a scalp electrode array placed according to the 10–20 system at C4, C2, C1, C3, Cz, and Cz + 6 cm. An alternative array consists of M4, M2, M1, and M3 located 1-cm anterior to C sites and Mz located 2-cm anterior to Cz. The triggering effect takes place mostly under the anode that should always be located over the cortical area to be activated. Consequently, stimulation circuits are designated as anode–cathode. Some activation under the cathode can occur at higher intensities. The right motor cortex is activated at C2 (hand and leg area) and C4 (hand area), and the left motor cortex is activated at C1 (hand and leg area) and C3 (hand area). The cathode is usually placed at Cz or in single cases at Cz + 6 cm (Fig. 5.27). By choosing a contralateral cathode and changing the polarity, the same electrodes can be used to stimulate different areas (e.g., C1–C2 for the left hand and leg area and C2–C1 for the right hand and leg area). This can be accomplished by switching the anode and cathode between consecutive trials, or with biphasic pulses.

Recording is usually done in the upper extremities from the abductor pollicis brevis and/or abductor digiti minimi muscles (Fig. 5.28) and in the lower extremities from the tibialis anterior, abductor hallucis, and sometimes gastrocnemius

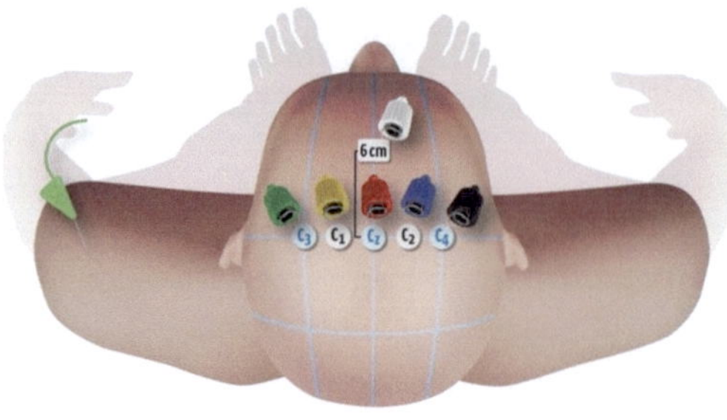

Fig. 5.27 Position of electrodes for transcranial stimulation of the motor cortex. © ARKANA Forum GmbH 2022. All Rights Reserved

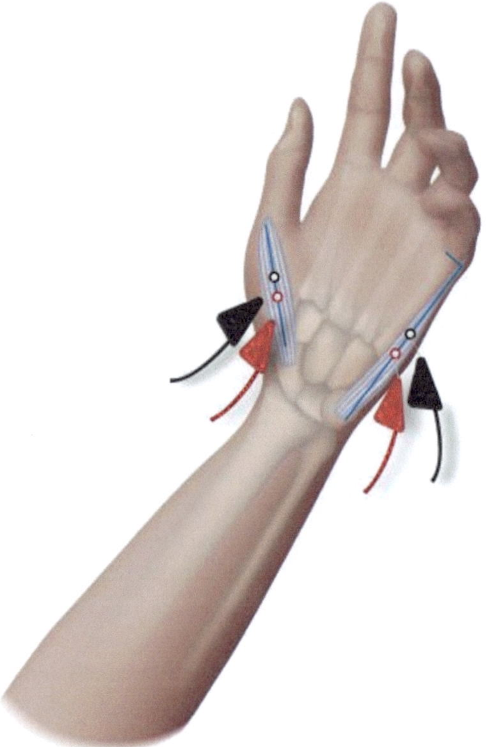

Fig. 5.28 Position of electrodes for recording MEPs from the upper extremities. M. abductor pollicis brevis (left) and M. abductor digiti minimi (right). © ARKANA Forum GmbH 2022. All Rights Reserved

muscles (Fig. 5.29). Signal acquisition is usually accomplished with needle electrodes inserted about 2–3 cm apart into the muscle belly. Depending on the surgical requirements, for

example, in spinal procedures, the muscles to be selected for recording should correspond to the level of the operation and the spinal nerves at risk (Table 5.28).

Transcranial stimulation excites pyramidal cell axons in the primary motor cortex. **The action potential** runs via the fast-conducting axons of the corticospinal tract (tractus corticospinalis, **first motoneuron**) through the posterior limb of the internal capsule to the upper brainstem and the medulla oblongata. In the lower medulla oblongata, the corticospinal tract crosses for the most part to the contralateral side (decussation or decussatio pyramidum) and passes from here downward in the lateral corticospinal tract (tractus corticospinalis lateralis). In the anterior horn, the action potential switches to the **second motoneuron** (α-motoneuron) at the level of its exit from the spinal cord and proceeds to the muscular end plate, excitation of which finally leads to contraction of the target muscles (Fig. 5.30).

Transcranial stimulation at C3/C4 can activate corticospinal axons deeply at the internal capsule or even more caudally. In addition, using biphasic pulses with C3/C4 or C1/C2 results in a loss of side selectivity. These techniques may be applicable to spinal surgery. However, applied for intracranial procedures, the pyramidal tract may be excited exclusively below the surgical site, so that no conclusion can be drawn about the functional status of the area actually at risk. Therefore, more superficial side-selective stimulation at C1–C2 and C2–C1 or C3–Cz and C4–Cz is indispensable for intracranial surgery [13]. Sometimes Cz–Cz + 6 cm is useful for focal bilateral leg area stimulation [14]. If the electrodes cannot be placed at the appropriate sites (e.g., due to craniotomy), direct cortical stimulation by means of a strip electrode should be preferred.

Fig. 5.29 Position of electrodes for recording MEPs from the lower extremities. M. abductor hallucis (upper), M. tibialis anterior (left) and M. gastrocnemius (right). © ARKANA Forum GmbH 2022. All Rights Reserved

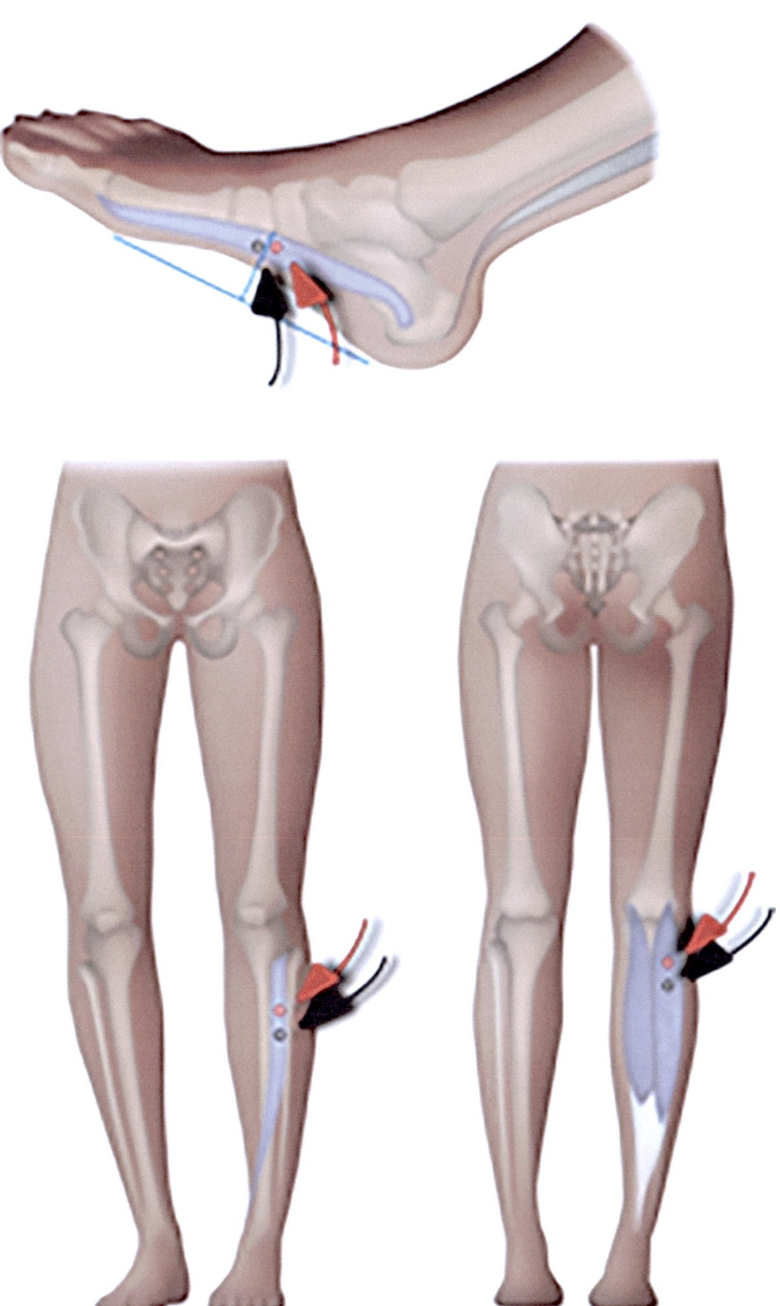

Typical responses are shown in Figs. 5.31 and 5.32. The contraction of the muscle results in a multiphasic wave. In contrast to SEPs, the shape of this multiphasic wave is not essential for interpretation. Therefore, the individual waves are not designated separately. Important parameters for interpretation include latency to the onset of the MEP signal, the peak-to-peak amplitude, and the intensity required to elicit the MEP. Table 5.14 presents typical onset latencies. The parameters commonly used for stimulation and recording are given in Table 5.15.

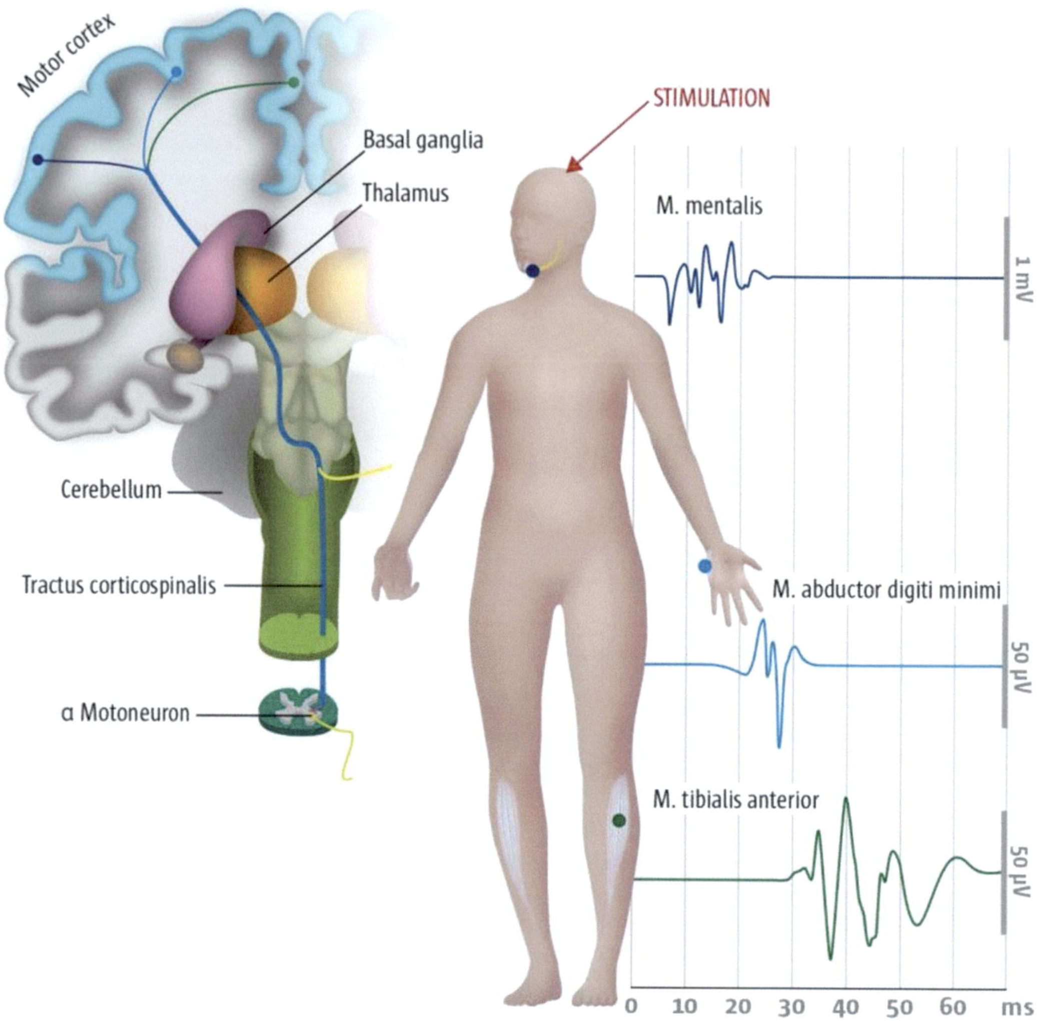

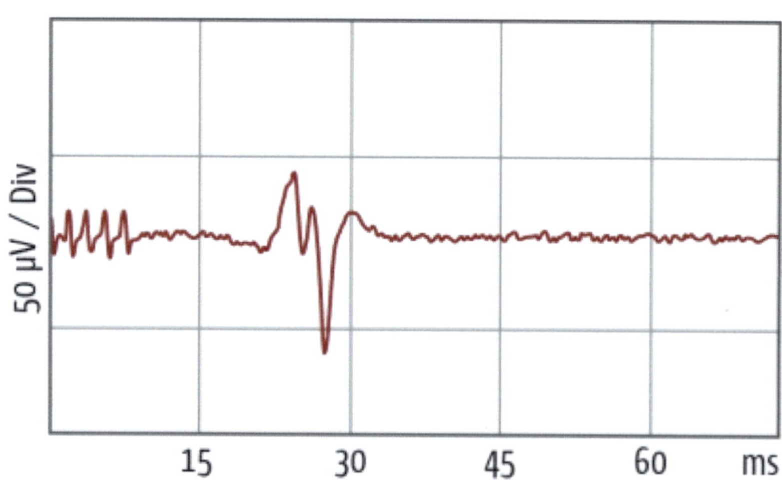

Fig. 5.30 Signal path of MEPs. © ARKANA Forum GmbH 2022. All Rights Reserved

Fig. 5.31 A typical transcranial MEP recorded from the M. abductor digiti minimi. © ARKANA Forum GmbH 2022. All Rights Reserved

Fig. 5.32 A typical transcranial MEP recorded from the M. tibialis anterior. © ARKANA Forum GmbH 2022. All Rights Reserved

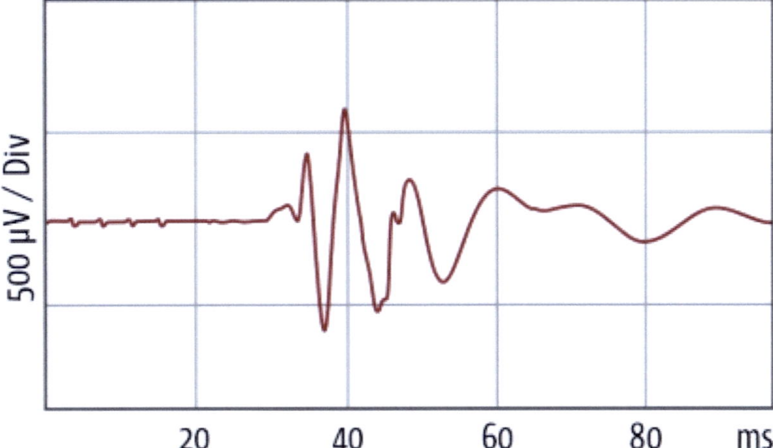

In creating MEP display montages, it is particularly helpful to arrange the muscles according to their position from cranial to caudal as well as from left to right. This order enhances interpretation and helps to avoid connection errors or to recognize them more quickly.

It is essential to use a soft bite block during transcranial electrical stimulation, since induced jaw muscle contractions risk bite injuries including tongue, lip, tooth, jaw, or endotracheal tube damage. Rolled-up gauze inserted between the molars of each side while keeping the tongue in the middle is proven effective for bite protection.

It is recommended to monitor at least two muscle groups per extremity. However, when the upper limbs serve as a control for thoracolumbar surgeries, one hand muscle is sufficient.

Although unilateral MEP monitoring of unilateral intracranial procedures is sufficient in principle, it is recommended to always record bilaterally in order to be able to interpret latency delays or amplitude reductions more quickly and reliably. This approach provides technical and systemic control: If deterioration occurs bilaterally, surgical manipulation seems unlikely as a cause. Similarly, for thoracic or more caudal spine operations indicating bilateral leg MEP monitoring, upper limb MEP controls should also be recorded.

The **D-wave** is of particular importance for monitoring motor function during intramedullary spinal cord surgery. It facilitates assessment of the integrity of the corticospinal tract, which may be at high risk, especially with intramedullary tumors.

Stimulation is usually performed at C1–C2 and C2–C1 or C3–C4 and C4–C3.

Recording is accomplished from the spinal cord by epidural electrodes. The recording electrode is located caudal to the lesion. A second electrode can be placed cranial to the lesion as a

Table 5.14 Typical latencies of transcranial MEPs recorded in anesthetized patients undergoing various spine surgeries [15]

	Onset latency (ms)
Hand	18–31
Foot	35–55

Table 5.15 Stimulation and recording parameters for transcranial MEPs (recommended starting values are marked in bold)

Stimulation current	40–250 mA
Stimulation frequency	0.5–2 Hz
Interstimulus interval	2–4 ms (**4 ms**)
Pulse form	**Monophasic** or biphasic rectangular pulse train
Train count	3–9 pulses (**5 pulses**)
Pulse duration	50–1000 μs (**500 μs**)[a]
Low-pass filter	1500–3000 Hz
High-pass filter	20 Hz
Time base	100–200 ms (**100 ms**)
Averaging	None

[a] Pulse duration choice is currently determined by stimulator design limitations. High-output stimulators require short pulses, while low-output devices require longer pulses. Future devices with maximum output adjusted to pulse duration may enable greater flexibility. If so, a duration of 200 μs that is near the estimated chronaxie could be optimal

control. D-waves can only be obtained from the cervical and thoracic spinal cord. They are too small to record or absent at the lumbosacral cord where the corticospinal tracts terminate.

Figure 5.33 shows a typical D wave. Common stimulation and recording parameters are listed in Table 5.16. Table 5.17 compares the postoperative motor status to be expected when D-waves or muscle MEPs deteriorate during intramedullary spinal cord surgery. The D-wave allows a more precise statement about *long-term* motor outcome. Specifically, if it is preserved above 50% of baseline amplitude, then no *persistent* motor deficit is likely even when muscle MEP loss predicts early weakness.

The electrodes for D-wave recordings are usually placed epidurally by the surgeon after opening. A few centers use subdural electrodes threaded up from a preoperative lumbar puncture.

5.4.2.2 Corticobulbar MEPs

Analogous to the corticospinal tract, the corticobulbar or corticonuclear tract (tractus corticobulbaris) innervates the **voluntary muscles**

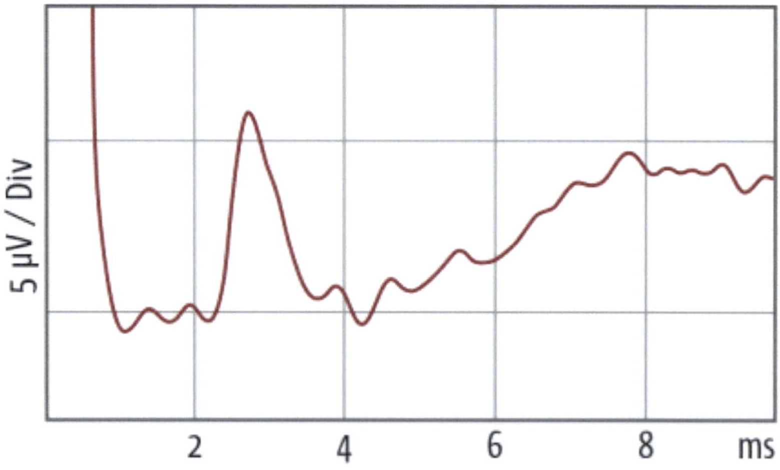

Fig. 5.33 A typical D-wave recording after transcranial stimulation. © ARKANA Forum GmbH 2022. All Rights Reserved

Table 5.16 Stimulation and recording parameters for transcranial D-waves (recommended starting values are marked in bold)

Stimulation current	40–150 mA
Stimulation frequency	0.4–2.1 Hz (select an odd divisor of 50 or 60 Hz)
Pulse form	Alternating-polarity monophasic or biphasic rectangular pulse[a]
Pulse duration	50–600 µs per phase (**500 µs**)
Low-pass filter	1500–2000 Hz
High-pass filter	0.2–2 or >100 Hz[b]
Time base	10–20 ms
Averaging	To medium–high reproducibility, usually 5–20 sweeps

[a] By alternating the polarity of monophasic pulses while averaging, or using biphasic pulses, one can ensure a bilateral D-wave and partially cancel out opposite-direction stimulus artifacts

[b] Stimulus artifact can overlap D-waves recorded with a 20–30 Hz high-pass filter. Opening the filter to 0.2–2 Hz can facilitate artifact/D-wave separation, but admits low-frequency interference. Alternatively, constraining the filter to >100 Hz (even 500 Hz) can also facilitate separation, but attenuates the response

Table 5.17 Validity of muscle MEPs vs. D-waves for prediction of motor outcome after intramedullary spinal cord tumor surgery (modified from [16])

D-wave	Muscle MEP	Expected motor outcome
Unchanged or <50% reduced	Unchanged or reduced but still present	Unchanged
Unchanged or <50% reduced	Unilateral or bilateral loss	Temporary motor deficit
>50% reduced	Loss	Long-term motor deficit

of the head (eye, face, mouth, throat) and **neck**. The corticobulbar tract starts from the cells of the motor cortex and runs in front of the corticospinal tract through the internal capsule to the brainstem. Most synapses are located in the basal nuclei of the pons. Corticobulbar MEPs facilitate continuous monitoring of **motor cranial nerves**. Because of the proximity between the stimulation and recording sites (stimulation of the motor cortex and recording from muscles in the face, mouth, throat or neck), a special stimulation technique is necessary.

Stimulation is done with C3–Cz for muscles on the right side and with C4–Cz for muscles on the left side.

Recording can be performed using paired needle or hookwire electrodes. Recording is feasible from the following muscles [17]:

- Rectus superior muscle, rectus inferior muscle, obliquus superior muscle, rectus lateralis muscle (N. III, IV, and VI)
- Masseter muscle (N. V)
- Orbicularis oculi muscle, orbicularis oris muscle, nasalis muscle, mentalis muscle (N. VII)
- Posterior pharynx, soft palate, vocalis muscle, crycothyroideus muscle (Nn. IX and X)
- Trapezius muscle (N. XI)
- Tongue muscles (N. XII)

When transcranial stimulation is too strong, spread of the electrical pulse will directly activate the peripheral part of the cranial nerve. Thus, monitoring could miss a compromise of the proximal nerve, brainstem, or motor cortex. Therefore, before or after using a **train**, stimulation with the same parameters but only with a **single pulse** should be performed. A single-pulse muscle response indicates direct activation of the peripheral cranial nerve and disqualifies the pulse train response from interpretation. On the other hand, a muscle response only after train stimulation is indicative of central activation at the level of the motor cortex, i.e., a true corticobulbar MEP. Another parameter to consider is the onset latency of the pulse train response. For facial MEPs, this should be >10 ms. If it is much shorter, then this may also indicate peripheral facial nerve excitation (the onset latency of a direct facial nerve stimulation CMAP is 5–7 ms, depending on the stimulus site on the nerve).

Figure 5.34 shows a typical corticobulbar MEP. Table 5.18 summarizes the commonly used stimulation and recording parameters.

5.4.2.3 Cortical Stimulation and Recording

Direct cortical stimulation for MEPs is performed with a strip electrode placed over the motor cortex. Alternatively, a hand-held probe can be used to scan the motor cortex.

Fig. 5.34 A typical transcranial corticobulbar MEP. The absence of a single-pulse response (left) rules out peripheral nerve activation. After train stimulation, the corticobulbar MEP is evident (right).© ARKANA Forum GmbH 2022. All Rights Reserved

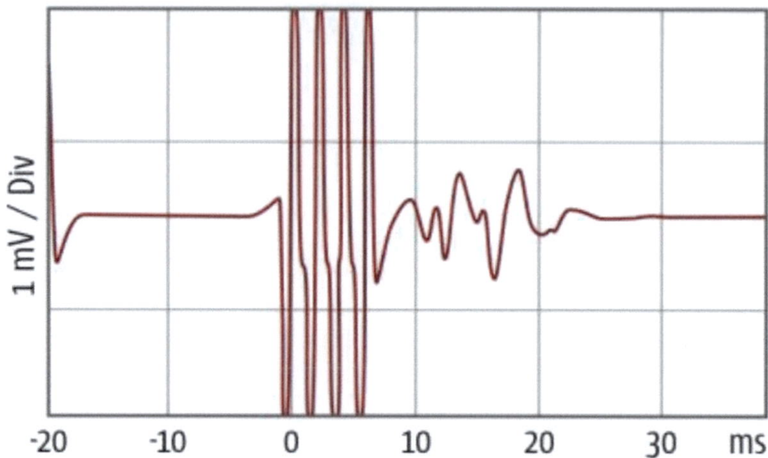

Table 5.18 Stimulation and recording parameters for transcranial corticobulbar MEPs (recommended starting values are marked in bold)

Stimulation current	40–120 mA
Stimulation frequency	0.5–2 Hz
Interstimulus interval	2–4 ms (**2 ms**)
Intertrain interval	20 ms (first single pulse, then train) 90 ms (first train, then single pulse)
Pulse form	Monophasic rectangular pulse train
Train count	3–6 pulses (**3 pulses**)
Pulse duration	50–1000 μs (**500 μs**)
Low-pass filter	1500–3000 Hz
High-pass filter	0.2–2 Hz or 50–150 Hz[a]
Charge reversal	Delayed (if available)[b]
Time base	40–80 ms (first single pulse, then train) 120 ms (first train, then single pulse)
Averaging	None

[a] Stimulus artifact can overlap corticobulbar MEPs recorded with a 20–30 Hz high-pass filter. Opening the filter to 0.2–2 Hz can facilitate artifact/MEP separation, but admits low-frequency interference. Alternatively, constraining the filter to 50–150 Hz may also facilitate separation, but can attenuate the response

[b] A charge-balancing reversal discharge of low current that decays slowly follows each pulse and contributes to stimulus artifact. A recent stimulator design reduces stimulus artifact by delaying charge reversal until after the response [18]

Recording of muscle MEPs is done in the same way as described for transcranial stimulation (see Sect. 5.4.2.1 "Transcranial Stimulation and Recording").

Figure 5.35 shows a strip electrode placed over the motor cortex. Table 5.19 presents the commonly used stimulation and recording parameters. The typical onset latencies correspond to those given for transcranial stimulation (see Table 5.14).

Direct stimulation of the motor cortex is accomplished by means of a strip electrode or a hand-held probe. For common monopolar technique, cortical stimulation is anodal (positive) and subcortical stimulation is cathodal (negative) [19]. The opposite-pole electrode is usually placed at the edge of the surgical field. Bipolar strip or probe stimulation can also evoke MEPs and can be more focal, but is less efficient.

5.4.3 Auditory Evoked Potentials (AEPs)

5.4.3.1 Brainstem Auditory Evoked Potentials (BAEPs)

Depending on the generators recorded from, there are **early, middle,** and **late AEPs**. Late

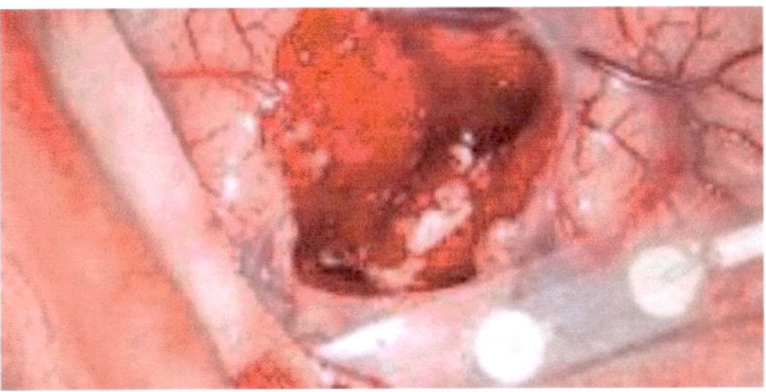

Fig. 5.35 Cortical stimulation using a strip electrode. © ARKANA Forum GmbH 2022. All Rights Reserved

Table 5.19 Stimulation and recording parameters for direct cortical stimulation MEPs (recommended starting values are marked in bold)

Stimulation current	4–25 mA
Stimulation frequency	0.5–2 Hz
Interstimulus interval	2–4 ms (**4 ms**)
Pulse form	Monophasic rectangular pulse train • Anodal for cortical stimulation • Cathodal for subcortical stimulation
Train count	3–6 pulse (**5 pulses**)
Pulse duration	100–1000 µs (**500 µs**)
Low-pass filter	1500–3000 Hz
High-pass filter	20 Hz
Time base	100–200 ms (**100 ms**)
Averaging	None

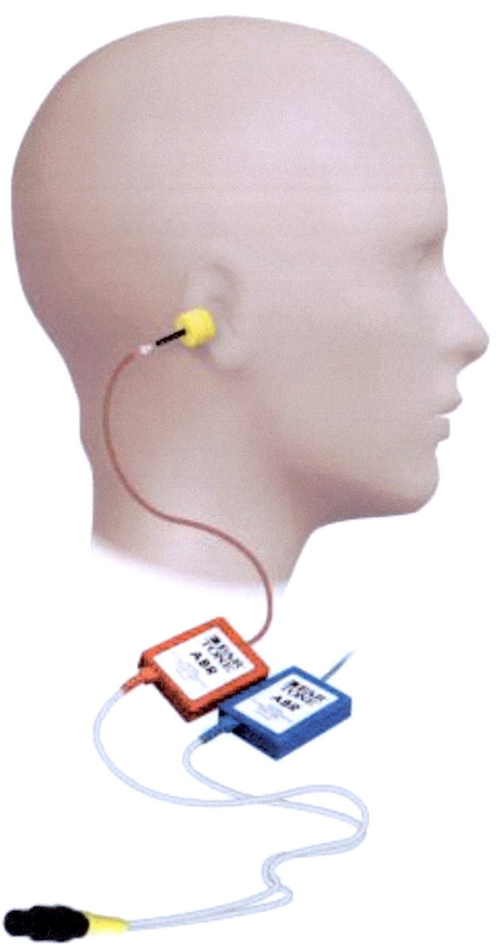

Fig. 5.36 Stimulator position for eliciting BAEPs. © ARKANA Forum GmbH 2022. All Rights Reserved

AEPs are absent under general anesthesia, and neuromonitoring primarily focuses on the evaluation of early AEPs, most commonly named brainstem auditory evoked potentials (**BAEPs**) or auditory brainstem responses. The BAEP provides objective information about peripheral and brainstem auditory pathway function and indicates the localization of impairment. It is used in particular during surgical interventions in the cerebellopontine angle or the brainstem.

Stimulation is performed by means of sound transducers connected via silastic tubes to soft earplugs surrounding a sound-conducting plastic tube. The earplugs are compressed and inserted into the external auditory canal where they expand to secure them in place (Fig. 5.36).

Recording electrodes are placed according to the 10–20 system. For the left BAEP, the electrode is placed at the left mastoid (A1), for the right BAEP at the right mastoid (A2); Cz is used as a common "reference" (Fig. 5.37). However, both electrodes are active, with A1 or A2 picking up a distal auditory nerve potential and Cz picking up brainstem signals. Due to the large distance between the recording electrodes and the generators in the brainstem, these far-field signals are very small (<1–2 µV). In addition, the long distance between recording electrodes enhances noise amplitude. Therefore, the SNR is very low and averaging 500–2000 sweeps is necessary to obtain reproducible potentials.

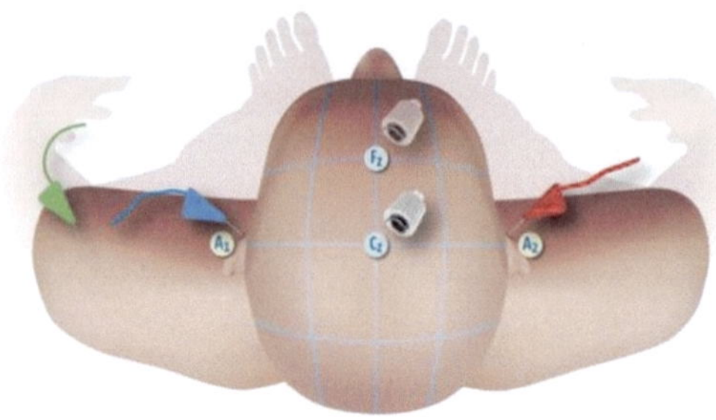

Fig. 5.37 Position of electrodes for recording BAEPs. © ARKANA Forum GmbH 2022. All Rights Reserved

Before inserting the earplug, the external ear canal should be inspected for secretions and cleaned if necessary. After insertion, the external ear canal must be well sealed to prevent fluid from entering during the surgical procedure. To avoid acoustic crossover to the opposite ear through bone, another earplug must be placed into the contralateral ear to deliver white noise masking.

The **sound** triggered by the stimulation causes

When SEP monitoring is performed in addition to BAEPs, Fz or CPz can be used instead of Cz for BAEPs.

the **tympanic membrane** to vibrate. The vibra-

If placement of the recording electrodes at the mastoid is not possible due to the planned surgical approach, the electrodes can be attached to the earlobe or positioned in front of the ear canal. Alternatively, tympanic electrodes can be used, which are placed into the ear canal and acquire signals directly from the tympanic membrane (electrocochleography).

tions are transmitted via the ossicles to the **oval window** and amplified along the way. From the oval window, the mechanical vibrations are trans-

mitted to the **basilar membrane** (Fig. 5.38). The vibrations of the basilar membrane lead to excitation of its **hair cells**. These convert the vibrations into **nerve impulses**, which are amplified at the same time.

From the hair cells, the **action potential** travels along the **cochlear nerve**, which unites with the vestibular nerve to form the vestibulocochlear nerve, until it reaches the **cochlear nuclei** (nuclei cochleares) in the brainstem. The anatomy of the auditory pathways in the brainstem is very complex and can be simplified for the AEP as follows: Most fibers cross through the **trapezoid body** (corpus trapezoideum) to the contralateral side. From here, the fibers ascend in the **lateral lemniscus** (lemniscus lateralis) to the **inferior colliculus** (colliculus inferior) of the midbrain. Some fibers remain ipsilateral and ascend via the **superior olivary complex** in the lateral lemniscus to the inferior colliculus. The pathways finally end in the **auditory area** of the cerebral cortex.

The BAEP consists of several waves numbered in the sequential order of their occurrence. Particularly important are waves I to V, which can be assigned to the following **generators** (Fig. 5.39):

- I: Distal part of the cochlear nerve
- II: Proximal part of the vestibulocochlear nerve and cochlear nuclei
- III: Lower part of the pons, or superior olivary complex
- IV/V: Lateral lemniscus/inferior colliculus

The following points can be helpful for **identifying and interpreting the individual waves**:

- The spatial proximity to the stimulation site often leads to a pronounced stimulation artifact that can overlay wave I. The artifact can be reduced using **alternating** stimulation.
- Wave I is absent in the contralateral recording.
- Absence of wave II is not necessarily pathological. Contralateral recording usually shows somewhat larger wave II amplitude and some-

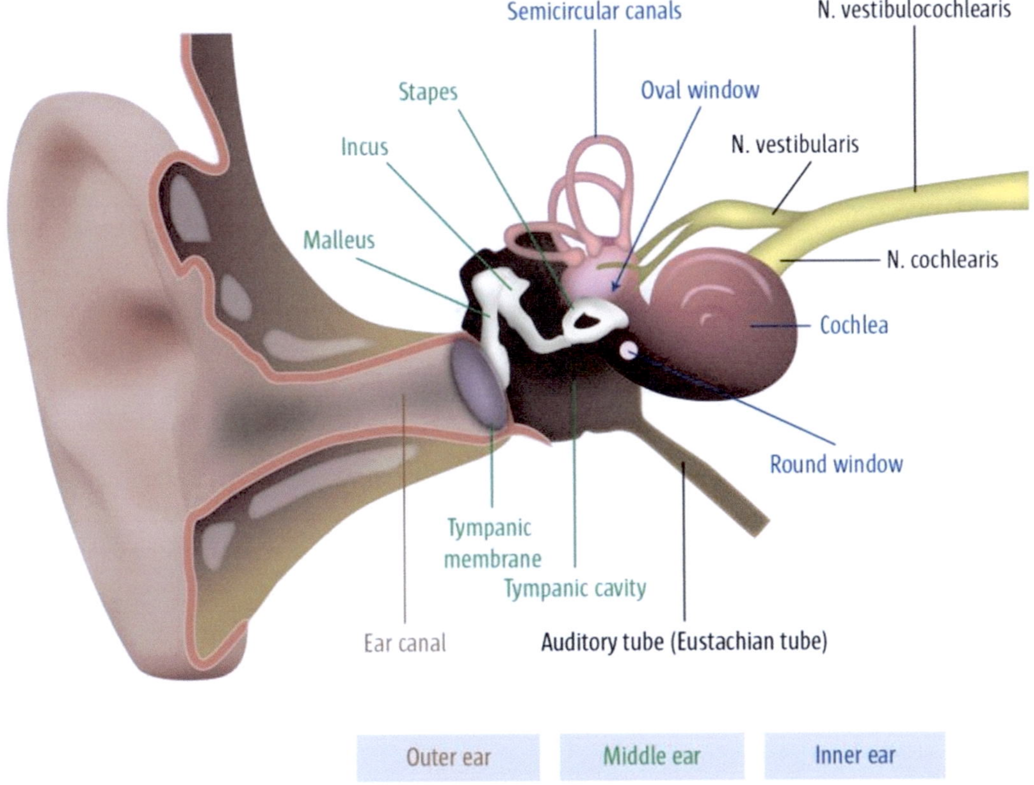

Fig. 5.38 Schematic illustration of the ear with the acoustic system (cochlea) and the vestibular system (semicircular canals). © ARKANA Forum GmbH 2022. All Rights Reserved

what shorter latency. There is no superposition with wave I.

- Waves IV and V often merge in the ipsilateral recording, but are usually separated in the contralateral recording. This wave complex can best be separated with rarefaction stimulation.
- The wave complex IV/V should have a length of 1.5 ms. A significantly shorter complex indicates absence of wave V.

For the **prediction of postoperative hearing**, the preservation of **wave V** is most important. If wave V is lost intraoperatively, the probability of postoperative complete hearing loss is 90%. Waves II and III, on the other hand, are very sensitive to manipulation of the nerve until it enters the brainstem, but have good recovery potential and thus represent a useful intraoperative early warning system. Deterioration of waves II and III can often be observed earlier than critical alterations of wave V [20].

Figure 5.40 depicts a typical BAEP. For rough comparison, mean latencies in awake normal controls are listed in Table 5.20. Note that latencies vary with head size and age. Furthermore, there are no normal values for the anesthetized state, and the length of the silastic tubes introduces an approximately 1 ms delay of peak latencies, while not affecting interpeak latencies. Table 5.21 shows the commonly used stimulation and recording parameters.

It should be noted that the mean latencies given in Table 5.18 *can only be used for functional assessment from the age of 4 years on.*

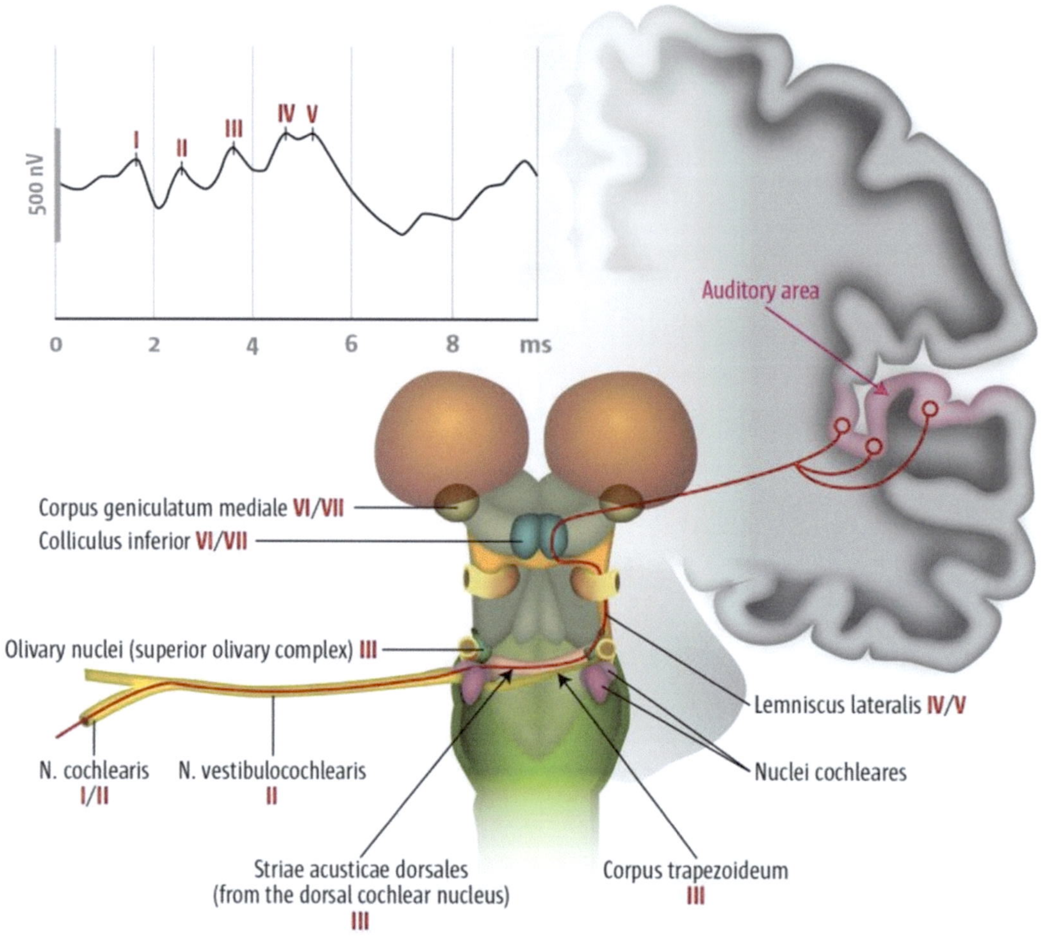

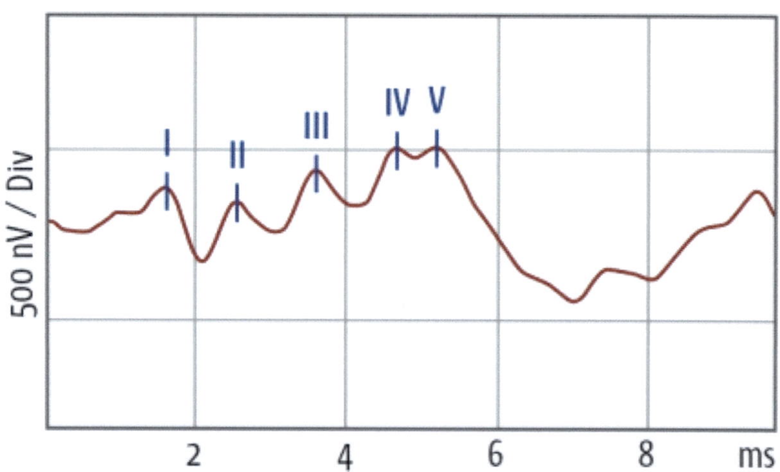

Fig. 5.39 Generators and waves I–V of the BAEP and VI–VII of the middle AEP. © ARKANA Forum GmbH 2022. All Rights Reserved

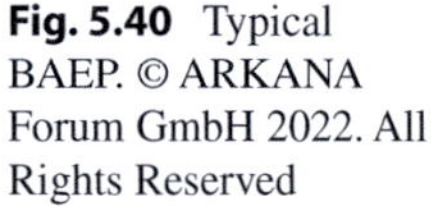

Fig. 5.40 Typical BAEP. © ARKANA Forum GmbH 2022. All Rights Reserved

Table 5.20 Mean BAEP absolute and interpeak latencies in normal awake control subjects [21]

	Latency (ms)
I	1.5
II	2.6
III	3.6
IV	4.7
V	5.5
I–III	2.0
III–V	1.8
I–V	3.9

Table 5.21 Stimulation and recording parameters for BAEPs (recommended starting values are marked bold)

Intensity	Maximum 95 dB HL (**75 dB** above hearing threshold)
Masking intensity	30 dB
Stimulation frequency	11.7–**49.1** Hz (select an odd divisor of 50 or 60 Hz)
Pulse type	**Click,** chirp, pulse, gaussian
Polarity	Condensation, rarefaction, **alternating**
Low-pass filter	**1500**–3000 Hz
High-pass filter	30–**150** Hz
Time base	10–20 ms (**15 ms**)
Averaging	500–2000 (**2000**)

5.4.3.2 Electrocochleography (ECochG)

Electrocochleography (ECochG) is an alternative technique for monitoring the auditory pathway.

Stimulation is performed with earplugs identical to the triggering of the BAEP.

Recording can be accomplished from the cochlea by a needle electrode inserted through the tympanic membrane (**transtympanic ECochG**). However, the needle can cause middle ear bleeding that disables recording. A non-invasive alternative is the **tympanic ECochG**. Here, a ball electrode connected to the earplug by a spring is placed on the tympanic membrane (Fig. 5.41). Since ECochG also uses a Cz reference, the recording picks up the same far-field brainstem signals as BAEPs. However, since the tympanic electrode is close to the cochlear nerve, ECochG registers a near-field wave I that is larger than with BAEP recording from the mastoid or earlobe [22].

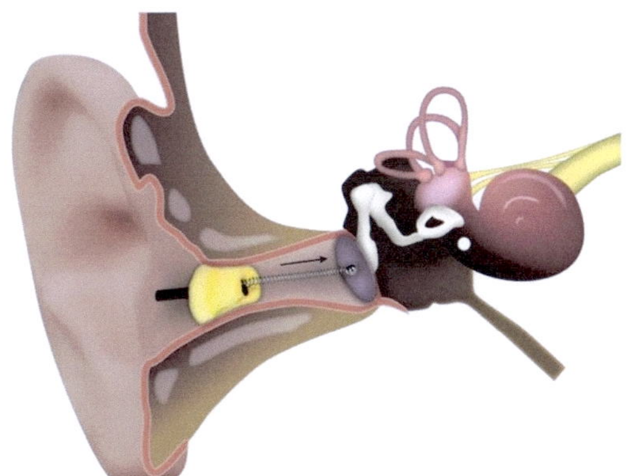

Fig. 5.41 Ball electrode on the tympanic membrane for ECochG recording. © ARKANA Forum GmbH 2022. All Rights Reserved

5.4.3.3 Compound Nerve Action Potentials (CNAPs)

Special electrodes allow recording of compound nerve action potentials (CNAPs) directly from the acoustic nerve [23].

After surgical exposure, a ball or cotton electrode is placed on the cochlear nerve. The reference is an electrode at Cz. The direct near-field nerve potential has substantially larger amplitude than BAEPs. Thus, no or minimal averaging (10–20 sweeps) is required to obtain reproducible potentials. However, the latency, amplitude, and shape of the CNAP depend on the location of the electrode, which can be positioned either close to the brainstem or more distally. Usually there is a positive-negative-positive CNAP roughly corresponding to wave I or II, and often there is a second smaller negative potential thought to volume conduct from the cochlear nucleus [23]. Since display sensitivity is reduced, later lower-amplitude BAEP waves from Cz are less apparent. Figure 5.42 shows a typical CNAP recorded from the cochlear nerve.

5.4.4 Visual Evoked Potentials (VEPs)

Visual evoked potentials are triggered by different visual stimuli that activate photoreceptors of

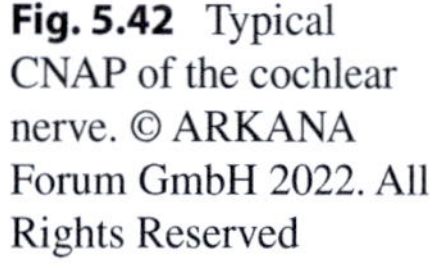

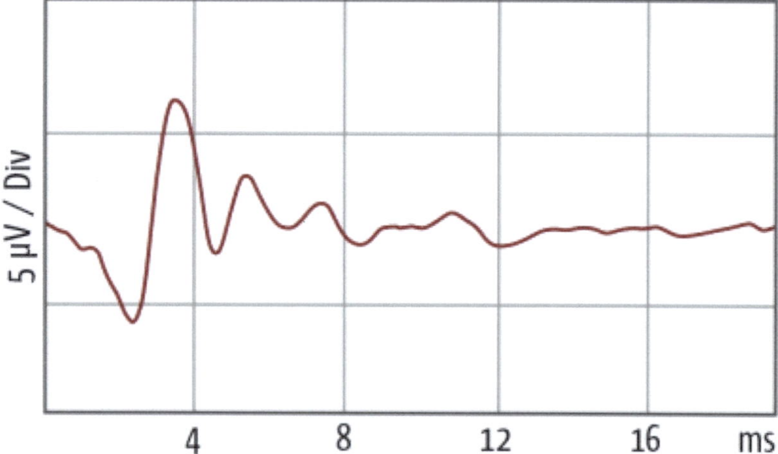

Fig. 5.42 Typical CNAP of the cochlear nerve. © ARKANA Forum GmbH 2022. All Rights Reserved

the retina. These photoreceptors are mainly divided into rods and cones. The **rods** are used for scotopic vision (vision under low light conditions). The **cones** are responsible for photopic vision (vision under high light conditions) and perceive changes in contrast, i.e., they mediate color vision in daylight.

Rods and cones can be activated separately by different **stimulation** techniques. Stimulation with flashes of light as used intra-operatively excites the light sensitive rods [21]. This can be accomplished with light emitting diode (LED) discs placed on the closed eyelids (Fig. 5.43).

There are still no generally accepted standards for the **recording** of intraoperative VEPs. It is recommended to place the electrodes near the visual cortex, i.e., over the occipital lobe. The corresponding 10–20 system sites are O1, O2, and Oz (Fig. 5.44). The reference can be Fz or Cz [24], or linked A1 and A2 [25]. For anterior visual pathway lesions, side-selective monocular stimulation and Oz–Fz recording is sufficient. For posterior visual pathway pathologies, side-selective recording can be done with O1–reference and O2–reference.

The photoreceptors of the retina activated by the flash convert the light into electrical

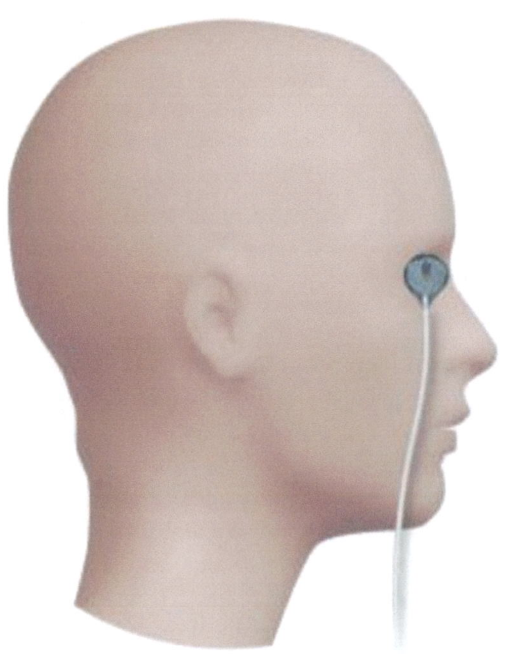

Fig. 5.43 Position of the LED disc for flash stimulation. © ARKANA Forum GmbH 2022. All Rights Reserved

impulses. The **action potential** travels along the optic nerve. In the optic chiasm, the nerve fibers of the nasally located sensory cells of the retina cross to the contralateral side, while

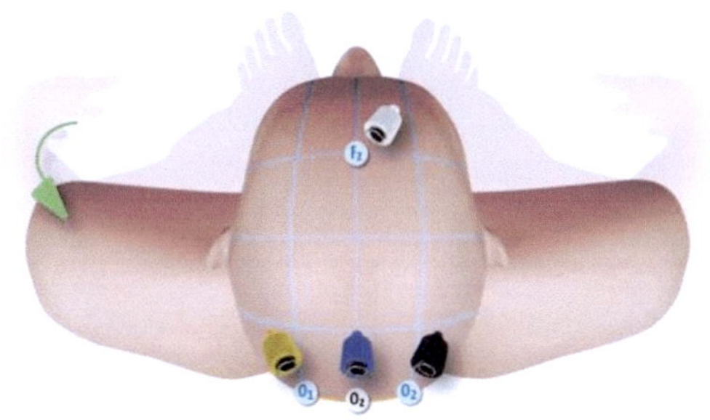

Fig. 5.44 Position of electrodes for VEP recording. © ARKANA Forum GmbH 2022. All Rights Reserved

the fibers of the temporally located sensory cells continue uncrossed. From the optic chiasm, the impulses travel via the optic tracts to the lateral geniculate body (corpus geniculatum laterale) and from there to the visual radiations, which ends in the visual cortex (Fig. 5.45).

The flash-triggered **responses** vary considerably between individuals with regard to latency, amplitude, and shape. Therefore, no generally accepted normal values are available.

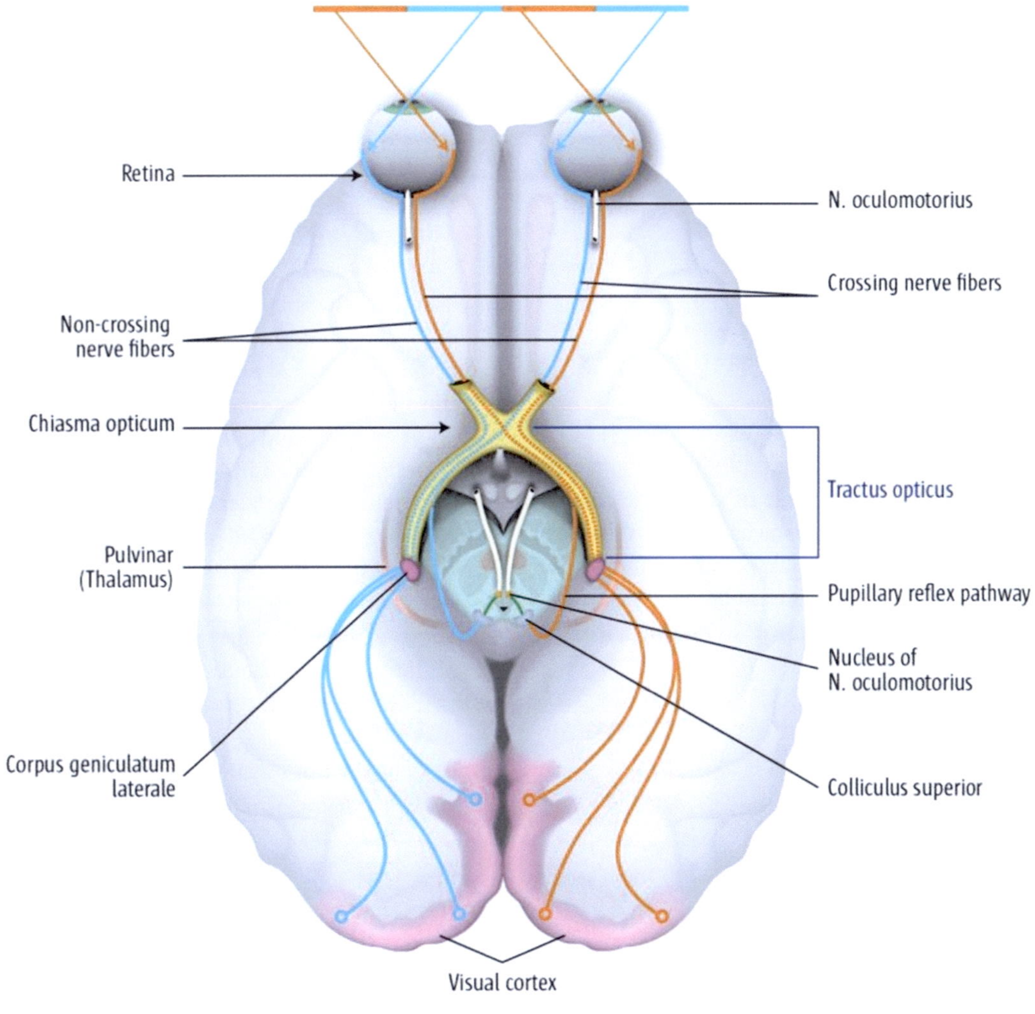

Fig. 5.45 Visual pathways and signal course of VEPs. © ARKANA Forum GmbH 2022. All Rights Reserved

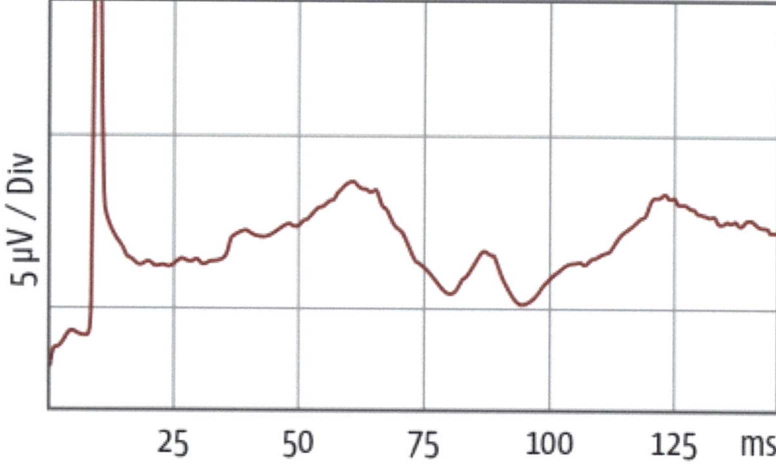

Fig. 5.46 A typical flash VEP. © ARKANA Forum GmbH 2022. All Rights Reserved

Table 5.22 Stimulation and recording parameters for flash VEPs

Intensity	3000–20,000 lux (**10,000 lux**)
Stimulation frequency	**1.1**–2.1 Hz (select an odd divisor of 50 or 60 Hz)
Low-pass filter	100 Hz
High-pass filter	**0.5**–1 Hz
Time base	**200**–300 ms
Averaging	25–300 sweeps (**100**)

Of particular importance for the interpretation of the signals are the intraindividual changes of the curves over the course of surgery. However, no clear results are yet available on the prognostic significance of flash VEP deterioration for postoperative visual function, particularly during surgeries risking posterior visual pathway damage [24].

An example of a VEP is shown in Fig. 5.46. Table 5.22 presents most frequently used stimulation and recording parameters.

5.5 Functional Topographic Mapping

5.5.1 Central Sulcus

Of particular importance for intraoperative localization of the central sulcus (sulcus centralis) is the median nerve **SEP phase reversal**.

Stimulation is performed on the median nerve of the left or right hand at the wrist.

Referential **recording** is done from the exposed cortex contralateral to the stimulation side using a strip electrode placed at a right angle across the suspected central sulcus.

When correctly placed, the postcentral contacts register SEPs with the usual negative polarity and largest amplitude at the primary sensory gyrus. The precentral contacts register signals reversed in polarity to positive, with largest amplitude at the primary motor gyrus. Therefore, the SEPs are phase reversed across the central sulcus (Fig. 5.47).

The reference should ideally be inactive for cortical SEPs. This makes Fz a questionable choice because it picks up the frontal P22 that is normally smaller than direct cortical SEPs, but could partially distort the results. Therefore, a forehead, mastoid, or wound margin reference away from frontoparietal cortex may be preferable. With a mastoid reference, a small subcortical P14 dip precedes the direct cortical responses.

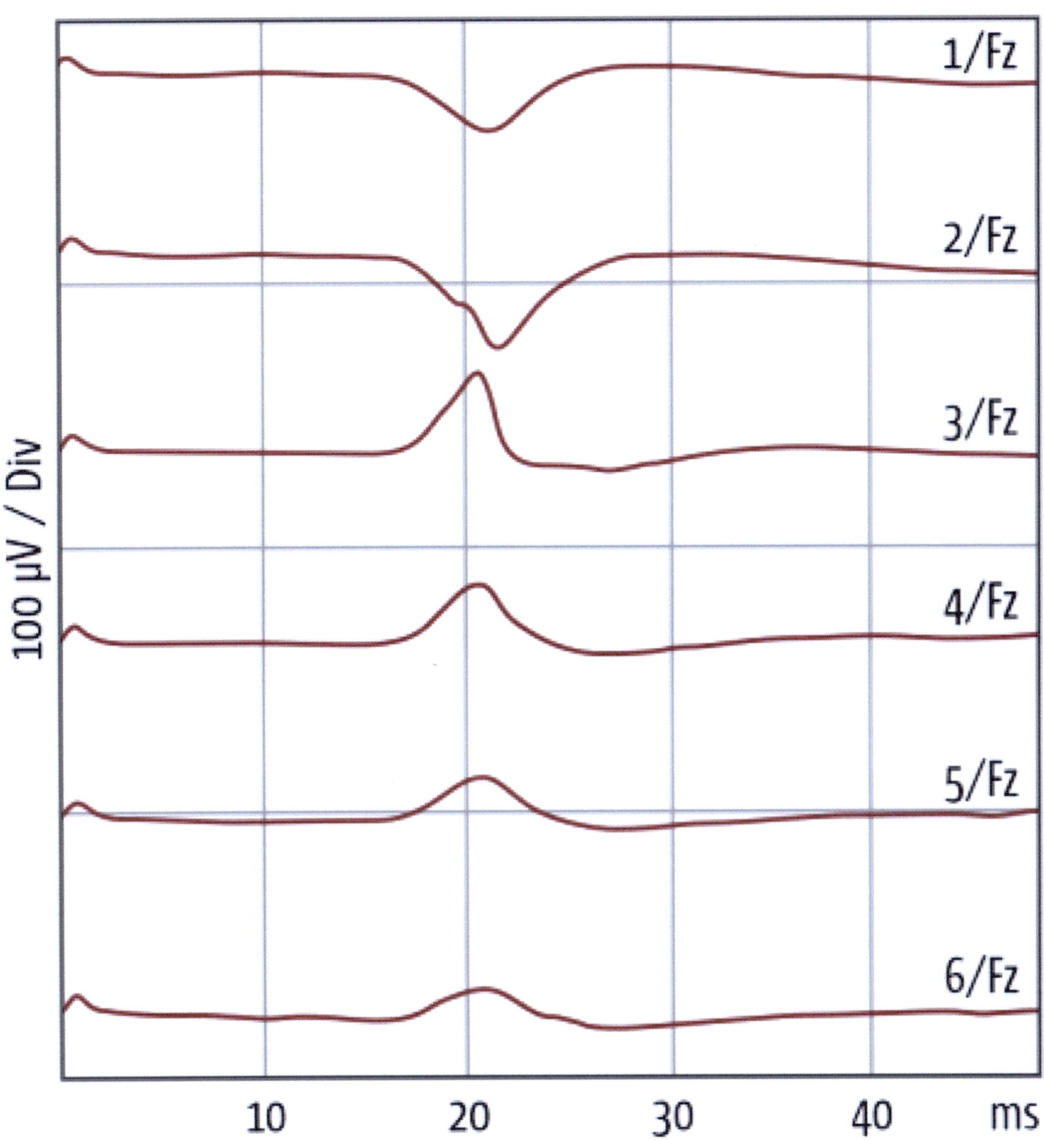

Fig. 5.47 Median nerve SEP phase reversal. Electrode contacts 1 and 2 (upper two traces) are precentral, and the remaining contacts (lower four traces) are postcentral. The central sulcus is located between contacts 2 and 3.© ARKANA Forum GmbH 2022. All Rights Reserved

5.5.2 Motor Cortex Mapping

With monopolar anodal pulse trains delivered through subdural strip electrodes or a hand-held probe, direct cortical stimulation MEPs can be used to localize the primary motor gyrus and map the motor homunculus (see Sect. 5.4.2.3 "Cortical Stimulation and Recording"). **Lowest MEP threshold** is a highly reliable localization criterion. This is important because strong stimuli can trigger MEPs from premotor and parietal cortex and thus be non-localizing. Furthermore, since median nerve SEP mapping is occasionally inaccurate for motor cortex identification, it is important to perform MEP mapping whenever primary motor cortex localization is critical. Once localized, modest suprathreshold intensity can be used to quickly find the hand, leg, and face areas of the motor homunculus and exclude the presence of primary motor cortex in other cortical regions or in pathological tissue.

5.5.3 Subcortical Corticospinal Tract Mapping

Combining the stimulation probe with a surgical instrument obviates the need for the surgeon to change the instrument, which is usually necessary prior to mapping. This allows for **continuous mapping** [26], a technique therefore also referred to as **dynamic mapping**.

Usually, the tip of the suction device serves simultaneously for monopolar stimulation (therefore also named mapping suction probe) facilitating continuous stimulation during the removal of a tumor and thus continuous control of the distance to the corticospinal tract without interrupting the surgical procedure. The lower the stimulation intensity required to trigger an MEP, the shorter the distance of the resection site to the corticospinal tract. Below a threshold of 1–3 mA, resection of the tumor is terminated because the risk of postoperative functional deficit is too high [26]. Figure 5.48 shows a typical example of dynamic mapping and monitoring using the mapping suction probe.

5.5.4 Language

Mapping of the language is possible **extraoperatively** via a previously implanted grid electrode, or **intraoperatively** during awake surgery.

Intraoperative stimulation is performed with a bipolar fork probe that is used to scan the

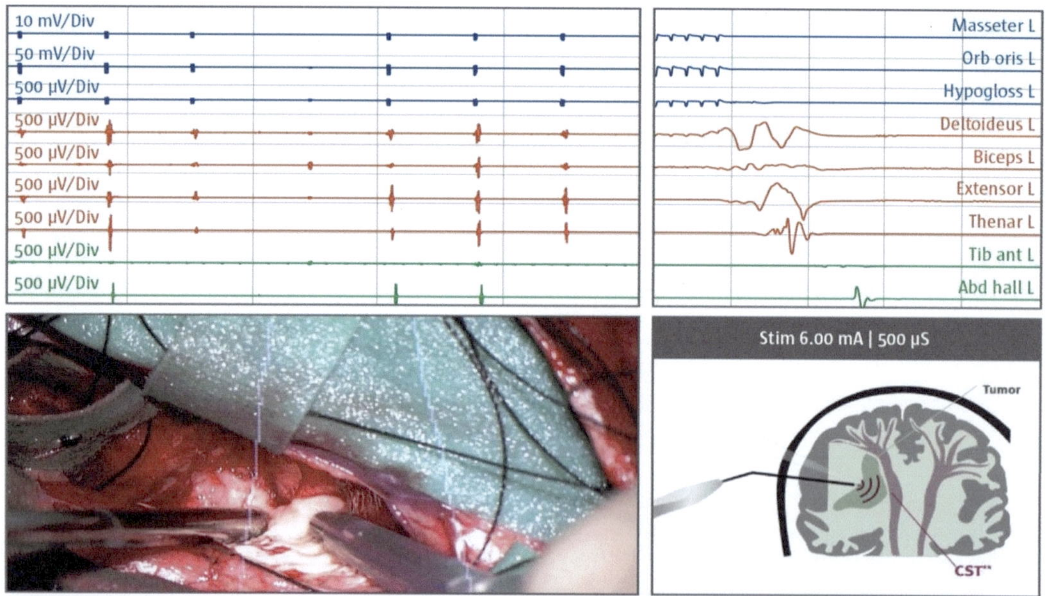

Fig. 5.48 Dynamic mapping and monitoring with monopolar stimulation through the tip of the suction device. Left: Surgical situs; right: Schematic representation. CST, corticospinal tract. Orb oris, orbicularis oris mucsle; Hypogloss, hypoglossal nerve, tongue muscle; Tib ant, tibialis anterior muscle; Abd hall, abductor hallucis muscle; L, left. © ARKANA Forum GmbH 2022. All Rights Reserved

expected language-relevant area. In contrast to MEP mapping, no response is triggered. Rather, language is blocked. The stimulation intensity should be below the threshold for triggering afterdischarges, since afterdischarges can be expected to transmit neuronal activity to distal areas, so that a neurological effect resulting from the stimulation can no longer be attributed exclusively to the stimulated area.

For intraoperative language mapping, only non-concentric bipolar hand probes are used.

If an epileptic seizure is triggered by direct cortical stimulation, it can be successfully interrupted with cold irrigation of the brain, using 4 °C isotonic saline solution or Ringer's solution.

During the stimulation periods, the patient is shown simple black-and-white graphics which he must **name**, always using the prefix sentence "This is a ...." If the patient is able to name the graphics correctly, it can be assumed that the stimulation probe was not placed at the language area. If the stimulation is followed by misnaming or speech inhibition, this area is involved in speech function.

Figures 5.49 and 5.50 show typical examples of language mapping. The commonly used stimulation parameters are given in Table 5.23. Table 5.24 explains various terms used in the context of language testing. Typical stimulation results are summarized in Fig. 5.51.

With direct cortical stimulation, care should be taken at high currents to ensure that the duration of stimulation does not exceed 4 s, as the risk of burns or seizures is significantly higher with prolonged stimulation [19].

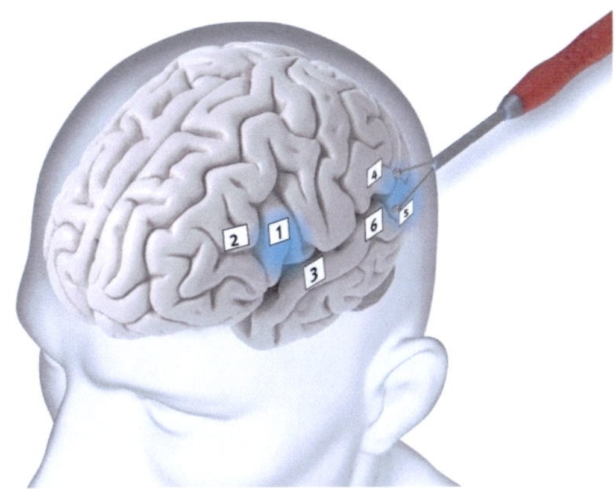

Fig. 5.49 Intraoperative mapping and monitoring of the language areas during awake surgery. © ARKANA Forum GmbH 2022. All Rights Reserved

Some centers perform more complex intraoperative language and cognitive mapping with various testing protocols.

5.5.5 Spinal Cord Mapping

In this section, we explore dorsal column and corticospinal tract mapping techniques that can be important for **intramedullary spinal cord surgery**, particularly when tumor or other pathology distorts the anatomy.

5.5.5.1 Dorsal Column Mapping
Dorsal midline myelotomy is the main surgical approach to the interior of the spinal cord. The surgeon tries to incise and enter the midline septum **between the gracile fasciculi** without injuring them. However, if the dorsal columns are displaced from the midline, then an anatomically centered myelotomy can damage them. In fact, **irreversible** tibial nerve **somatosensory evoked potential (SEP) deterioration** commonly follows myelotomy at any level, and median nerve SEPs may also deteriorate with cervical myelotomy (Fig. 5.52). These patients may have postoperative **discriminative touch and proprioceptive deficits** that can impede rehabilitation. Nevertheless, since motor evoked potentials (MEPs) and motor strength are unaffected, the surgery will continue.

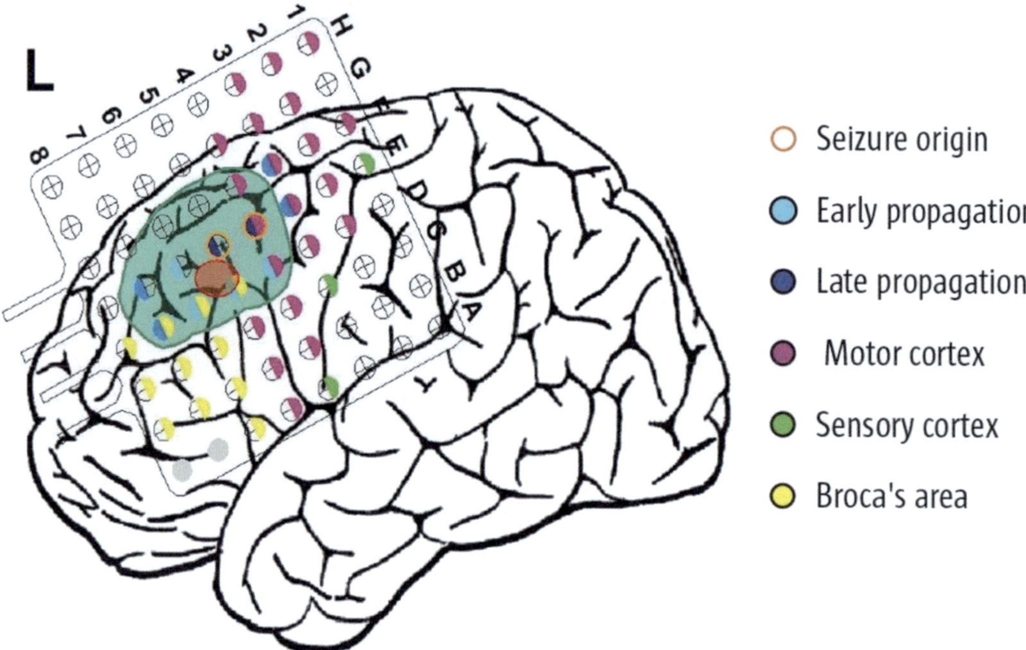

Fig. 5.50 Recording of the EEG and extraoperative mapping of language areas and sensorimotor cortex; from [27], with permission. © ARKANA Forum GmbH 2022. All Rights Reserved

Table 5.23 Stimulation parameters for mapping language areas [19]

Stimulation current	4–20 mA
Stimulation frequency	50–60 Hz
Stimulation duration	1–4 s
Pulse form	Biphasic rectangular pulses
Pulse duration	100–1000 µs

Table 5.24 Different terms used in language testing

Speech arrest	No verbal utterance
Speech disturbance	Incomprehensible utterance of prefix sentence and object name
Aphasic speech arrest	Error-free utterance of the prefix sentence, no object naming
Paraphasic misnaming	Error-free utterance of the prefix sentence, incorrect object naming

The main goal of dorsal column mapping in this context is to guide the surgeon to the **physiologic midline** and thereby **reduce the risk of dorsal column injury** during myelotomy. There are two basic approaches: spinal cord recording or spinal cord stimulation.

Spinal Cord Recording

The recording method employs a **miniature 8-contact electrode** laid horizontally across the exposed dorsal cord after dural opening [28–30]. The contacts are thin stainless-steel wires embedded with 1 mm spacing into a 1 cm wide silastic strip. One records polyphasic near-field travelling potentials called **dorsal column volleys (DCVs)** after stimulating one tibial nerve at the ankle and then the other using supramaximal pulses of 0.2 ms duration at up to 13.3 Hz. A 50 ms time base, 50–1700 Hz bandwidth, and averaging of 100–200 sweeps are appropriate. The contacts show a DCV **amplitude gradient**, and the one with **largest amplitude** is closest to the activated gracile fasciculus. The midline is between the two contacts showing greatest amplitude to left and right tibial nerve stimulation (Fig. 5.53).

This technique is effective for the **cervical** and **thoracic** spinal cord where other potentials do not obscure the small tibial nerve DCV [29]. It breaks down in the lumbar cord where the larger stationary N22 potential from gray matter con-

Fig. 5.51 Results of the stimulation for language testing. © ARKANA Forum GmbH 2022. All Rights Reserved

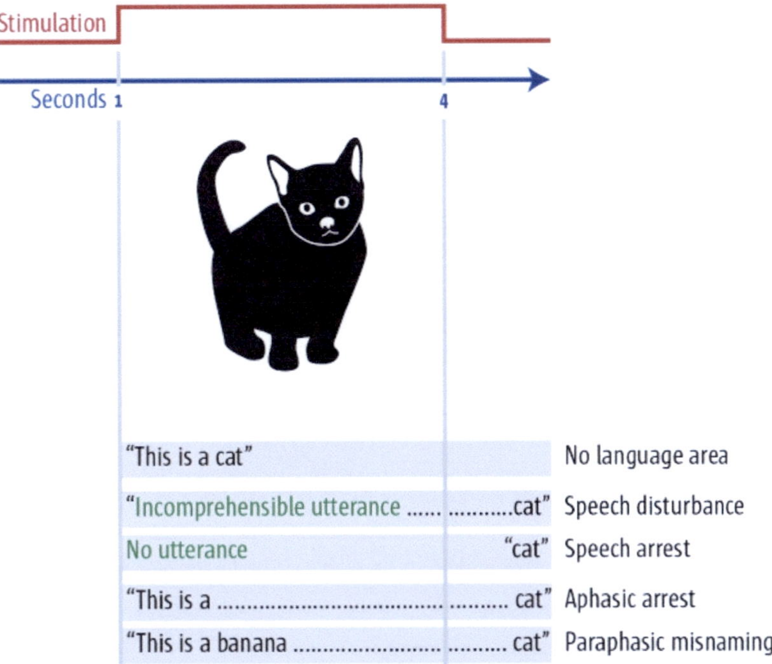

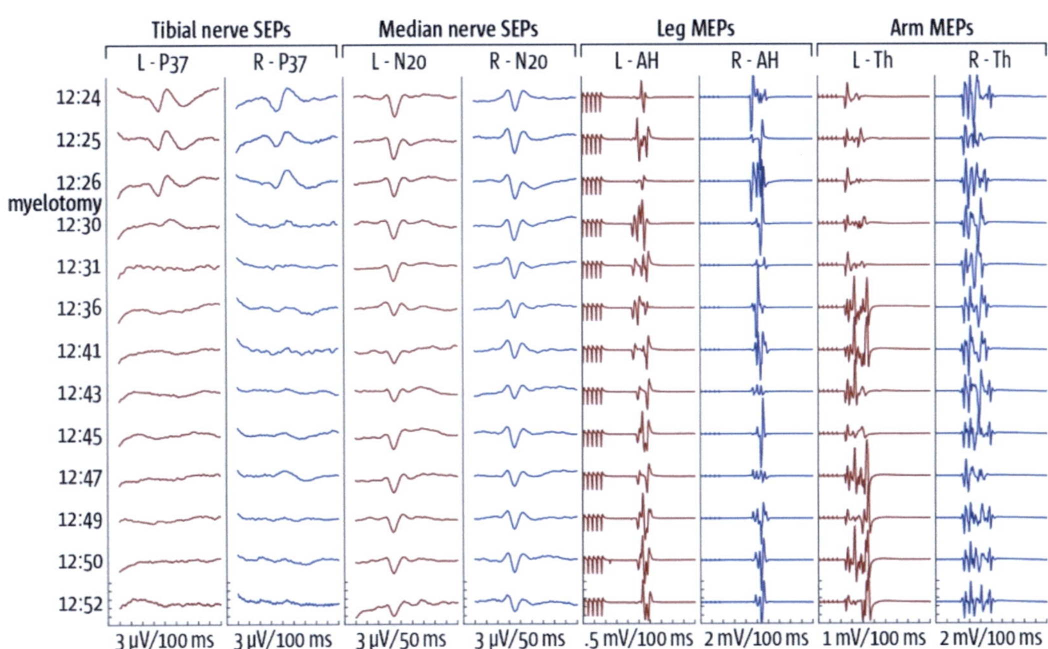

Fig. 5.52 Bilateral tibial nerve cortical P37 disappearance and slight median nerve cortical N20 reduction after cervical midline myelotomy. *L* left, *R* right, *AH* abductor hallucis muscle, *Th* thenar muscle. Modified from [6], with permission

ceals the DCV. Similarly, with median nerve stimulation, the stationary cervical N13 potential obscures cuneate fasciculus DCVs.

Although this method may help reduce the incidence of dorsal column injury, it has not gained much use outside of a few centers. This

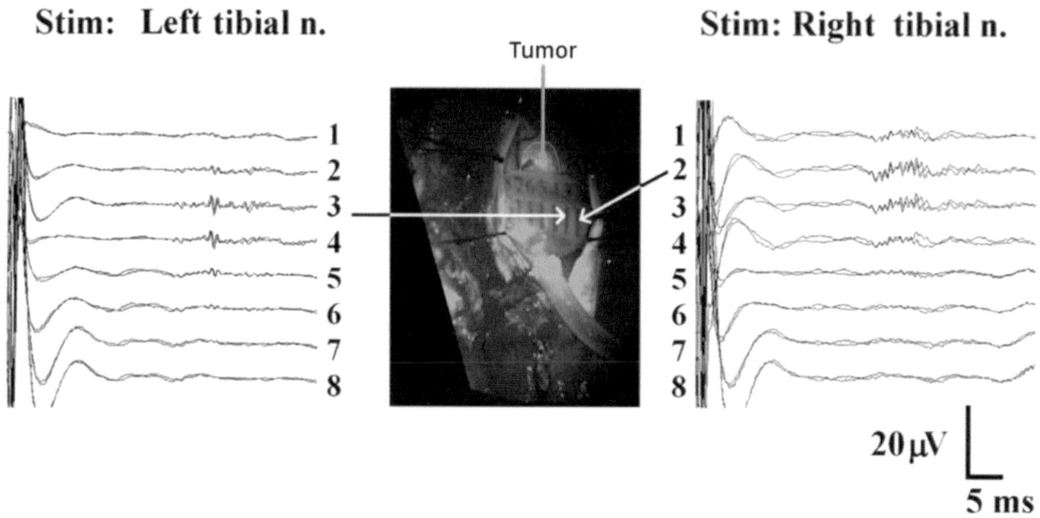

Fig. 5.53 Dorsal column volleys showing the midline between contacts 2 and 3 and displaced laterally by tumor. From [30], with permission

may be partly due to a lack of commercially available miniature recording electrodes.

Spinal Cord Stimulation

Direct **stimulation of the gracile fasciculus** with a hand-held probe initiates orthodromic and antidromic action potential volleys. A **bipolar** probe facilitates focal stimulation and may be concentric or forked with 2–3 mm tip separation keeping the cathode in the direction of the intended action potentials.

Peripheral Nerve Recording

Antidromic impulses descend the dorsal columns and then without synapse the Ia afferent fibers of peripheral nerves, where they are recordable. In the original report, the stimuli were 0.2 ms duration pulses of 3–8 mA intensity delivered at 9.1 Hz, and recordings were made over the posterior tibial nerve at the ankle using a 100 ms time base, 30–300 Hz bandwidth, and averaging of 50–100 sweeps [31]. By recording bilaterally, one can identify unilateral responses indicating **left or right gracile fasciculus** activation, and the stimulus sites producing **greatest response amplitude** are closest to the gracile fasciculi. The **midline** septum is the site in

between where stimulation evokes **little or no response** (Fig. 5.54). Again, this technique is not widely employed.

Scalp Recording

Orthodromic impulses ascend the gracile fasciculus and, after synaptic relays in the gracile nucleus and thalamus, reach the contralateral mesial leg area primary **sensory cortex**. This produces a dipolar cortical SEP analogous to the tibial nerve P37/N37, but with much shorter peak latency of 8–20 ms, depending on the stimulated level [32, 33]. The scalp response is normally positive at the centroparietal midline and ipsilateral scalp, with an approximately simultaneous contralateral scalp negative pole. By recording **CP3–CP4, left gracile fasciculus** stimulation produces a **positive** deflection (positivity at CP3–negativity at CP4), while **right gracile fasciculus** stimulation produces a **negative** deflection (negativity at CP3–positivity at CP4). Thus, there is a **phase reversal** between left and right gracile fasciculus stimulation. With stimulation in the **midline,** there is either **no response**, or bilateral activation causing **cancellation** of the opposite-polarity responses. Recording from **CPz to Fz** can distinguish between these possibilities: it is

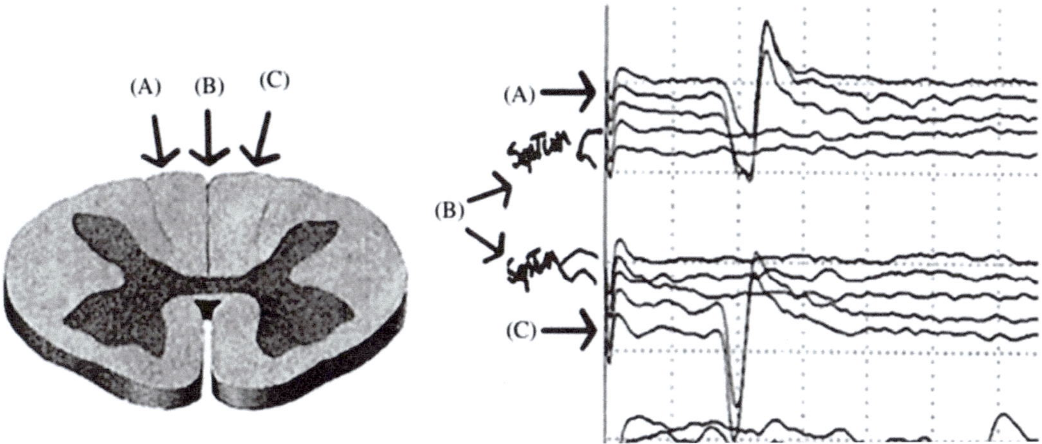

Fig. 5.54 Dorsal column stimulation with posterior tibial nerve recording at the ankle. (*A*) Right gracile fasciculus. (*B*) Midline septum. (*C*) Left gracile fasciculus. Modified from [29], with permission

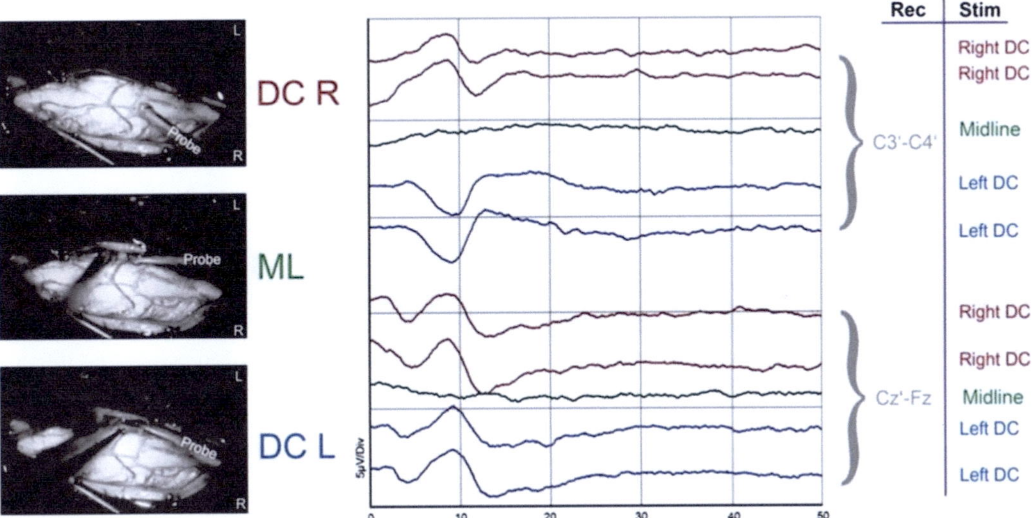

Fig. 5.55 Gracile fasciculus stimulation with scalp potential phase reversal. CP3–CP4 (C3′–C4′) shows a phase reversal between right (R) and left (L) dorsal column (DC) stimulation, and no response with midline (ML) stimulation. CPz–Fz (Cz′–Fz) shows no phase reversal (the negative deflections suggest mistaken Fz–CPz recording). From [29], with permission

also **flat** if there is **no response**, or shows a **positive** deflection if there is **bilateral activation** with cancellation in CP3–CP4 (Fig. 5.55).

The stimuli are 0.2 ms pulses of 0.2–0.5 mA intensity at up to 4.7 Hz frequency. A 50 ms time base, 30–300 Hz bandwidth, and averaging of 10–20 sweeps are appropriate for recording. This rapid method is currently the preferred dorsal column mapping technique and may help reduce the incidence of dorsal column injury. As yet unknown is how it will perform with variations of scalp SEP topography (see Sect. 5.4.1.2 "Tibial Nerve SEPs"). It should work with rare nondecussation that would still show a phase reversal, but with reversed polarity of the left and right gracile fasciculus responses.

5.5.5.2 Corticospinal Tract Mapping

Reliable corticospinal tract mapping is of even greater clinical interest because **avoiding a permanent motor deficit** is a major surgical objective. There are two basic approaches: combined transcranial and spinal cord stimulation or spinal cord stimulation.

Combined Transcranial and Spinal Cord Stimulation

The combined stimulation technique depends on **D-wave collision** [29, 34]. A single-pulse transcranial stimulus evokes a descending D-wave recorded with an epidural spinal electrode just above the surgical level. Simultaneously, one applies a single-pulse spinal cord stimulus with a hand-held probe. If this activates corticospinal axons, then antidromic ascending corticospinal action potentials collide with the descending ones at some point above the epidural electrode. In this case, the **D-wave amplitude drops**. The magnitude of the drop varies because (1) the D-wave is bilateral to some unknown extent, while the spinal cord stimuli are unilateral, and (2) the lesion may locally block conduction of some corticospinal axons that therefore cannot be activated by spinal cord stimuli. If the D-wave amplitude is unaltered, then spinal cord stimulation did not activate any conducting corticospinal fibers. Thus, it is possible to **identify functional corticospinal tract axons** by showing a **reduction of rostral D-wave amplitude**. This method is not widely used, possibly due to its being somewhat complex.

Spinal Cord Stimulation

It would be simpler to stimulate the spinal cord to find the corticospinal tract by showing a motor nerve or muscle response. However, there is a **problem with motor selectivity**. Specifically, dorsal column stimulation can also evoke motor responses through a **central H-reflex** due to retrograde activation of Ia afferent collaterals that synapse on lower motor neurons.

Peripheral Nerve Recording

One idea was to record **neurogenic "MEPs"** from peripheral motor nerves, such as the tibial nerve in the popliteal fossa. However, it turned out that these responses are predominantly **antidromic sensory potentials** of dorsal column origin [35]. Consequently, this method failed.

Muscle Recording After Single-Train Stimulation

Another idea is to stimulate the spinal cord with 60 Hz trains while recording **muscle responses** [31], or single 3-pulse trains while recording **muscle MEPs** [36]. Either must indicate **lower motor neuron activation**, but one cannot assume corticospinal tract specificity, because a central H-reflex could be the source.

Muscle Recording After Double-Train Stimulation

Fortunately, a recent modification consisting of low-intensity (0.2–2 mA) **double-train** stimulation with a **60 ms intertrain interval** apparently **resolves the motor selectivity problem** [29, 37]. The first train evokes a muscle MEP with corticospinal tract or dorsal column stimulation. The second train evokes a nearly identical second MEP with corticospinal tract stimulation, but either no response or a clearly dissimilar (smaller or larger) MEP with dorsal column stimulation (Fig. 5.56).

The reason for the difference is that the corticospinal synaptic **refractory period** is short, while the dorsal column synaptic refractory period is normally >60 ms. Thus, with corticospinal tract stimulation, the second train **after the refractory period** evokes a nearly identical second MEP. With dorsal column stimulation in neurologically intact patients, the second train **during the refractory period** elicits no response. However, in patients with antecedent spasticity that variably alters the central H-reflex, the second train can elicit a second MEP, but of substantially different amplitude than the first.

Thus, for the first time there seems to be a spinal cord stimulation technique to identify the corticospinal tracts and differentiate them from the dorsal columns. However, we need more experience to determine the ultimate value of this new method.

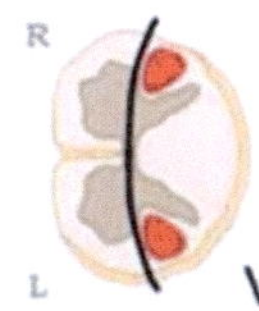

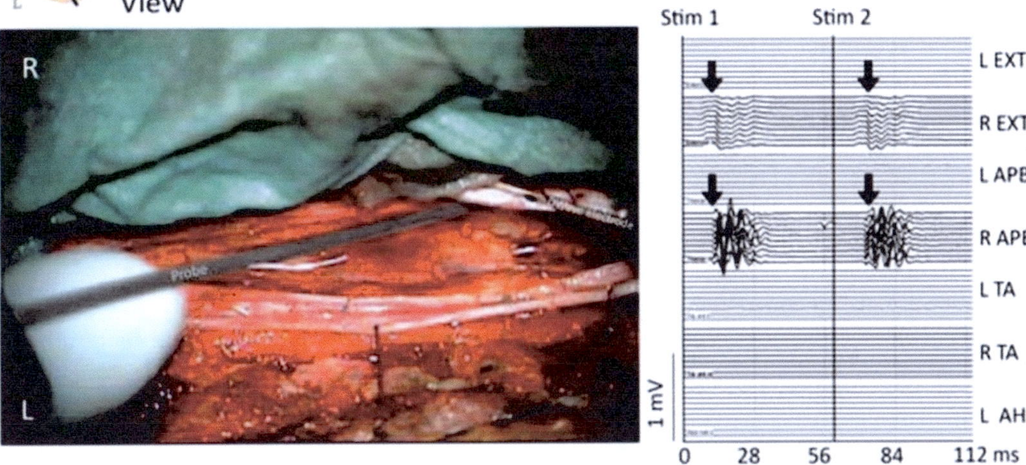

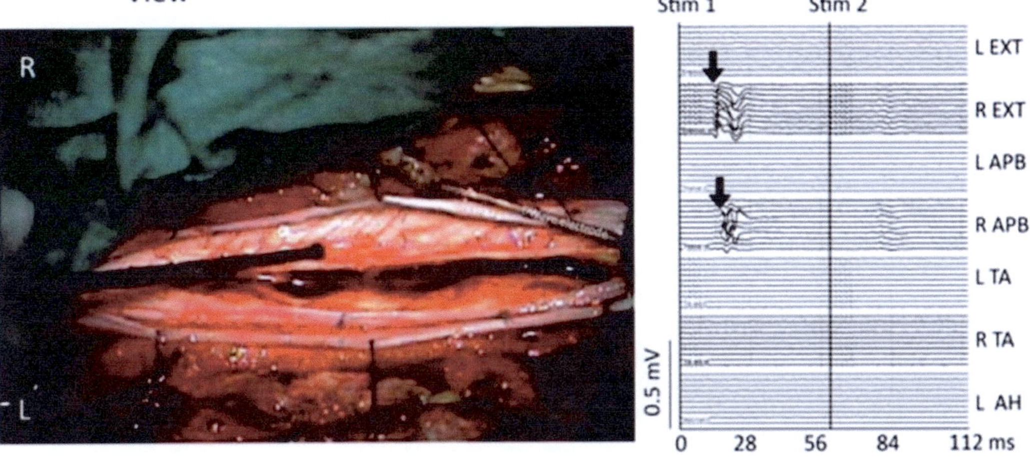

Fig. 5.56 Double-train spinal cord stimulation and muscle recording. With corticospinal tract stimulation, the first and second train (Stim 1 and Stim 2) evoked nearly identical responses. With dorsal column stimulation, Stim 2 produced a much smaller response than Stim 1. *R* right, *L* left, *EXT* extensor digitorum muscle, *APB* abductor pollicis brevis muscle, *TA* tibialis anterior muscle, *AH* abductor hallucis muscle. From [37], with permission

5.5.5.3 Conclusion

Spinal cord stimulation with scalp SEP phase reversal recording is emerging as a preferred dorsal column mapping technique to quickly find the physiological dorsal midline. Double-train spinal cord stimulation with muscle recording promises to enable rapid corticospinal tract mapping. Such techniques might ultimately improve neurologic outcome after intramedullary spinal cord surgery.

5.6   Cranial Nerves

Methods for functional examination of some cranial nerves, such as the optic nerve or the cochlear nerve, have already been described. The following is an **overview** on the modalities and techniques for intraoperative electrophysiological assessment of cranial nerves. This topic is especially relevant since cranial nerve mapping and monitoring has become a standard in many fields, such as neurosurgical interventions in the cerebellopontine angle, ENT surgeries on the parotid gland (parotid surgery), and general surgical procedures in the area of the thyroid gland (struma surgery).

Modalities used are based on the function of the respective cranial nerves: motor, sensory, or mixed. Identification and monitoring of the motor cranial nerves are performed using continuous EMG and triggered CMAPs. Triggered CMAPs are recorded using a pair of electrodes placed in the indicator muscle. For monitoring sensory cranial nerve function, evoked potentials in particular are available, for example, the SEP of the trigeminal nerve.

Table 5.25 and Figs. 5.57, 5.58, 5.59, 5.60, 5.61, 5.62, and 5.63 provide an overview of the modalities and techniques used for cranial nerve monitoring. In Table 5.26, the recommended stimulation parameters for direct activation of motor cranial nerves are given.

When placing the electrodes for monitoring cranial nerves III, IV, and VI, one thinks of the eye as a clock (Fig. 5.64):

- *The electrodes for monitoring the oculomotor nerve (III) are placed at 6 o'clock.*
- *For monitoring the trochlear nerve (IV) and the abducens nerve (VI), the side is important: On the right side, the recording electrodes for monitoring the trochlear nerve (IV) are placed at 2 o'clock and for monitoring the abducens nerve (VI) at 9 o'clock. On the left side, the constellation is as follows: trochlear nerve (IV) monitoring at 10 o'clock and abducens nerve (VI) monitoring at 3 o'clock.*

Table 5.25 Overview of cranial nerve monitoring

No.	Name	Function	Fiber type	Monitoring
I	N. olfactorius	Smell	Sensory	Not possible
II	N. opticus	Vision	Sensory	VEP
III	N. oculomotorius	Eye movements, pupil function	Somatomotor, parasympathetic	M. rectus superior, M. rectus inferior
IV	N. trochlearis	Eye movement	Somatomotor	M. obliquus superior
V	N. trigeminus	Muscles of mastication, sensitivity face	Somatomotor, sensory	M. masseter
VI	N. abducens	Eye movement	Somatomotor	M. rectus lateralis
VII	N. facialis	Facial muscles	Somatomotor, parasympathetic, sensory	M. orbicularis oculi, M. orbicularis oris, M. nasalis, M. frontalis, M. mentalis
VIII	N. vestibulocochlearis	Hearing and balance	Sensory	AEP
IX	N. glossopharyngeus	Throat muscles, taste	Somatomotor, parasympathetic, sensory	Soft palate, M. stylopharyngeus
X	N. vagus	Throat muscles, laryngeal muscles, vegetative functions	Somatomotor, parasympathetic, sensory	M. vocis, M. crycothyroideus
XI	N. accessorius	Neck rotation	Somatomotor	M. trapius
XII	N. hypoglossus	Tongue muscles	Somatomotor	Tongue muscles

- *Special care should be taken at the following positions of the right eye: At 3 o'clock is the nasolacrimal duct, and at 10 to 11 o'clock is the lacrimal gland. On the left eye, these zones are located at 1 to 2 o'clock and 9 o'clock, respectively. Electrodes must not be applied at these points.*

Monitoring of the **recurrent laryngeal nerve** is of particular importance during operations in the area of the **thyroid gland**. This nerve runs behind the thyroid gland and innervates the laryngeal muscles (Fig. 5.65). Injury to the recurrent laryngeal nerve results in vocal cord paralysis.

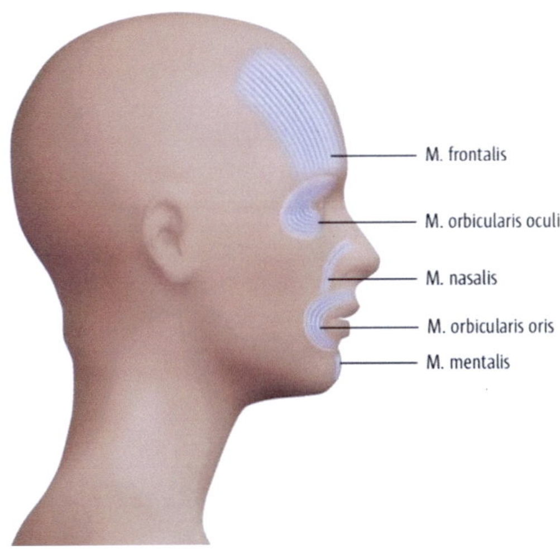

Fig. 5.58 Facial muscles. © ARKANA Forum GmbH 2022. All Rights Reserved

Fig. 5.57 Eye muscles. © ARKANA Forum GmbH 2022. All Rights Reserved

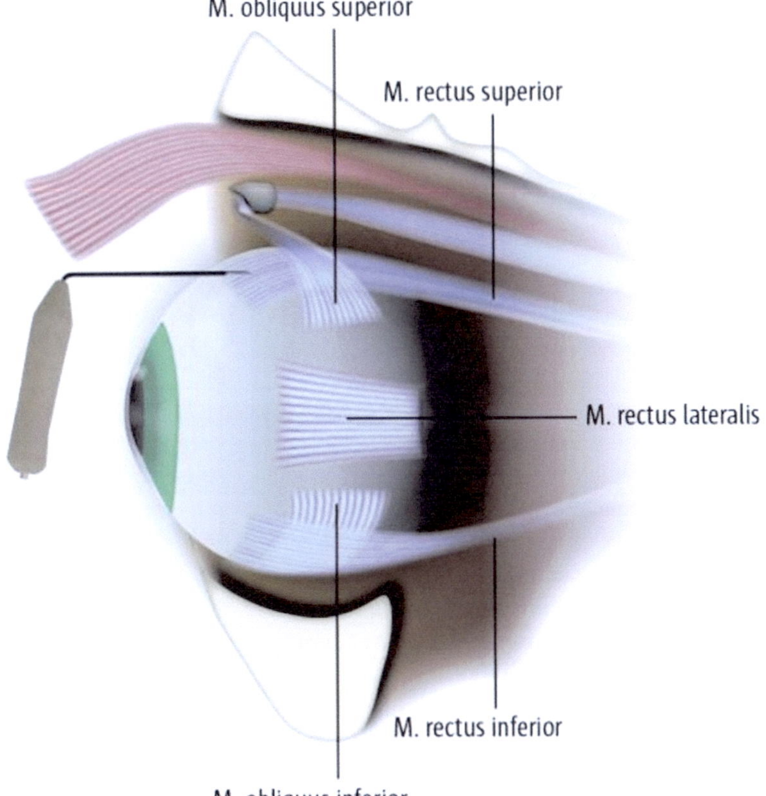

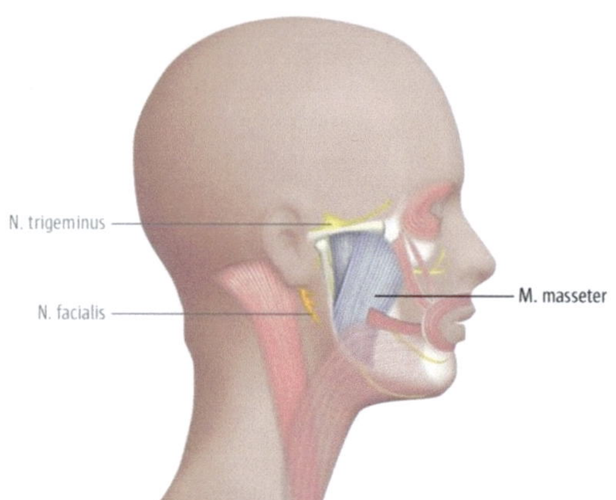

Fig. 5.59 M. masseter. © ARKANA Forum GmbH 2022. All Rights Reserved

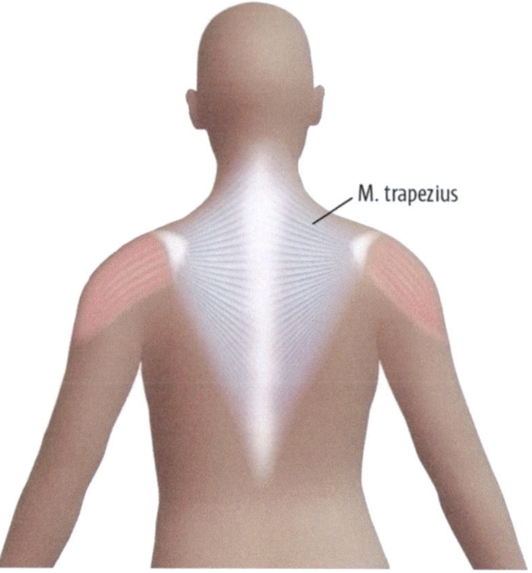

Fig. 5.61 M. trapezius. © ARKANA Forum GmbH 2022. All Rights Reserved

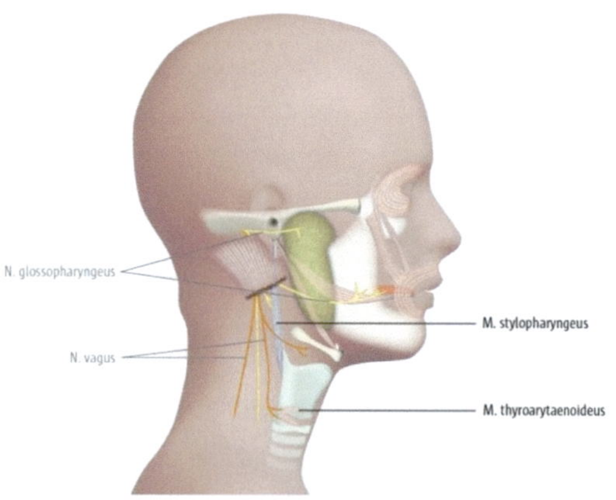

Fig. 5.60 M. stylopharyngeus. © ARKANA Forum GmbH 2022. All Rights Reserved

Unilateral injury to the nerve causes hoarseness, while bilateral injury leads to closure of the glottis and consequent respiratory distress.

Stimulation of the recurrent laryngeal nerve can be accomplished directly in a monopolar or bipolar fashion. As a rule, bipolar stimulation is preferred. In either case, however, the nerve is assessed only intermittently. In order to ensure continuous control, stimulation of the vagus nerve has been developed. To do this, a stimulation electrode is looped around the vagus nerve (Fig. 5.66). By this electrode, which remains in situ until the end of the operation, the vagus nerve can be continuously stimulated at a low frequency (e.g., 1 Hz).

Recording is done from the vocalis muscle evaluating CMAPs. Until now, needle electrodes have been used for this, which are inserted through the cricothyroid ligament into the ipsilateral vocalis muscle. Currently, non-invasive recording is preferred using surface electrodes applied to the endotracheal tube (e.g., adhesive tube electrodes). During intubation, the electrode leads come into contact with the vocal cords and can thus indicate contraction-related changes in the EMG.

Figure 5.67 shows a typical response of the vocalis muscle. Mean values for amplitudes and latencies are given in Table 5.27.

The recurrent laryngeal nerve is a branch of the vagus nerve (cranial nerve X) that runs around the subclavian artery on the right side and around the aortic arch on the left side and passes behind the thyroid gland to the laryngeal musculature. The course around the aortic arch on the left side results in a significantly longer latency after stimulation of the vagus nerve compared to stimulation on the right side.

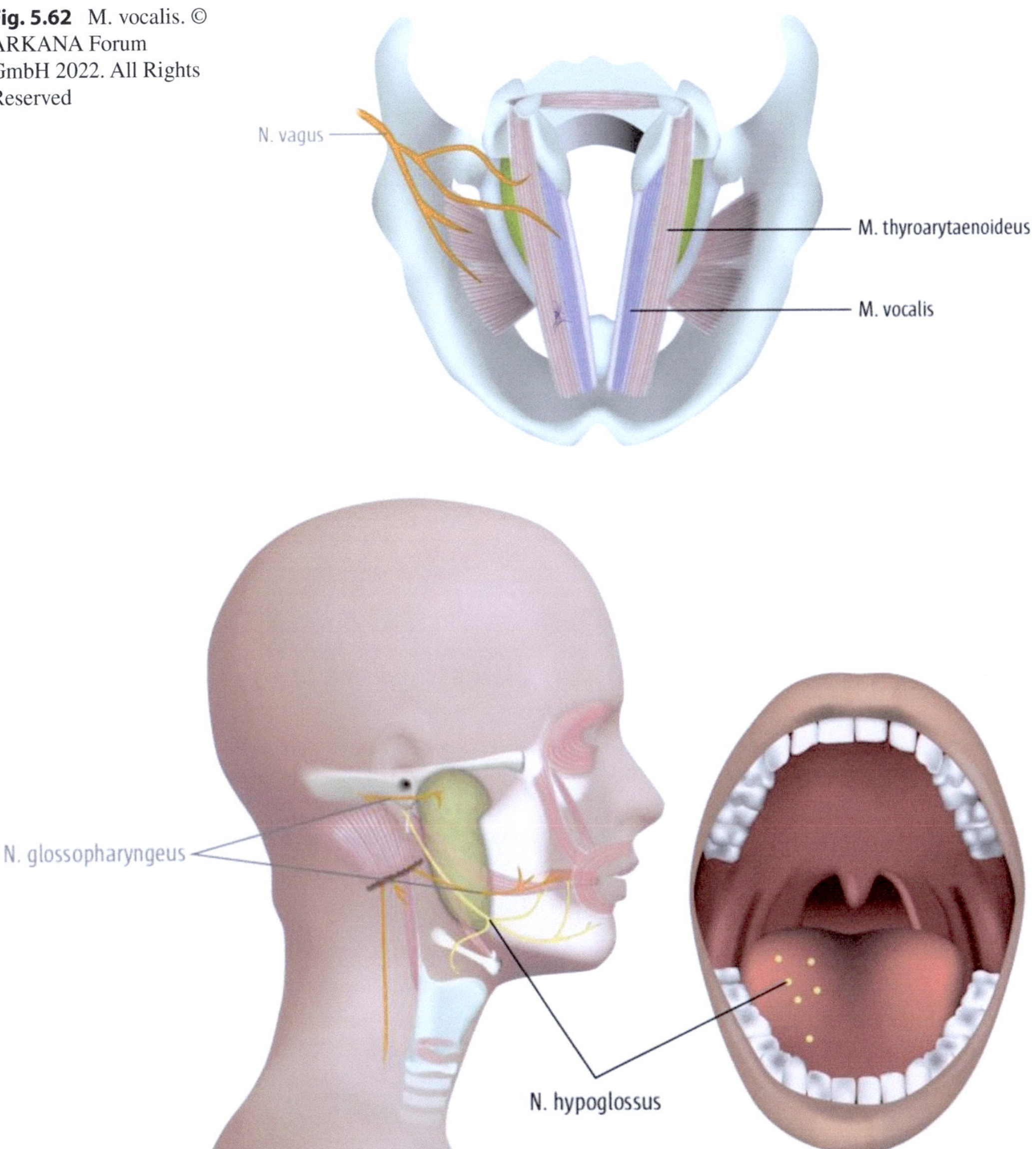

Fig. 5.62 M. vocalis. © ARKANA Forum GmbH 2022. All Rights Reserved

Fig. 5.63 Soft palate and tongue muscles. © ARKANA Forum GmbH 2022. All Rights Reserved

Table 5.26 Stimulation and recording parameters for mapping and monitoring motor cranial nerves (recommended starting values are marked in bold)

Stimulation current	0.01–2 mA (**0.1 mA**)
Stimulation frequency	1.5–3 Hz
Pulse form	Monophasic rectangular pulse, cathodal
Pulse duration	50–300 µs (**200 µs**)
Low-pass filter	1500–2000 Hz
High-pass filter	20–30 Hz

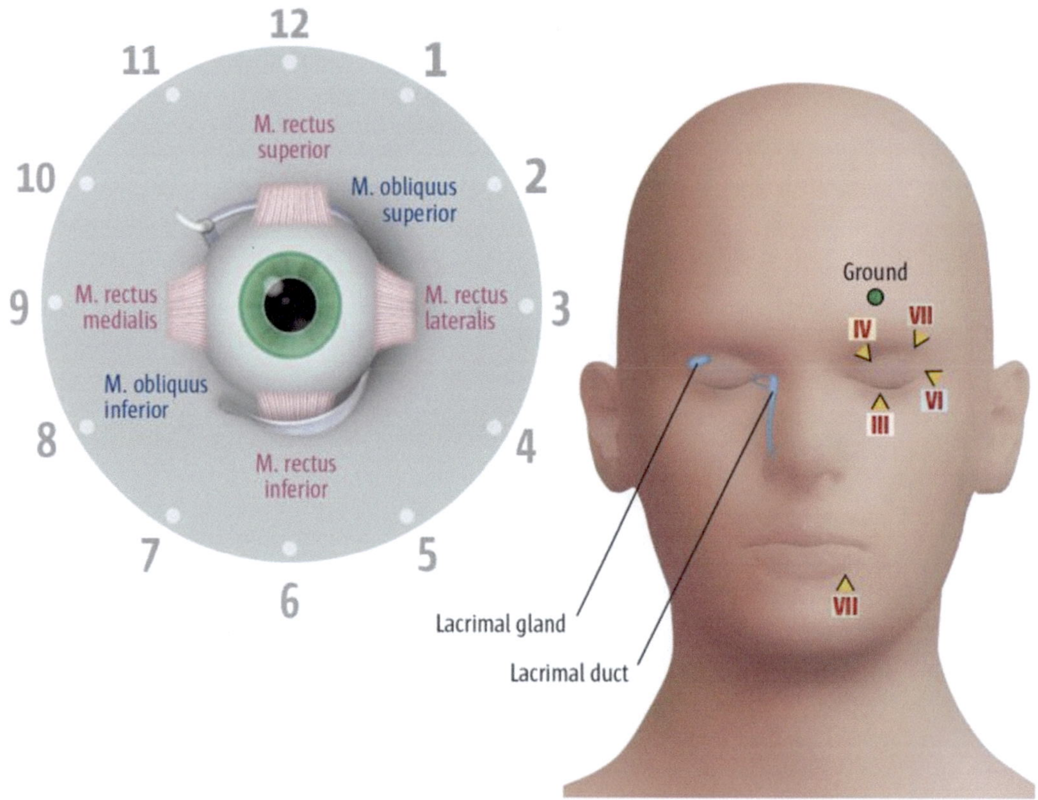

Fig. 5.64 Electrode placement at left eye muscles. © ARKANA Forum GmbH 2022. All Rights Reserved

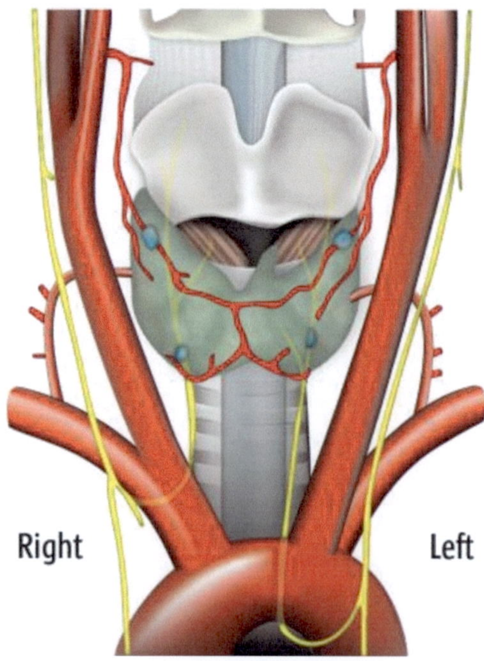

Fig. 5.65 Course of the recurrent laryngeal nerve in dorsal view. © ARKANA Forum GmbH 2022. All Rights Reserved

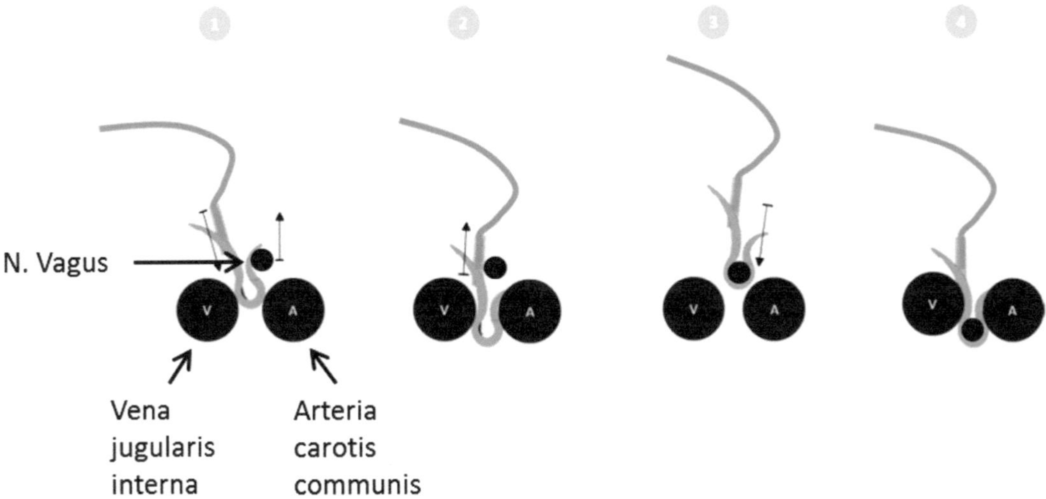

Fig. 5.66 Schematic illustration of placing the electrode for continuous stimulation of the vagus nerve. © ARKANA Forum GmbH 2022. All Rights Reserved

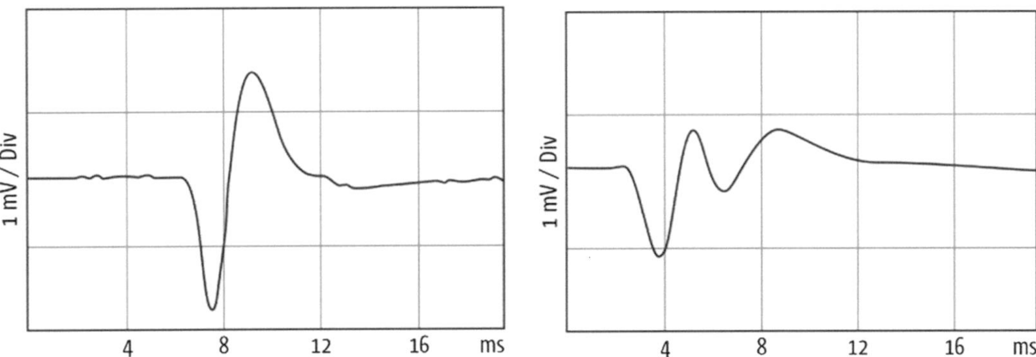

Fig. 5.67 Vocalis CMAP after stimulation of the vagus nerve (left) and the recurrent laryngeal nerve (right). © ARKANA Forum GmbH 2022. All Rights Reserved

Table 5.27 Mean and standard deviation values for amplitudes and latencies of vocalis CMAPs after stimulation of the vagus and laryngeal recurrent nerve [38]

	Amplitude in µV	Latency in ms
N. vagus left	420 ± 255	7.7 (6.1–10)
N. vagus right	717 ± 479	6.8 (4.3–9.5)
N. laryngeus recurrens left	604 ± 504	3.7 (2.5–4.3)
N. laryngeus recurrens right	783 ± 512	3.2 (2.5–4.3)

5.7 Spinal Nerves

Spinal nerve monitoring has already been briefly addressed in the presentation of the modalities to assess ascending and descending pathways by means of SEPs and MEPs. The following is an **overview** on the options for intraoperative electrophysiological assessment of the spinal nerves. These monitoring techniques have proven to be helpful during surgical treatment of spinal tumors, particularly of intramedullary tumors. They have also found widespread use during placement of pedicle screws [39, 40]. In addition, spinal nerve monitoring is frequently applied in selective dorsal rhizotomy for the treatment of pain and spasticity. In all these applications, predominantly the motor parts of the nerves are monitored.

Stimulation to identify the nerves is accomplished using a hand-held probe.

Recording of the CMAP is done by means of a pair of electrodes placed in the indicator muscle(s). Additionally, the irritation of nerves can be continuously assessed by observing the spontaneous activity of the EMG.

Table 5.28 provides an overview of the spinal nerves and their respective indicator muscles. Figures 5.68, 5.69, 5.70, and 5.71 illustrate the indicator muscles in the cervical, thoracic, lumbar, and sacral spine.

Table 5.28 Overview of spinal nerves and indicator muscles (the muscles recommended for monitoring are marked in bold)

Segment	Designation	Indicator muscle	Spinal nerve
Cervical	C2	**M. sternocleidomastoideus**	**N. accessorius**
		M. trapezius	N. accessorius
	C3	**M. trapezius**	**N. accessorius**
		M. sternocleidomastoideus	N. accessorius
	C4	**M. trapezius**	**N. accessorius**
		M. supraspinatus	N. suprascapularis
	C5	**M. deltoideus**	**N. axillaris**
		M. biceps	N. musculocutaneus
	C6	**M. brachioradialis**	**N. radialis**
		M. biceps	N. musculocutaneus
		M. deltoideus	N. axillaris
		M. flexor carpi radialis	Median nerve
		M. triceps	N. radialis
	C7	**M. triceps**	**N. radialis**
		M. flexor carpi radialis	Median nerve
	C8	**M. abductor digiti minimi**	**N. ulnaris**
		M. abductor pollicis brevis	Median nerve
Thoracic	T 1	M. abductor digiti minimi	N. ulnaris
		M. abductor pollicis brevis	N. medianus
	T 2	**M. intercostalis, between 2nd and 3rd rib**	**2nd N. intercostalis**
	T 3	**M. intercostalis, between 3rd and 4th rib**	**3rd N. intercostalis**
	T 4	**M. intercostalis,** between 4th and 5th rib	4th N. intercostalis
	T 5	**M. rectus abdominis, upper part**	**5th N. intercostalis**
		M. intercostalis, between 5th and 6th rib	5th N. intercostalis
	T 6	**M. rectus abdominis, upper part**	**6 th N. intercostalis**
		M. intercostalis, between 6th and 7th rib	6th N. intercostalis
	T 7	**M. rectus abdominis, middle part**	**7th N. intercostalis**
		M. intercostalis, between 7th and 8th rib	7th N. intercostalis
	T 8	**M. rectus abdominis, middle part**	**8th N. intercostalis**
		M. intercostalis, between 8th and 9th rib	8th N. intercostalis
	T 9	**M. rectus abdominis, lower part**	**9th N. intercostalis**
		M. intercostalis, between 9th and 10th rib	9th N. intercostalis
	T 10	**M. rectus abdominis, lower part**	**10th N. intercostalis**
		M. intercostalis, between 10th and 11th rib	10th N. intercostalis
	T 11	**M. rectus abdominis, lower part**	**11th N. intercostalis**
		M. intercostalis, between 11th and 12th rib	11th N. intercostalis
	T 12	**M. rectus abdominis, lower part**	**N. subcostalis**

Table 5.28 (continued)

Segment	Designation	Indicator muscle	Spinal nerve
Lumbar	L1	**M. iliopsoas**	**N. femoralis**
		M. sartorius	N. femoralis
	L2	**M. sartorius**	**N. femoralis**
		M. vastus medialis	N. femoralis
		M. rectus femoris	N. femoralis
		M. adductor magnus	N. obturatorius
	L3	**M. rectus femoris**	**N. femoralis**
		M. sartorius	N. femoralis
		M. vastus medialis	N. femoralis
		M. adductor magnus	N. obturatorius
	L4	**M. rectus femoris**	**N. femoralis**
		M. vastus medialis	N. femoralis
		M. tibialis anterior	N. fibularis profundus (N. peroneus)
		M. adductor magnus	N. obturatorius
	L5	**M. tibialis anterior**	**N. fibularis (peroneus) profundus**
		M. fibularis longus (M. peroneus longus)	N. fibularis (peroneus) superficialis
Sacral	S1	**M. gastrocnemius**	**N. tibialis**
		M. abductor hallucis	N. plantaris medialis from N. tibialis
		M. tibialis anterior	N. fibularis (peroneus) profundus
		M. fibularis longus (M. peroneus longus)	N. fibularis (peroneus) superficialis
	S2	**M. abductor hallucis**	**N. plantaris medialis from N. tibialis**
		M. gastrocnemius	N. tibialis
		M. sphincter ani externus	N. pudendus
	S3	**M. sphincter ani externus**	**N. pudendus**
	S4	**M. sphincter ani externus**	**N. pudendus**

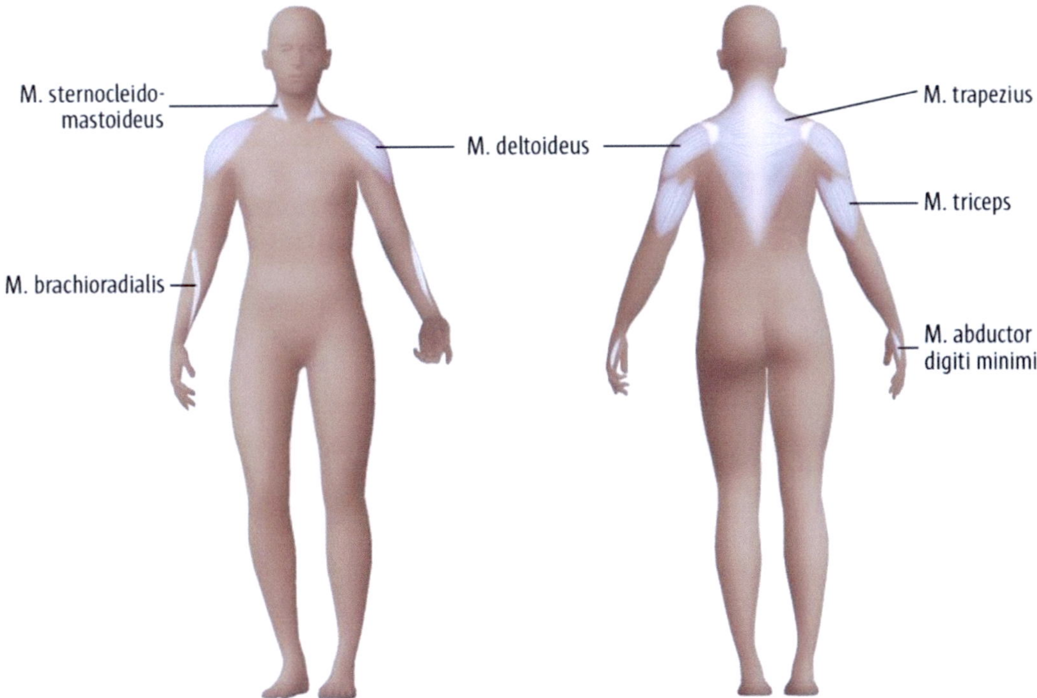

Fig. 5.68 Indicator muscles for the cervical spine. © ARKANA Forum GmbH 2022. All Rights Reserved

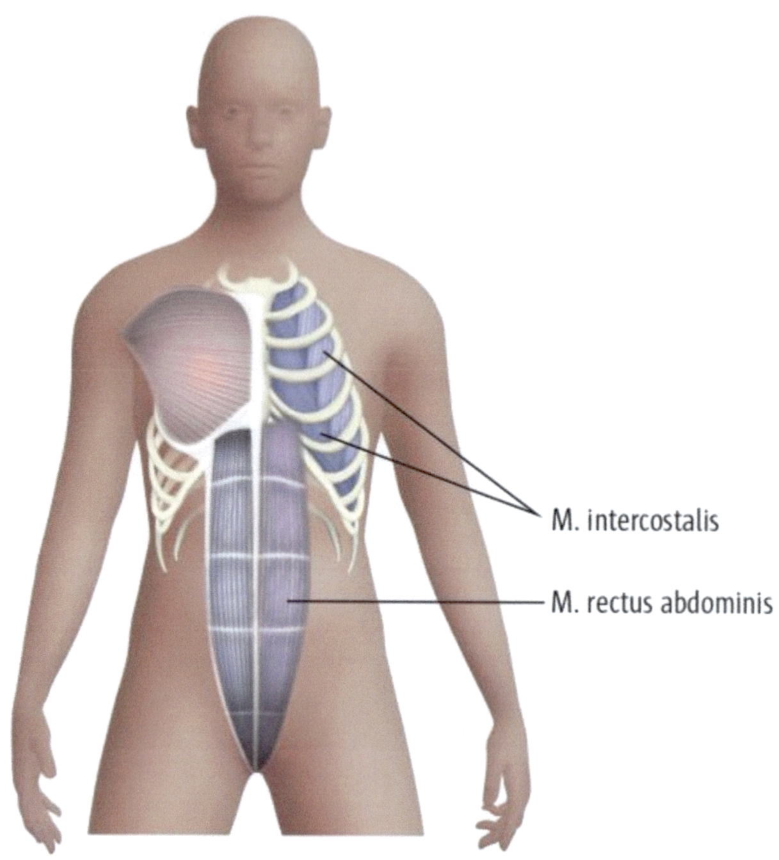

Fig. 5.69 Indicator muscles for the thoracic spine. © ARKANA Forum GmbH 2022. All Rights Reserved

Figure 5.72 shows a typical CMAP recorded from the vastus medialis muscle. In Table 5.29, commonly used stimulation and recording parameters for spinal nerve monitoring are summarized.

5.7.1 Implantation of Pedicle Screws

Spinal nerve monitoring in pedicle screw implantation has now become widely used. This application is based on the threshold stimulation current required to trigger a response in the muscle innervated by the endangered spinal nerve and to compare the result to a defined current threshold. To do this, stimulation is applied in the drill hole in which the pedicle screw is to be inserted. The current intensity is gradually increased. From the intensity required to trigger a CMAP, the proximity of the spinal nerve and the likelihood of pedicle breach can be estimated.

If the required stimulation current for triggering an EMG signal is **below** the defined **current threshold**, the orientation of the drill hole should be changed, as there is a risk of pedicle perforation and impairment of the spinal nerve by insertion of the screw. However, if the required stimulation current is **above** the defined **current threshold**, the orientation of the burr hole with respect to the nerve is safe and the pedicle screw can be inserted or remain in this position. Impairment of the nerve or breakthrough of the medial pedicle wall is not to be expected.

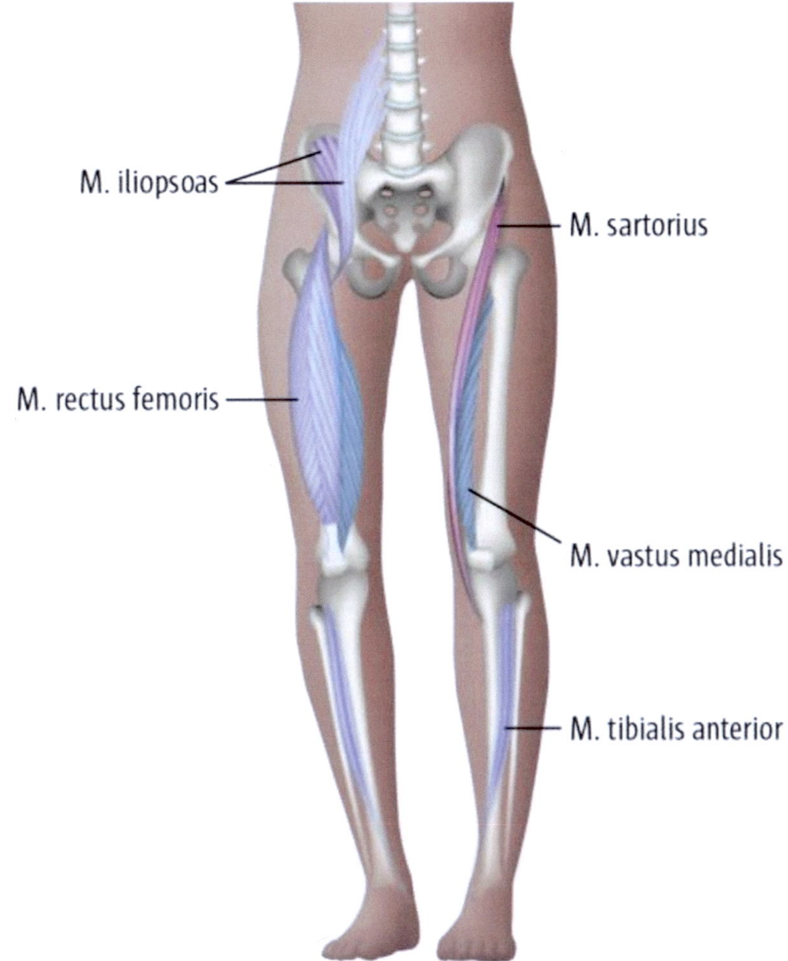

However, there is still controversy about the exact **threshold values** of the stimulation current. Evidence-based values are available only for lumbar pedicle stimulation [39, 40] (Table 5.30). Table 5.31 gives some rough criteria for interpretation of the stimulation current required to trigger a CMAP in thoracic pedicle implantation.

In the meantime, systems have been developed that are capable of stimulation and interpretation of the signals **semi-automatically**. Responses are automatically classified, and as a function of the stimulation current necessary to activate the nerve, feedback is given to the surgeon by different color signals (Table 5.32).

Depending on the type of the surgical procedure, SEP and MEP monitoring in addition to pedicle stimulation may be advisable. Especially in the surgical treatment of scoliosis, monitoring of the ascending and descending pathways is indispensable due to the expected stretching and compression of the spinal cord and supplying arteries.

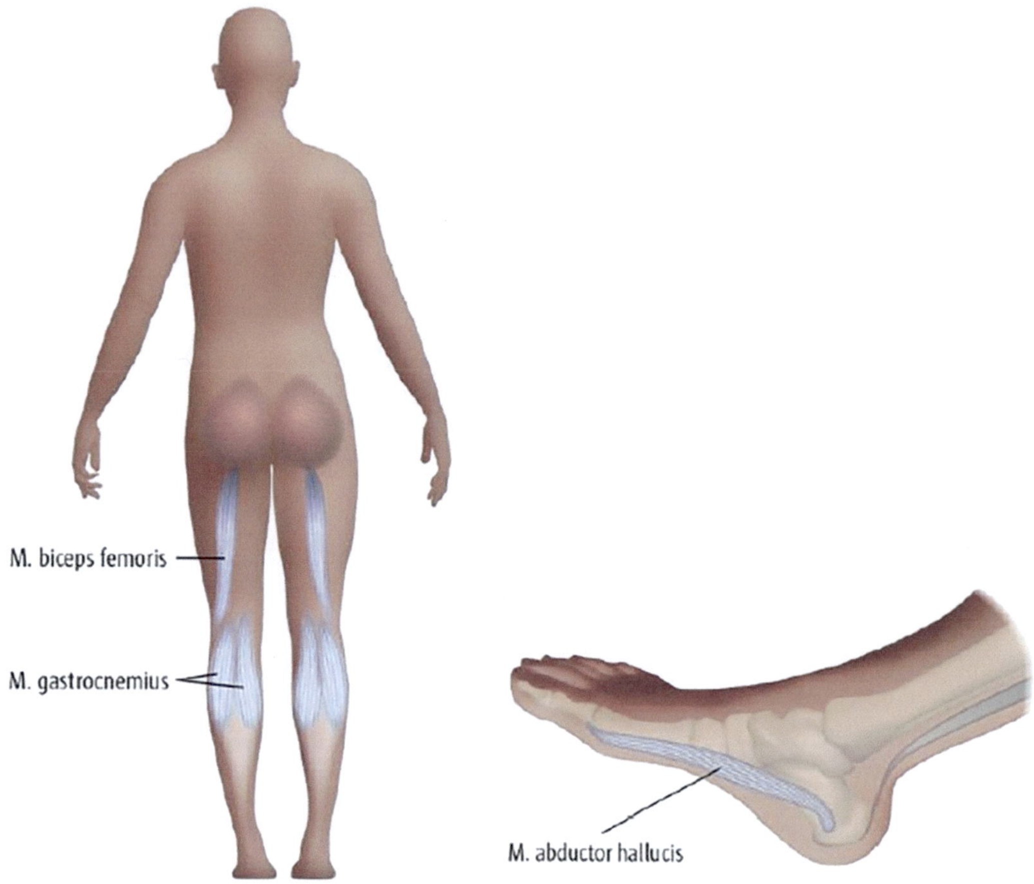

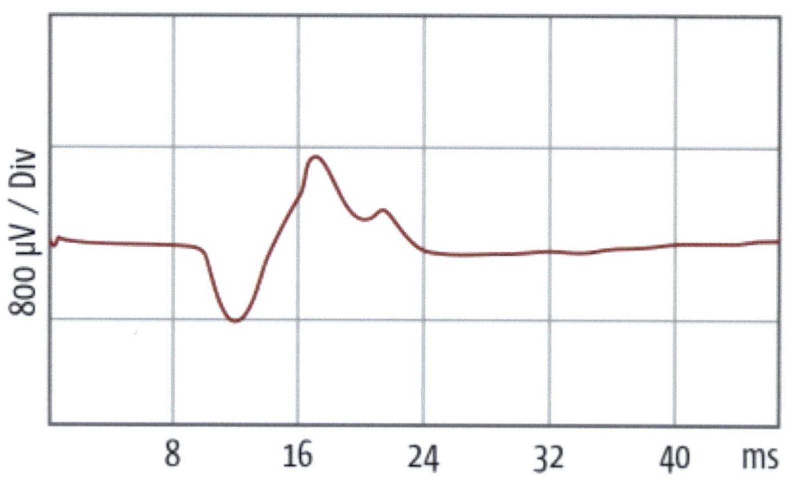

Fig. 5.71 Indicator muscles for the sacral spine. © ARKANA Forum GmbH 2022. All Rights Reserved

Fig. 5.72 Typical CMAP after spinal nerve stimulation, recorded from vastus medialis muscle. © ARKANA Forum GmbH 2022. All Rights Reserved

Table 5.29 Stimulation and recording parameters for spinal nerve monitoring (recommended starting values are marked in bold)

Stimulation current	0.01–2 mA
Stimulation frequency	1.5–3 Hz
Pulse form	Monophasic rectangular pulse, cathodal
Pulse duration	100–300 µs (**200 µs**)
Low-pass filter	1500–2000 Hz
High-pass filter	20 Hz

Table 5.30 Stimulation current and probability of pedicle perforation in the lumbar spine [40]

Stimulation current (mA)	Probability of medial pedicle perforation (%)
>8	0.31
4–8	17.4
<4	54.2
<2.8	100

Table 5.31 Stimulation current and probability of pedicle perforation in thoracic spine [39]

Stimulation current	Probability of medial pedicle perforation
>6 mA	0%
<6 mA and more than 60% lower than the mean value of all other thresholds in the respective patient	High probability

Table 5.32 Stimulation current and color signals in automated detection

Cervical		Lumbar	
Stimulation current (mA)	Display	Stimulation current (mA)	Display
1–4	Red	2–7	Red
>4	Yellow	7–10	Yellow
		>10	Green

5.8 Reflexes

Reflexes represent involuntary, rapid responses to specific stimuli that always occur in the same way. Because the reflex arc does not cross the cortex, the state of consciousness does not matter. Nevertheless, reflexes are influenced by anesthesia. The following reflex tests are used in the context of IONM, whereby the sensory and motor parts of the reflex arc can be assessed.

5.8.1 Blink Reflex

The blink reflex, also known as the corneal reflex, is a physiological blinking of the eyelids elicited by stimulation (e.g., touching by a foreign body) of the cornea. The sensory component is represented by the trigeminal nerve, the motor component by the facial nerve.

Stimulation is performed at the supraorbital nerve above the eyebrow with needle or surface electrodes. Train stimulation is necessary for reproducible responses intraoperatively. The use of four pulses has proven to be optimal for this application [41].

Recording is accomplished from the orbicularis oculi muscle with needle or surface electrodes (Fig. 5.73).

Figure 5.74 illustrates the **signal path** of the blink reflex. In the awake patient, two signal components can be recorded ipsilaterally to the stimulus, resulting from two different pathways, while contralaterally only the second component can be obtained. The **first component (R1)** is generated by an oligosynaptic circuit between the sensory part of the trigeminal nerve and the motor part of the facial nerve in the pons. The reflex circuit of the **second component (R2)** runs polysynaptically across the lateral medulla oblongata. Under general anesthesia, only the first component (R1) is recordable, presumably due to the influence of the anesthetics on the polysynaptic circuitry [41].

A typical potential is shown in Fig. 5.75. Commonly used stimulation and recording parameters are given in Table 5.33.

The blink reflex is very sensitive to anesthetics. With total intravenous anesthesia, the administration of boluses should be avoided in critical phases. Under inhalation anesthesia, stable potentials can only be obtained at low doses [41].

5.8.2 Bulbocavernosus Reflex

The bulbocavernosus reflex (BCR) represents an oligosynaptic reflex involving the sacral spinal cord. It is used intraoperatively to monitor the afferent and efferent fibers of the **pudendal nerve** and the reflex center located at level **S2–S4** in the gray matter of the spinal cord. Indirectly, the BCR can also be applied to monitor bladder and rectal function, which pass through the pudendal nerve. Simultaneous monitoring of the BCR and the SEP of the pudendal nerve allows differentiation between disorders in the afferent and efferent parts of the reflex arc [42].

Stimulation is performed via a pair of electrodes. In females, the cathode is placed at the clitoris and the anode at the adjacent labia [43]. In males, two cup electrodes are placed 2–3 cm apart on the dorsal penis. The cathode is located at the base of the penis (see also Sect. 5.4.1.4 "Pudendal Nerve SEPs").

Recording is accomplished with hookwire, needle [44], or surface [43] electrodes from the

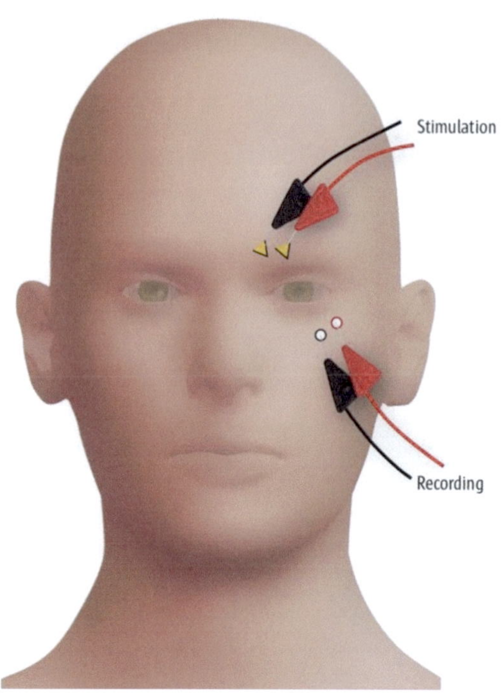

Fig. 5.73 Electrode placement for the blink reflex. © ARKANA Forum GmbH 2022. All Rights Reserved

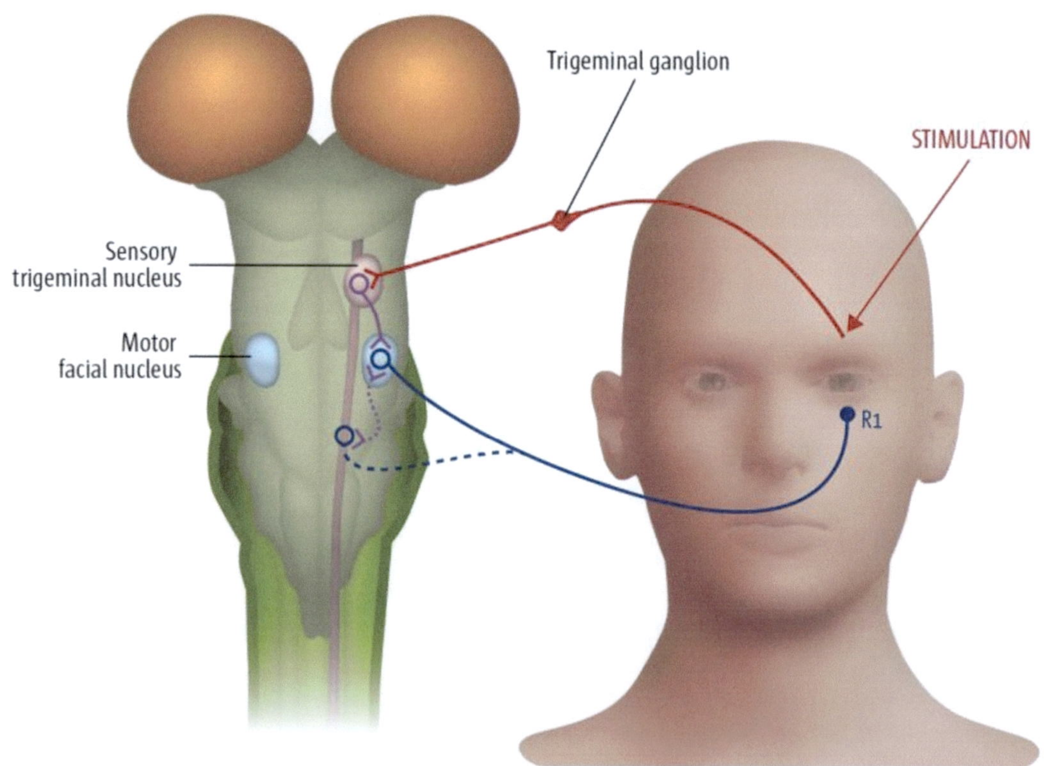

Fig. 5.74 Signal path of the blink reflex. © ARKANA Forum GmbH 2022. All Rights Reserved

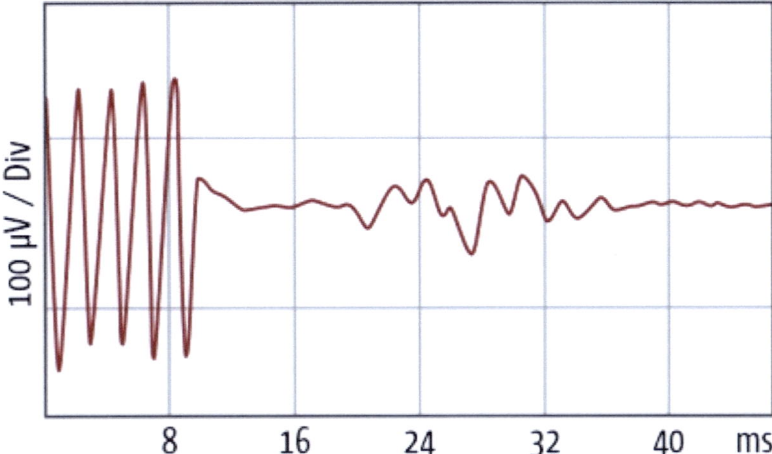

Fig. 5.75 Typical blink reflex, recorded intraoperatively. © ARKANA Forum GmbH 2022. All Rights Reserved

Table 5.33 Stimulation and recording parameters for the blink reflex (recommended starting values are marked in bold)

Stimulation current	20–40 mA
Stimulation frequency	0.4 Hz
Pulse form	Monophasic rectangular pulse, single or train
Train count	1–**4**
Pulse duration	200–400 µs (**400 µs**)
Low-pass filter	2–3 kHz
High-pass filter	20–30 Hz
Time base	100 ms
Averaging	None

external anal sphincter. Reproducible signals can be obtained—comparable to MEPs – with trains of two to five pulses [44] (Fig. 5.76).

The stimulus **activates** the sensory fibers of the dorsal nerves of the clitoris and penis, respectively. The fibers enter the spinal canal at the level of S2–S4 and the spinal cord at the level of the conus medullaris (T12/L1), each via the posterior roots. There, the excitation is switched to the somatomotor fibers of the pudendal nerve through a few synapses. These fibers exit the conus medullaris and the spinal canal through the corresponding anterior roots to reach the external anal sphincter. Figure 5.77 shows the signal path of the bulbocavernosus reflex.

In **response** to stimulation, a polyphasic CMAP can be recorded from the external anal sphincter. The amplitude of this wave, which par-

ticularly depends on the position of the recording electrode, is not assessed. Attention is rather paid to latency and reproducibility of the response over the course of the operation [42].

Figure 5.78 shows a typical response signal. Commonly used stimulation and recording parameters are given in Table 5.34.

> *Anesthesia has a major influence on the bulbocavernosus reflex. Especially under inhalation anesthesia, triggering the reflex may be difficult or even impossible. Therefore, total intravenous anesthesia without muscle relaxants is recommended [43].*

5.8.3 Motor Reflexes

Motor reflexes can be triggered by **mechanical** or **electrical** stimulation. The mechanically activated motor reflex is called **muscle stretch reflex**. The path of the muscle stretch reflex can be monitored by **electrical** stimulation of the corresponding nerve. Thereby, two waves can be recorded: First, a typical CMAP, here also called the **M-wave,** and later the **H-wave (Hoffmann reflex)**. The H-reflex can be used to assess proximal nerve segments and the excitability of the α-motoneuron. It represents a monosynaptic reflex which has some relevance for intraoperative monitoring in hip surgery.

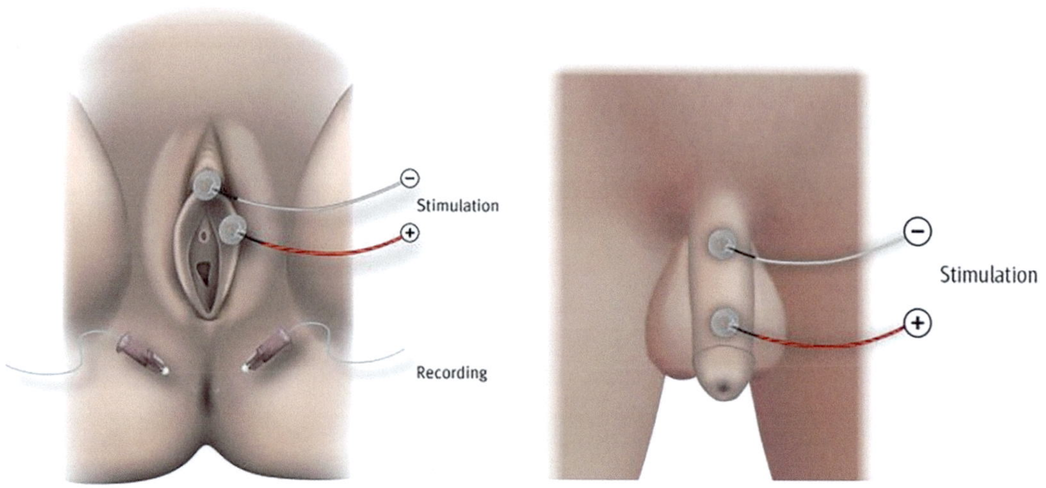

Fig. 5.76 Position of electrodes for monitoring the bulbocavernosus reflex (left: females; right: males). The recording electrodes are placed in the identical position in both genders.© ARKANA Forum GmbH 2022. All Rights Reserved

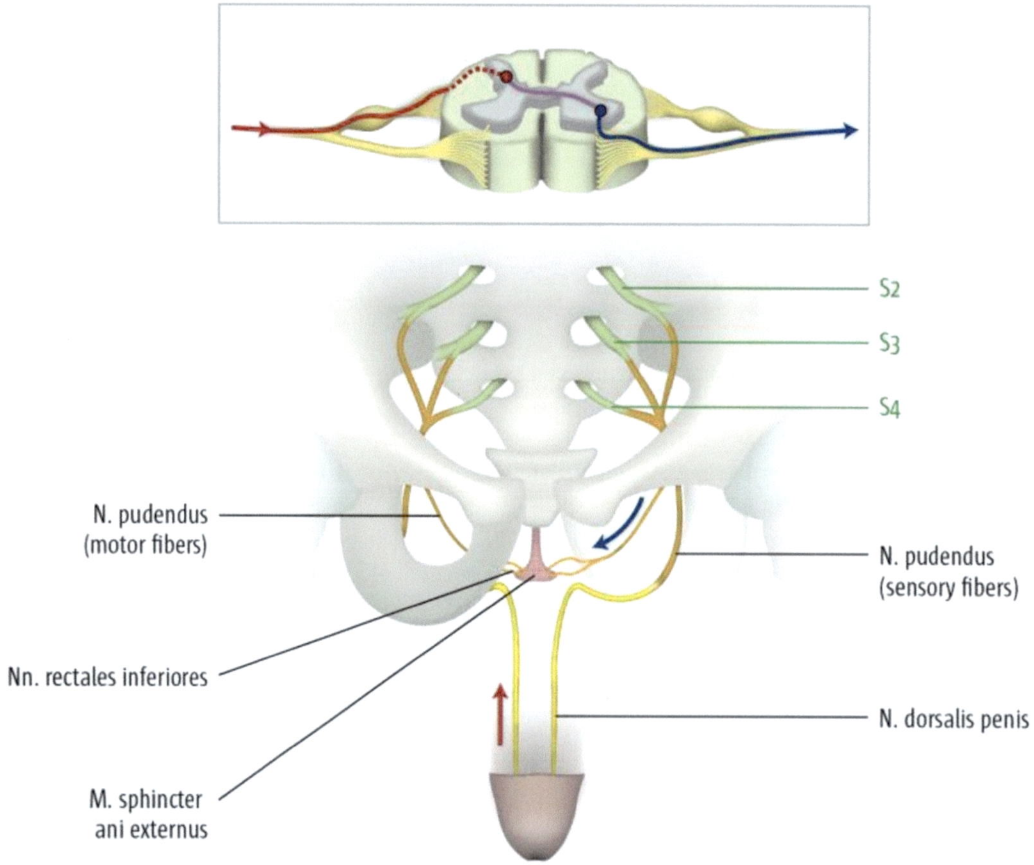

Fig. 5.77 Signal path of the bulbocavernosus reflex in males. © ARKANA Forum GmbH 2022. All Rights Reserved

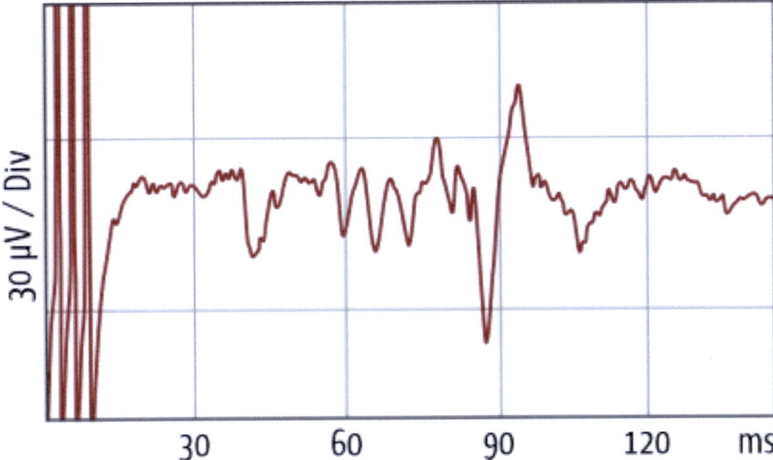

Fig. 5.78 Typical BCR recorded from the external anal sphincter in a young male. © ARKANA Forum GmbH 2022. All Rights Reserved

Table 5.34 Stimulation and recording parameters for the BCR [45] (recommended starting values are marked in bold)

Stimulation current	20–40 mA
Stimulation frequency	2.3 Hz
Pulse form	Monophasic rectangular pulse, single or train
Train count	1–5 pulses (**3 pulses**)
Pulse duration	200–500 µs (**200 µs**)
Low-pass filter	2000–3000 Hz
High-pass filter	20–30 Hz
Time base	150–200 ms
Averaging	1–4 sweeps

The H-reflex should not be confused with the **F-wave**. An electrical impulse propagates in motor nerves both distally (orthodromic) and proximally (antidromic). The distally propagating excitation causes contraction of the muscle and allows recording of the M-wave. The proximally running excitation is reflected in the anterior horn in an unknown way, so that the excitation runs distally again and enables the recording of another later wave from the muscle, the F-wave [42]. Thus, the F-wave represents a rebound wave from the α- motoneuron and not a reflex. F-waves are not relevant for intraoperative monitoring.

Stimulation to elicit the **H-reflex** is typically done in mid to distal sections of peripheral nerves (classically the tibial nerve at the popliteal fossa with recording from the soleus muscle and, more rarely, the median nerve at the level of the cubital fossa with recording from the flexor carpi radialis muscle). When stimulating more proximally (e.g., directly over the cauda equina), the **posterior root muscle response** (**PRMR**) and the **anterior root muscle response** (**ARMR**) can be elicited. For stimulation of the cauda equina, large surface electrodes are placed at the third lumbar intervertebral space (anode) and the navel (cathode) (Fig. 5.79).

Recording is done from the quadriceps femoris muscle (1), tibialis anterior muscle (2), triceps surae muscle (3), abductor hallucis muscle (4), and extensor digitorum communis brevis muscle (5), each on both sides (Fig. 5.80). In case of limited availability of lead channels, monitoring of the contralateral side can be limited to a subset of the abovementioned muscles.

The **H-reflex** is based on the particular feature of some peripheral nerves in which afferent fibers are thicker than motor axons. Since the thicker axons can be excited with lower current, a range in which predominantly afferent fibers are activated can be reached by slowly increasing the stimulus intensity. In this range, the H-reflex can be recorded. In the case of the **PRMR**, afferent parts of the nerve roots are stimulated. The stimulus is switched monosynaptically at the spinal level, resulting in a muscle response. There is a long refractory period of about 50 ms. Only

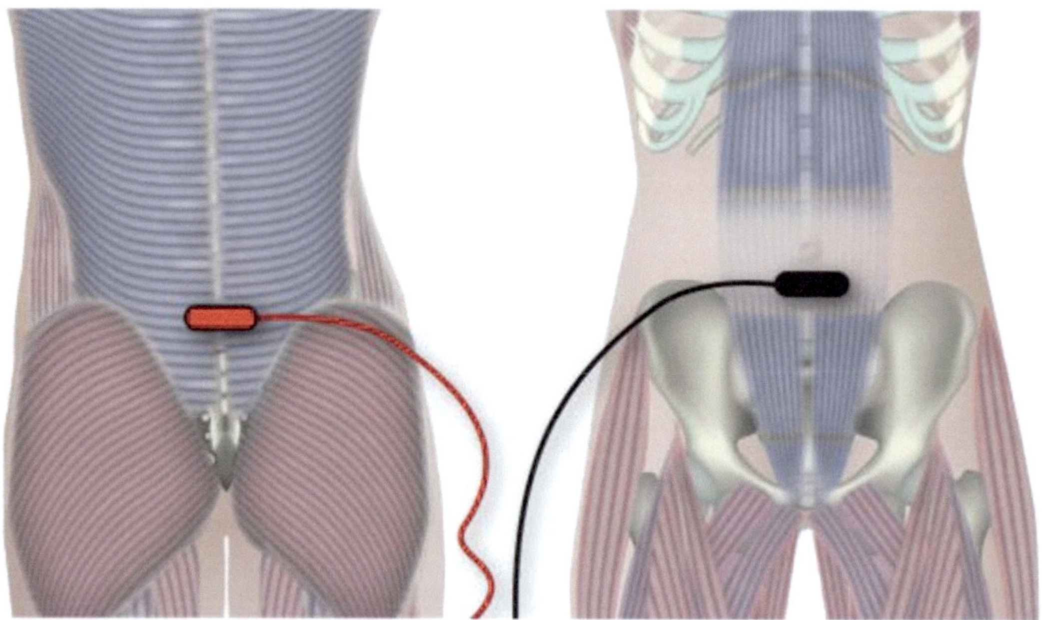

Fig. 5.79 Position of electrodes for triggering the PRMR and ARMR. © ARKANA Forum GmbH 2022. All Rights Reserved

thereafter, a new stimulus can trigger another response via the α-motoneuron. With the **ARMR**, direct stimulation of the motor root leads to a muscle response, and hence there is no (or a much shorter) refractory period [46]. These differences can be used to determine whether the contraction of the muscle was caused by the PRMR or the ARMR, which is not possible evaluating shape, amplitude, or latency of the response. Stimulation is performed with two pulses delivered at a short interval of 50 ms. If a response is seen only after the first pulse, it was transmitted via the PRMR. However, if a response is also seen after the second stimulation pulse, the ARMR has been triggered, more specifically reflecting the motor axons of the lumbosacral plexus. Therefore, the component after the second stimulus is crucial for monitoring. Of partic-

ular importance is the reproducibility of the results over the course of the operation.

Double stimulation can be realized technically by using the facilitation function. Thereby, the same output channel must be selected for the facilitation and the actual stimulation pulse.

The signal path of PRMR and ARMR is demonstrated in Fig. 5.81. A typical response is shown in Fig. 5.82. Standard values of latencies and amplitudes are not yet available. The commonly used stimulation and recording parameters are summarized in Table 5.35.

Fig. 5.80 Target muscles for recording the PRMR and ARMR. © ARKANA Forum GmbH 2022. All Rights Reserved

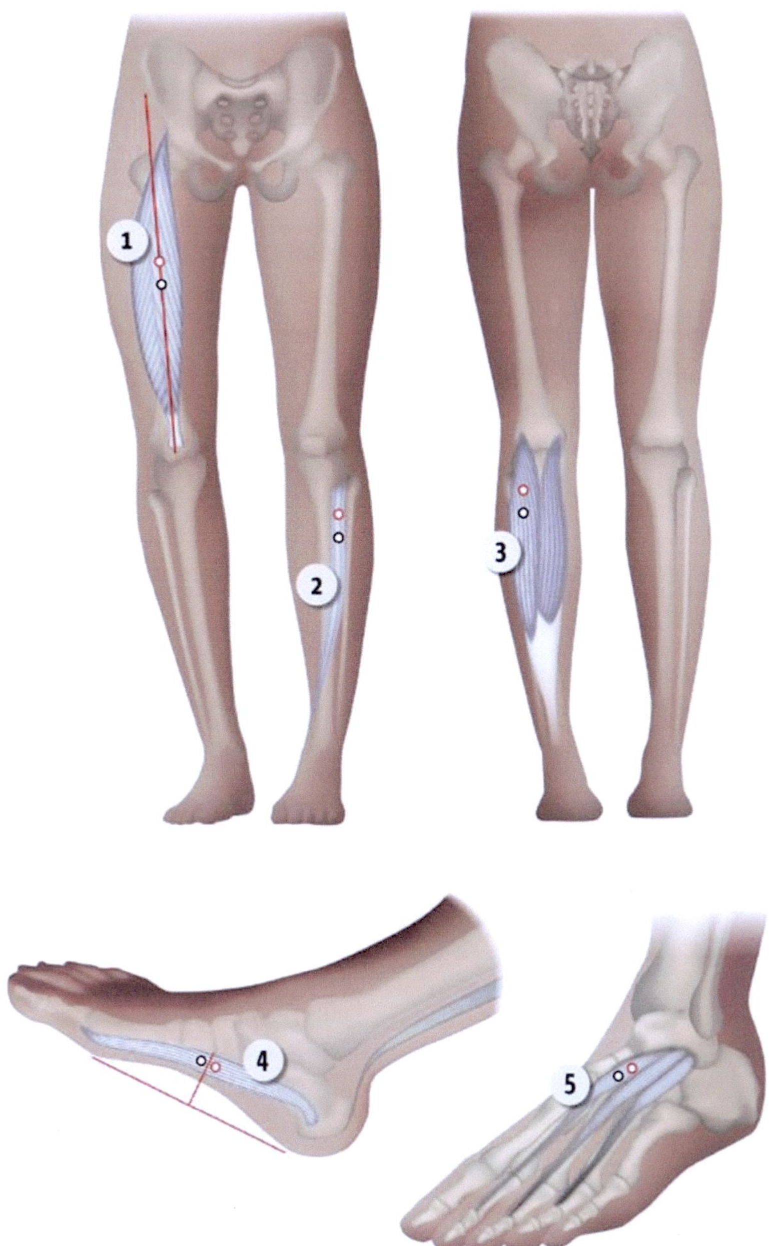

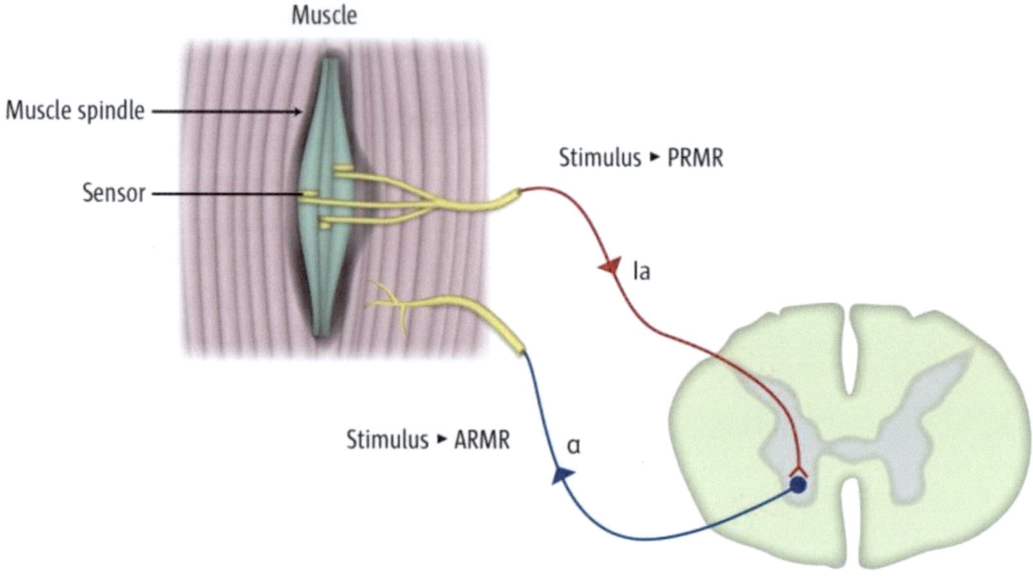

Fig. 5.81 Signal path of the PRMR and ARMR. © ARKANA Forum GmbH 2022. All Rights Reserved

Fig. 5.82 Typical ARMR during monitoring in hip surgery, recorded from the triceps surae muscle. Responses are seen after both the first and second stimulation pulse 50 ms later. © ARKANA Forum GmbH 2022. All Rights Reserved

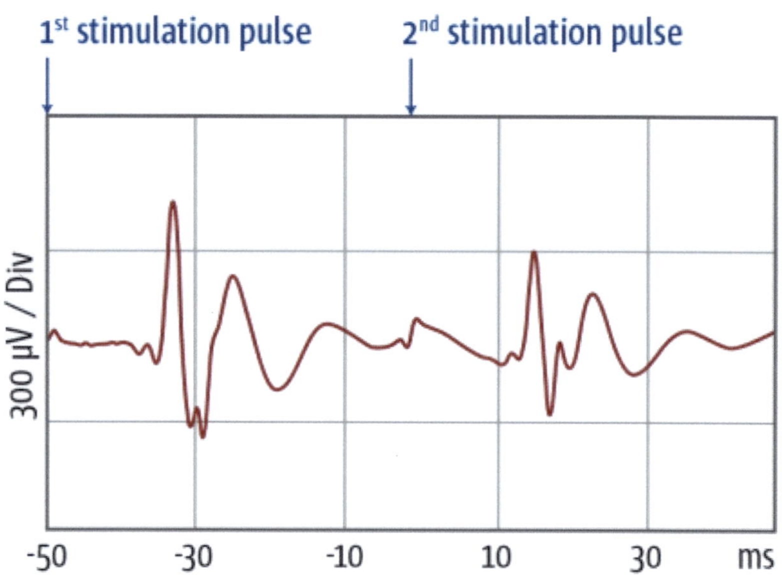

Table 5.35 Stimulation and recording parameters for the ARMR and PRMR (recommended starting values are marked in bold)

Stimulation current	**40**–200 mA
Stimulation frequency	0.5–2 Hz
Intertrain interval	50 ms, 2 pulses
Pulse form	Monophasic rectangular pulse, cathodal
Pulse duration	1000 μs
Low-pass filter	1000 Hz
High-pass filter	10 Hz
Time base	100 ms
Averaging	None

5.9 Autonomic Nervous System

Autonomic nervous system monitoring can be used in all surgeries, where the autonomous nerves of the pelvis minor are at risk. However, it has been established mainly in **rectal surgery**. During these pelvic procedures, the autonomic nerves, such as those of the inferior hypogastric plexus and the pelvic splanchnic nerves, may be injured, resulting in disturbances of anorectal and urogenital functions. Neurophysiologic mapping and monitoring are accomplished by recording the **EMG of the internal anal sphincter** and **intravesical pressure measurement**.

Stimulation is performed with a bipolar hand-held probe. To induce a change in the baseline tone of the target muscles, longer stimulation trains must be used. For this, rectangular pulses of 200 μs duration are applied at a frequency of 30 Hz. The current intensity usually ranges between 8 and 12 mA. Stimulation is possible at the inferior hypogastric plexus and the pelvic splanchnic nerves (N. splanchnici pelvici). In individual patients, it has been noted that stimulation of the superior hypogastric plexus and the hypogastric nerve (N. hypogastricus) can also trigger contraction of the detrusor muscle [47].

Recording is done from involuntarily innervated smooth muscles. The first target muscle is the **internal anal sphincter (IAS)** (M. sphincter ani internus), the EMG of which is recorded either by a bipolar needle electrode or a surface rectal electrode. It is recommended to place the needle electrode under ultrasound guidance. The second target muscle, the **detrusor muscle** (M. detrusor vesicae), a smooth muscle in the wall of the bladder, is recorded indirectly by measuring the internal bladder pressure. For this, a connection set containing a pressure sensor and a syringe for filling the bladder is placed between the bladder catheter and the urine bag. The pressure sensor is connected to the monitoring system, thus allowing parallel registration of the EMG of the IAS and the bladder pressure. Immediately before the measurement, the bladder is filled with 200 ml of Ringer's solution. This basic filling is necessary in order to facilitate contraction of the detrusor muscle by the electrical stimulation. In addition, the **external anal sphincter (EAS)** (M. sphincter ani externus) is monitored as a relaxation control. This is done with either a bipolar needle electrode or a surface rectal electrode.

The **stimulus travels** to the target muscles through the fine neural network of the lesser pelvis. In contrast to the monitoring of voluntary nerves and muscles, no evoked response to a defined stimulus is triggered here. Rather, electrical stimulation modulates the resting tone of the smooth muscles.

Figure 5.83 illustrates the position of electrodes for monitoring the autonomic nerves of the lesser pelvis. In Fig. 5.84, nerves and plexus in the lesser pelvis are depicted. Table 5.36 summarizes the commonly used stimulation and recording parameters.

> *Since the detrusor muscle contracts slowly, a stimulation period of at least 5 s is necessary.*

Successful stimulation **results** in an increase in the bladder pressure and/or an EMG response of the IAS (Fig. 5.85). The reference is the baseline muscle tone before stimulation, which can also be measured in the relaxed patient under anesthesia.

An increase in bladder pressure of 1 cm H_2O is regarded as a positive reaction. With the IAS, only signal changes are evaluated. Standard values for the amplitude are not available. The monitoring technique as described facilitates prediction of the postoperative anorectal and urogenital function already with a one-sided positive response [47, 48]. In addition, positive signals on both sides of both modalities allow a statement about the sexual function to be expected postoperatively [49].

> *In order to ensure that the electrophysiological signals are recorded from smooth and not skeletal muscles and thus only autonomic nerves are assessed, it is*

advised to use a muscle relaxant during the measurement. If the patient is not relaxed and responses corresponding to the typical patterns of skeletal muscles are

seen on the EAS channel, it should be visually verified that not the entire pelvic floor is twitching, which could overlay the signal of the IAS.

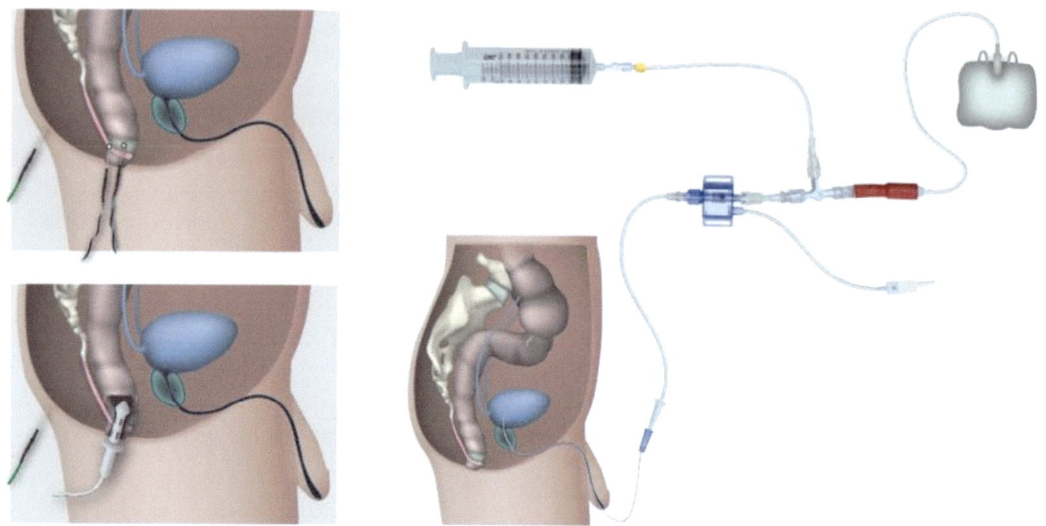

Fig. 5.83 Position of electrodes for monitoring the autonomic nerves of the pelvis minor. © ARKANA Forum GmbH 2022. All Rights Reserved

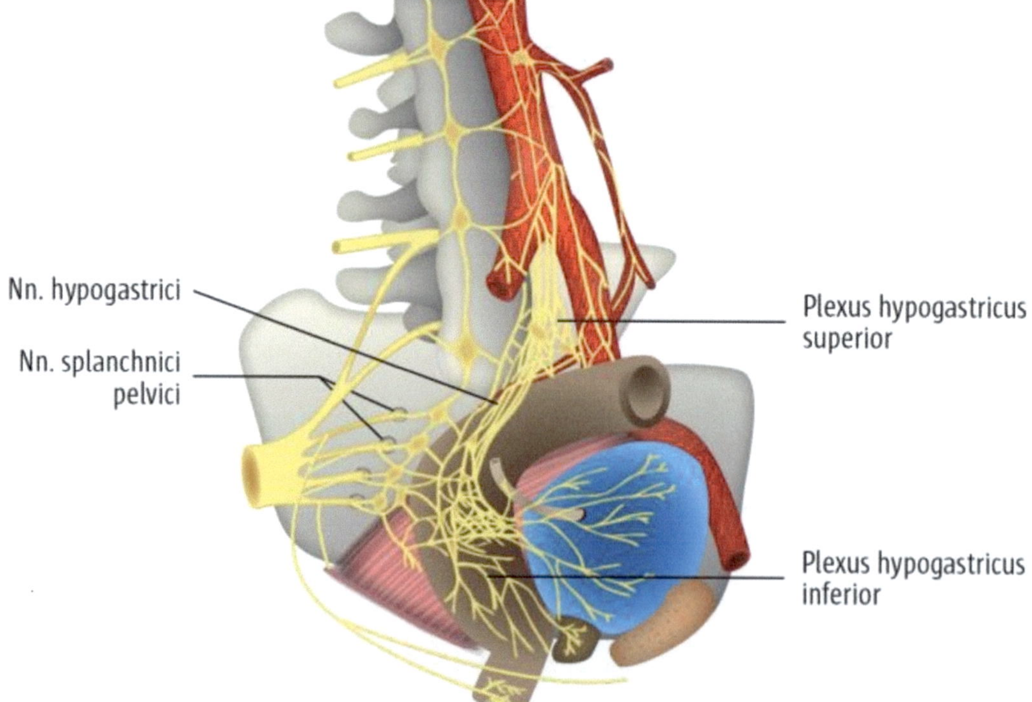

Fig. 5.84 Nerves and plexus in the pelvis minor. © ARKANA Forum GmbH 2022. All Rights Reserved

Table 5.36 Stimulation and recording parameters for pelvic monitoring (recommended starting values are marked in bold)

Stimulation current	**8–12 mA**
Stimulation frequency	30 Hz
Pulse form	Monophasic rectangular pulse, bipolar
Pulse duration	200 μs
Stimulation period	At least 5 s
Low-pass filter	Internal anal sphincter: 25 Hz External anal sphincter: 3000 Hz
High-pass filter	Internal anal sphincter: 5 Hz External anal sphincter: 0.5 Hz
Averaging	None

This IONM technique can be used in all surgeries, where the autonomous nerves innervating the detrusor and internal anal sphincter muscles are at risk. This involves, for example, urogenital or gynecological interventions, but also neurosurgical procedures of the conus/cauda and sacral spinal nerves. In these cases, the setup for bladder pressure and IAS monitoring can be attached parallel to further IONM techniques such as EMG monitoring and mapping of the motor nerves. The connection set is placed between the bladder and the urine bag, and needle electrodes are placed in the IAS. For stimulation of sacral spinal nerves, a smaller bipolar stimulation probe (e.g., bipolar concentric probe) should be used.

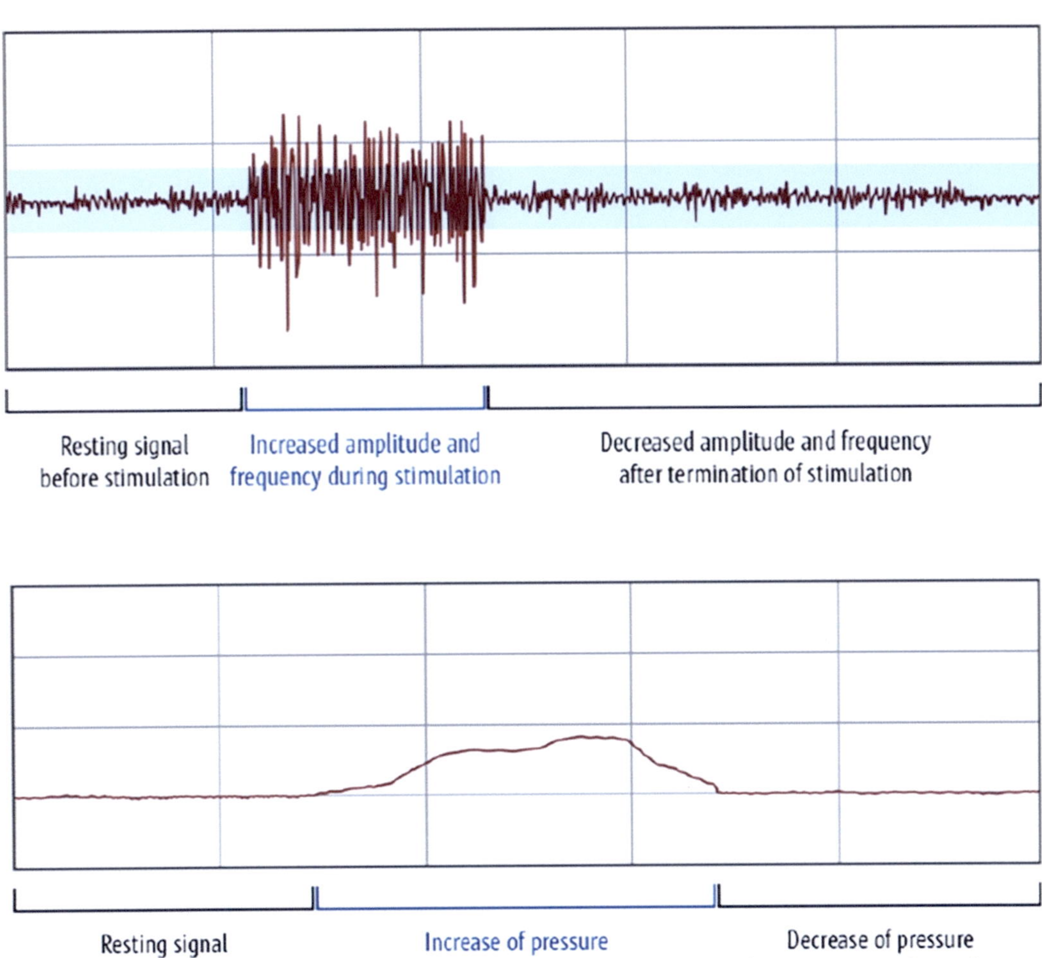

Fig. 5.85 Signals during monitoring autonomic nerves of the pelvis minor. © ARKANA Forum GmbH 2022. All Rights Reserved

For mapping the autonomous nerves, the stimulation parameters should be set to 30 Hz and low intensities (starting with 0.5 mA). For parallel use of triggered EMG, this means that the stimulation parameters have to be adjusted according to the nerves stimulated: Lower frequency for motor nerves and higher frequency for autonomous nerves. Signal interpretation of detrusor and IAS responses is done as described above. When triggered EMG or MEPs are used as well, relaxation of the patient is not possible. In these cases, EAS responses must be taken in account as well, since very large deflections here can overlay IAS responses so that they cannot always be interpreted unambiguous and stimulation intensity should be reduced.

> *When using the detrusor monitoring technique in children, the amount of Ringer's solution filled into the bladder has to be adjusted to the volume of the bladder respectively.*

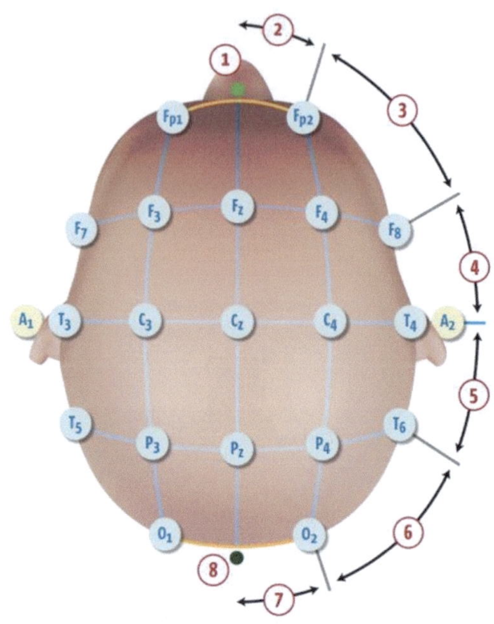

Fig. 5.86 Test question—The 10–20 system from top view. © ARKANA Forum GmbH 2022. All Rights Reserved

5.10   Test Questions

1. Which electrode placement scheme is the basis for the recording of the EEG as well as evoked potentials?
2. How are the two basic lines for electrode placement defined in this system?
3. Please complete the numbered labels in the following Fig. 5.86.
4. Which term is represented by the abbreviation CMAP?
5. Which type of spontaneous EMG activity should the surgeon be informed of immediately and why?
6. Which electrodes and probes are commonly used for neurography?
7. Complete the following text:
   Evoked potentials are elicited by a ________________ at a defined location. The response is ________________ to the stimulus and can be recorded as a typical wave from the various nervous structures or from the musculature. Individual waves of the signal obtained can be assigned to different ________________.
8. Which parameters play an important role in the evaluation of an evoked potential? Label the numbers in the following Fig. 5.87 accordingly.
9. When and for what purpose is averaging used in the recording of evoked potentials and what is the number of averaged sweeps based on?
10. What is the major disturbance variable that affects the recording of evoked potentials and how can its influence be minimized?
11. What is monitored by SEPs?
12. What adverse changes of the SEP are considered critical and must be reported to the surgeon?
13. Where are the electrodes for traditional recording of median nerve SEPs, tibial nerve SEPs and trigeminal nerve SEPs placed?
14. Where are the stimulation electrodes for median nerve SEPs placed?

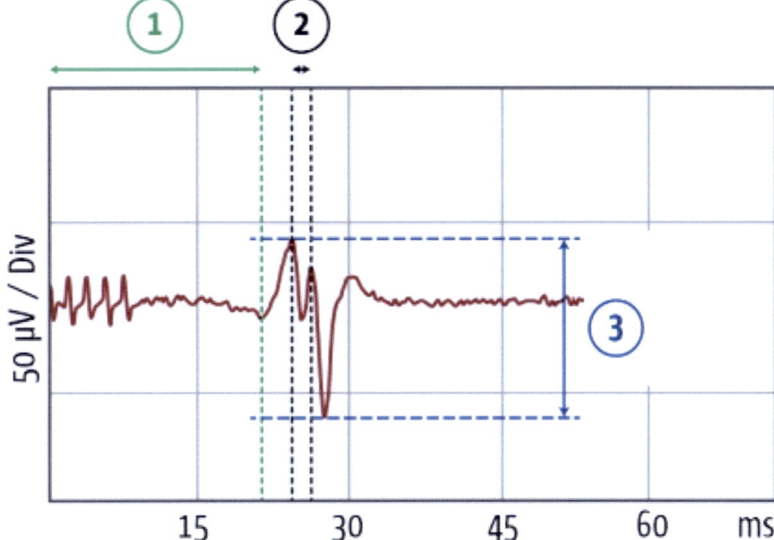

Fig. 5.87 Test question—Analysis of an evoked potential. © ARKANA Forum GmbH 2022. All Rights Reserved

Table 5.37 Test question—SEP onset latencies

	Latency (ms)
Median nerve	
Tibial nerve	

15. Complete in the Table 5.37 the usual latencies of median and tibial nerve cortical SEPs recorded at the scalp.
16. Complete the following text on tibial nerve SEPs:

    The ______________ triggered by stimulation initially runs along the tibial nerve. At the lumbosacral junction (L5/S1), it enters the spinal canal and, at the level of the conus medullaris (T12/L1), it reaches the spinal cord via the ________________. From there, the signal rises in the dorsal column (________________) to the dorsal column nucleus (________________) in the inferior medulla oblongata (first neuron). There the second neuron begins, crossing to the opposite side in the ________________ and continuing to ascend to the nucleus ventralis posterior of the thalamus. Here, the signal switches to the third neuron, which reaches the primary sensory cortex in the ______________ gyrus.

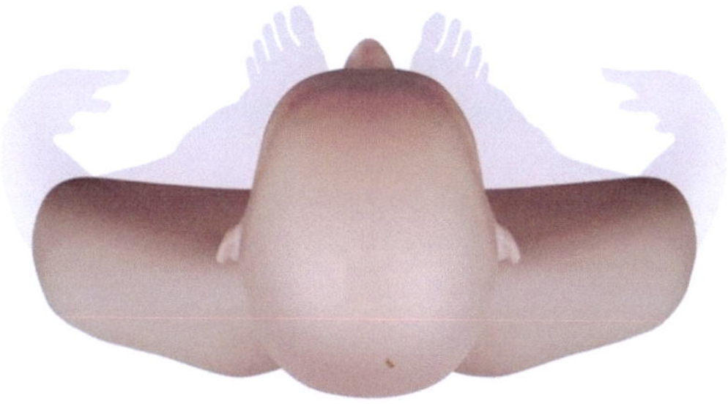

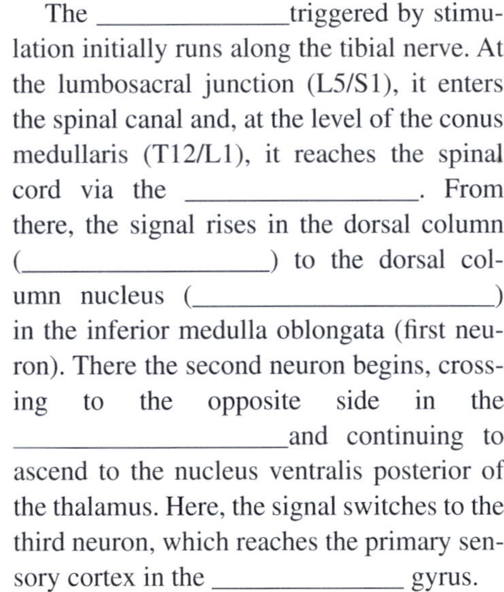

Fig. 5.88 Test question—Position of electrodes for transcranial stimulation of the motor cortex. © ARKANA Forum GmbH 2022. All Rights Reserved

17. Which sensory nerves can be stimulated in the upper extremity for SEP monitoring as an alternative to the median nerve?
18. In which cases are trigeminal SEPs usually recorded?
19. In which cases are pudendal nerve SEPs usually recorded?
20. Which stimulation and recording sites are used for pudendal nerve SEPs?
21. Sketch in the Fig. 5.88 the possible electrode positions for eliciting transcranial MEPs.
22. Which type of activation is most effective in transcranial stimulation for muscle MEPs? Under which electrode does the stimulation effect mostly take place?

23. Where can the stimulation electrodes for right limb MEP monitoring in spinal surgery be placed? Where is the anode, where is the cathode?

24. Name in the Fig. 5.89 the muscles for the recording of MEPs according to the respective electrode positions.

25. What is the difference in the selection of transcranial MEP stimulation sites between spine surgery and brain surgery?

26. What is the minimum number of muscle groups that should be monitored per limb?

27. Complete the following text:

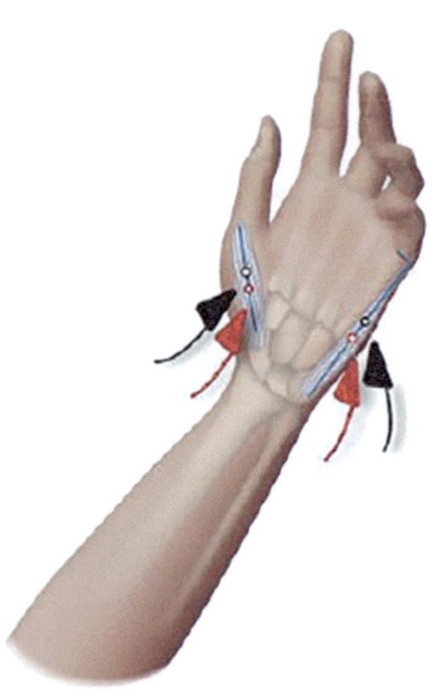

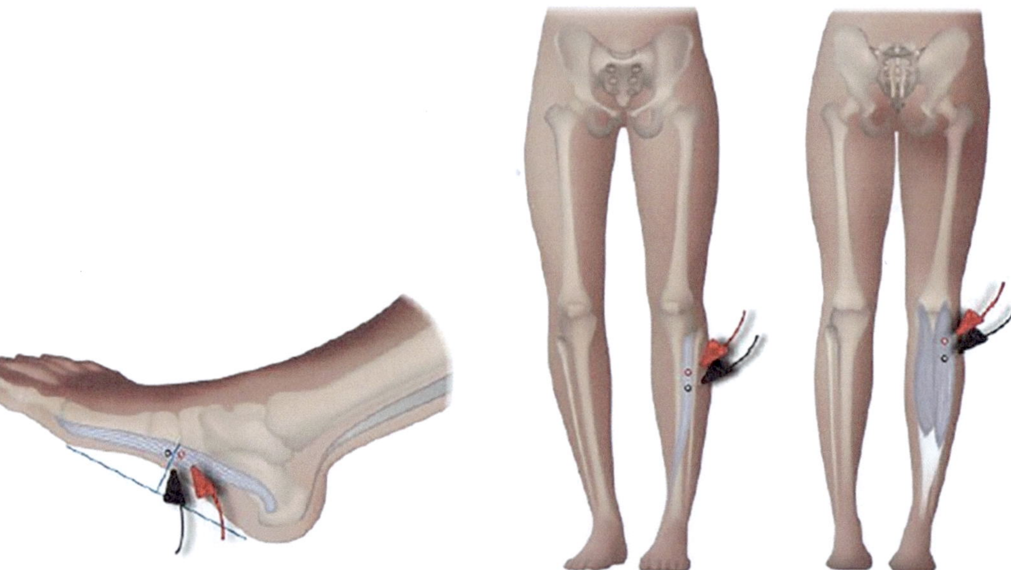

Fig. 5.89 Test question—Electrode positions for recording of MEPs from the upper and lower extremities. © ARKANA Forum GmbH 2022. All Rights Reserved

Transcranial stimulation excites the ___________________________ in the primary motor cortex. The action potential runs via fast conducting axons of the ___________________ (first motoneuron) through the posterior limb of the internal capsule to the upper part of the brainstem and the medulla oblongata. In the lower medulla oblongata, the corticospinal tract crosses for the most part to the contralateral side (___________________) and passes from here downward in the ________________ corticospinal tract. In the ______________, the action potential switches to the second motoneuron (____________) at the level of its exit from the spinal cord and proceeds to the muscular end plate, excitation of which finally leads to contraction of the target muscles.

28. What are the usual latencies of MEPs recorded from the hand and foot?

29. Which are important parameters for the interpretation of MEPs?

30. Complete the following Table 5.38 on the expected postoperative motor status based on muscle MEP and D-wave monitoring.

31. Which special stimulation technique must be used for the recording of corticobulbar MEPs?

32. Interpret the following Fig. 5.90.

33. Which types of AEP do you know and which are used intraoperatively?

34. Where are the electrodes placed for intraoperative BAEP recording?

35. Label the waves and name the corresponding generators of each wave in the Fig. 5.91:

36. Complete the following Table 5.39 on peak latencies of BAEP.

37. Where are the electrodes placed for the recording of VEPs?

38. Complete the following text:

The ___________________________ of the retina activated by the flash convert the light into electrical impulses. The action potential travels along the ___________________________. In the ___________________________ (optic nerve crossing), the nerve fibers of the ___________________________ located sensory cells of the retina cross to the contralateral side, while the fibers of the ___________________________ located sensory cells continue uncrossed. From the optic chiasm, the transmission of stimuli leads via the ___________________ to

Table 5.38 Test question—Validity of muscle MEPs vs. D-waves for prediction of postoperative motor outcome

D-wave	Muscle MEP	Expected motor status
Unchanged or reduced <50%	Preserved or reduced, but still present	
Unchanged or reduced <50%	Unilateral or bilateral loss	
>50% reduced	Loss	

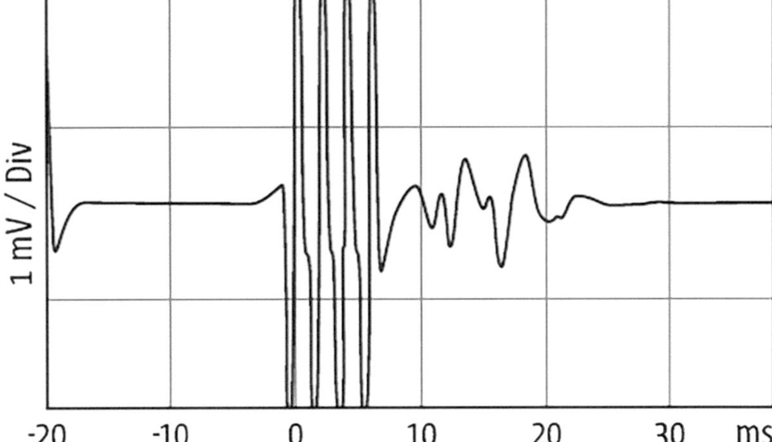

Fig. 5.90 Test question—Typical transcranial corticobulbar MEP. © ARKANA Forum GmbH 2022. All Rights Reserved

Fig. 5.91 Test question—Typical BAEP. © ARKANA Forum GmbH 2022. All Rights Reserved

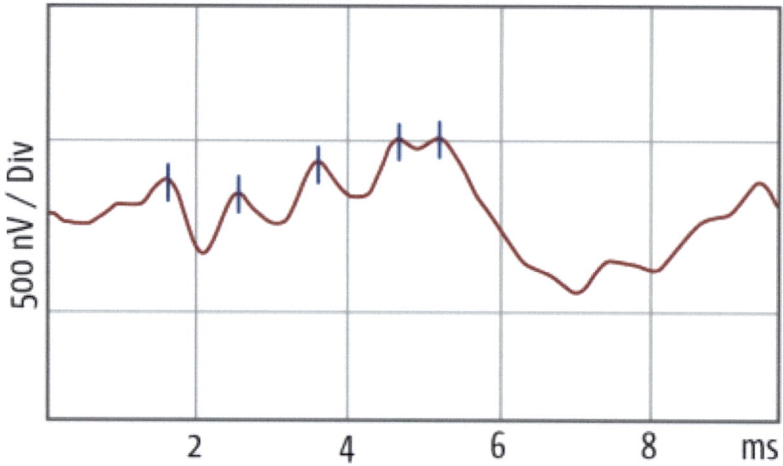

Table 5.39 Test question—Mean latencies of waves I to V of the BAEP in awake normal control subjects

	Latency (ms)
I	
II	2.6
III	
IV	4.7
V	

the lateral geniculate body (corpus geniculatum laterale) and from there to the visual radiation, which ends in the _______________.

39. Which nerve is stimulated for recording the SEP phase reversal?
40. Interpret the following curves (Fig. 5.92).
41. Which type of surgery indicates spinal cord mapping?
42. What is the main goal of dorsal column mapping, and why?
43. What are the available dorsal column mapping techniques, and which is currently preferred?
44. What is the purpose of corticospinal tract mapping?
45. List the available corticospinal tract mapping techniques.
46. How would you perform the D-wave collision mapping technique?
47. Why is there a motor selectivity problem with spinal cord stimulation?
48. Which spinal cord stimulation technique can overcome the motor selectivity problem, and why?
49. Name the numbered muscles in the following Figs. 5.93 and 5.94.
50. Complete the following Table 5.40 on cranial nerve monitoring.
51. Sketch the needle placement for right-sided monitoring of the oculomotor nerve, trochlear nerve and abducens nerve in the Fig. 5.95.
52. Complete the following Table 5.41 on spinal nerve monitoring.
53. The branches of which nerves can be monitored using the blink reflex?
54. Sketch the electrode placement for monitoring the blink reflex in the Fig. 5.96.
55. In which operations is monitoring of the BCR useful?
56. Where are stimulation and recording done for the BCR?
57. Name the numbered labels in the Fig. 5.97:

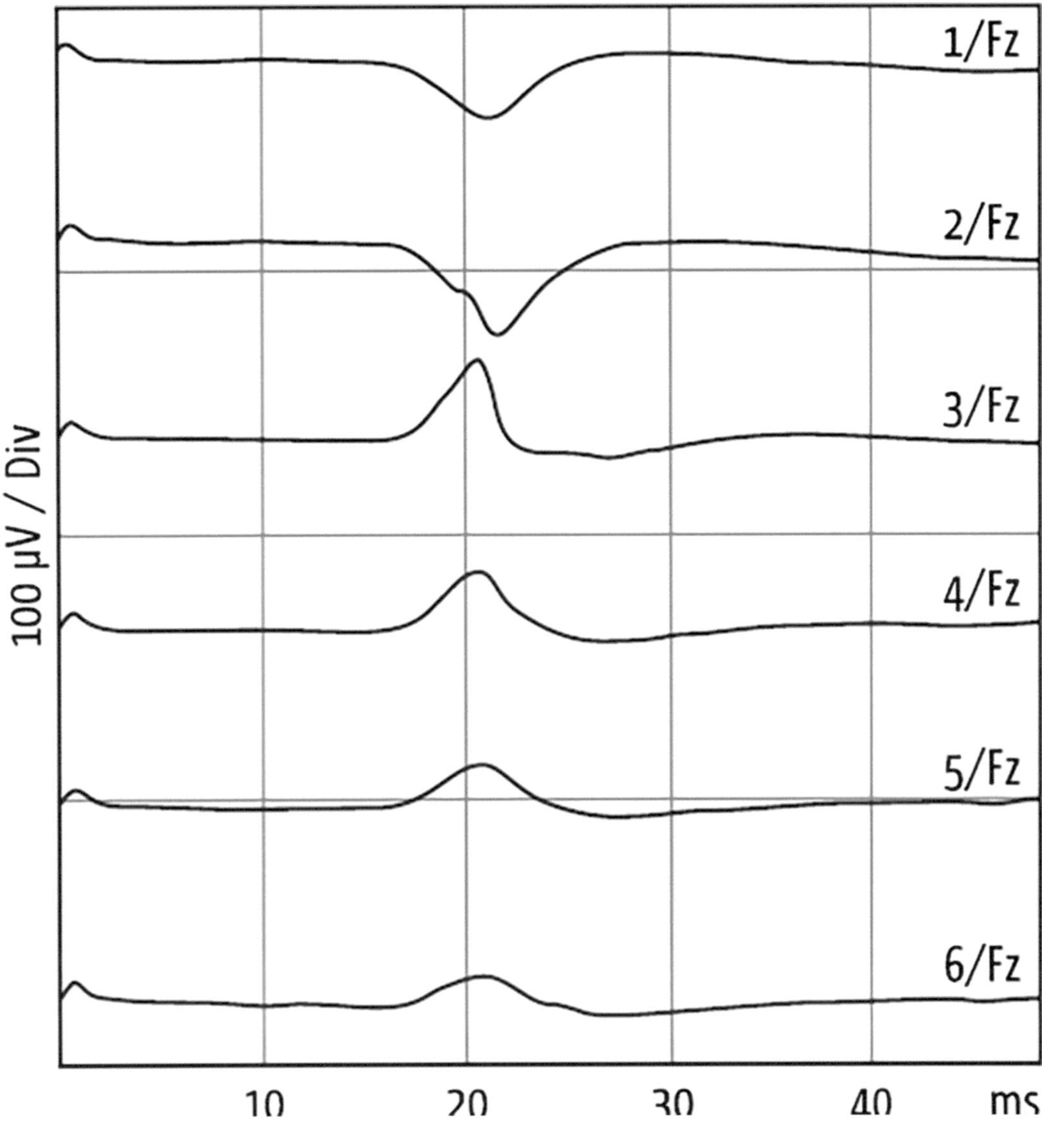

Fig. 5.92 Test question—SEP phase reversal. © ARKANA Forum GmbH 2022. All Rights Reserved

58. Which muscles can be selected for monitoring of the PRMR/ARMR?
59. Interpret the Fig. 5.98 (PRMR/ARMR).
60. Which nerves are stimulated for monitoring the autonomic nervous system in the lesser pelvis and from which muscles are responses recorded and how?
61. What is the special feature of the muscles recorded in autonomic nervous system monitoring, and how is the stimulation of the autonomic nerves accomplished?
62. Which statements about outcome can be made on the basis of autonomic nervous system monitoring in the lesser pelvis?

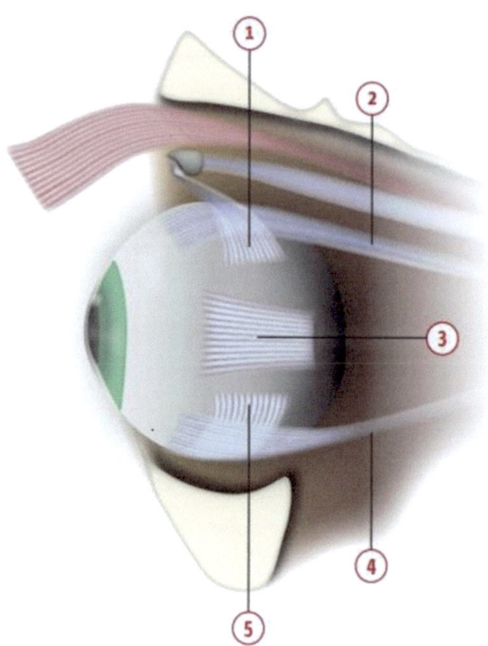

Fig. 5.93 Test question—Eye muscles. © ARKANA Forum GmbH 2022. All Rights Reserved

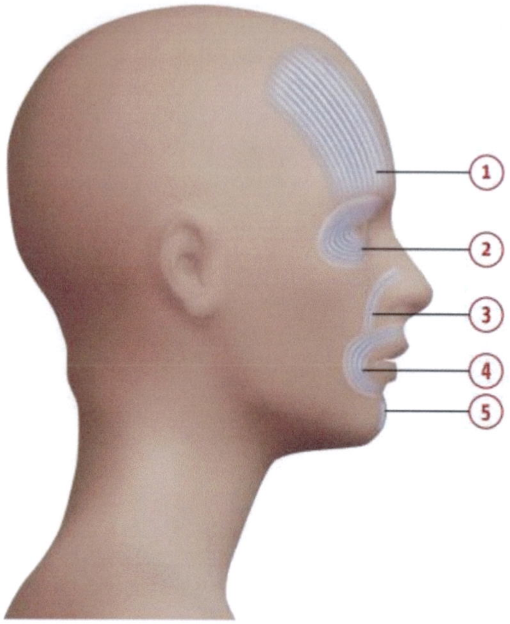

Fig. 5.94 Test question—Facial muscles. © ARKANA Forum GmbH 2022. All Rights Reserved

Table 5.40 Test question—Cranial nerve monitoring

No.	Name	Monitoring
I	N. olfactorius	Not possible
II	N. opticus	
III	N. oculomotorius	
IV		M. obliquus superior
V		M. masseter
VI	N. abducens	
VII		
VIII	N. vestibulocochlearis	
IX		Soft palate, M. stylopharyngeus
X		
XI	N. accessorius	
XII		Tongue muscles

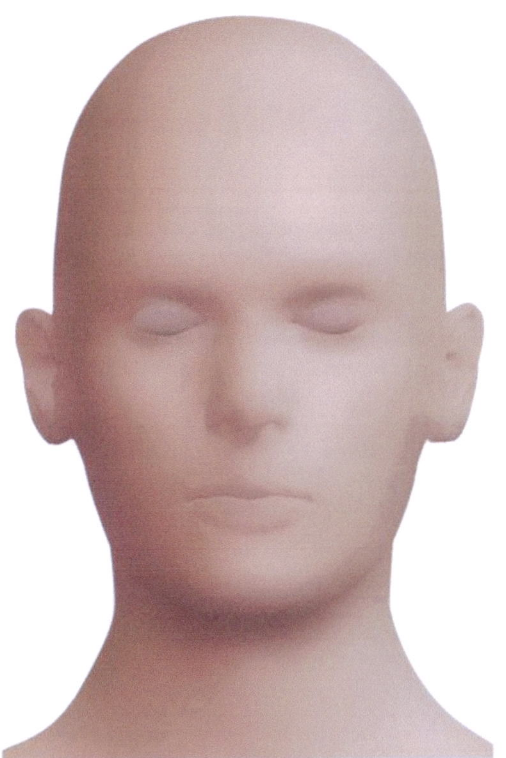

Fig. 5.95 Test question—Electrode placement at right eye muscles. © ARKANA Forum GmbH 2022. All Rights Reserved

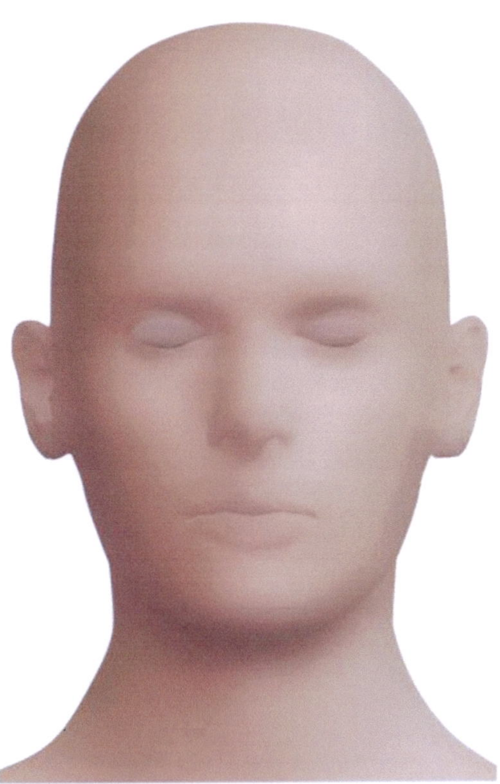

Fig. 5.96 Test question—Electrode placement for monitoring the blink reflex. © ARKANA Forum GmbH 2022. All Rights Reserved

Table 5.41 Test question—Cervical spinal nerves and indicator muscles

Segment	Designation	Monitoring	Nerve
Cervical	C2	M. sternocleidomastoideus	
	C3		
	C4		
	C5	M. deltoideus	N. axillaris
	C6		N. radialis
		M. biceps	
	C7		N. radialis
	C8		N. ulnaris
		M. pollicis brevis	

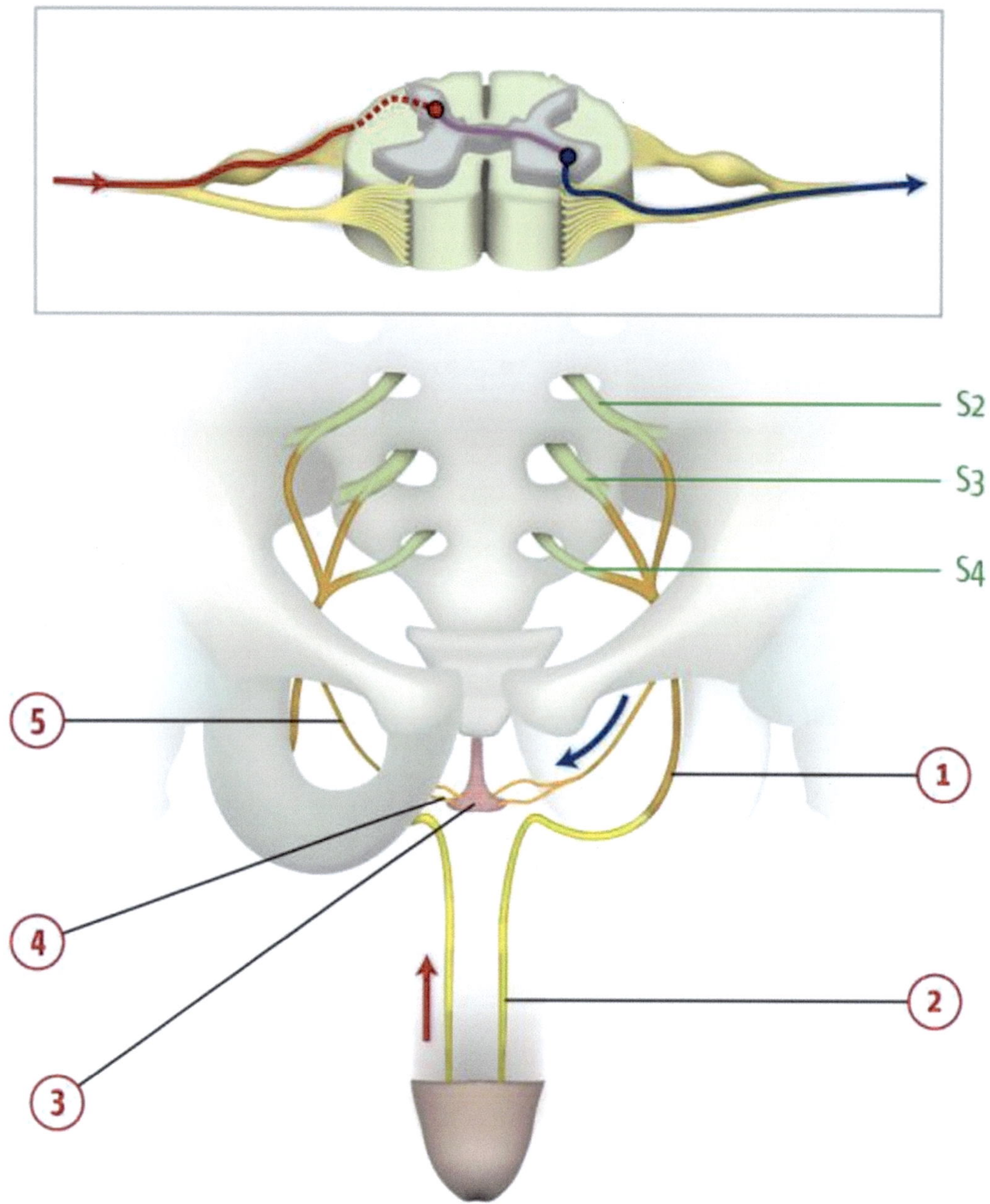

Fig. 5.97 Test question—Signal path of the bulbocavernosus reflex in males. © ARKANA Forum GmbH 2022. All Rights Reserved

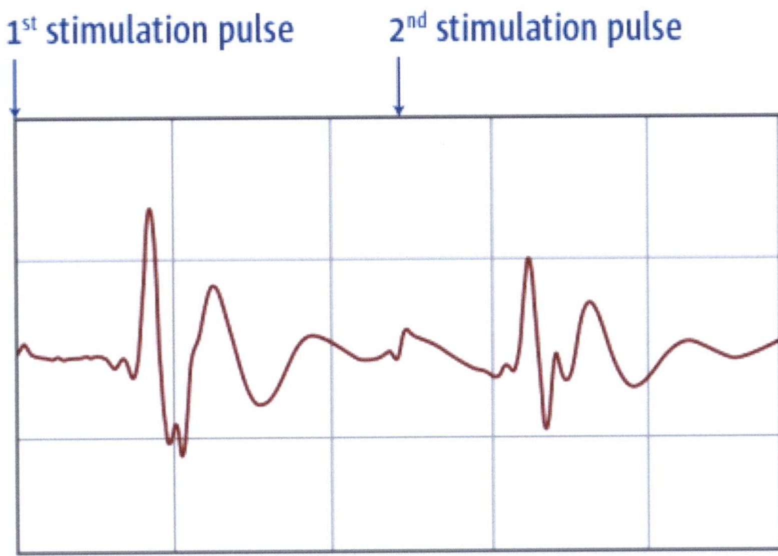

Fig. 5.98 Test question—Typical ARMR during monitoring in hip surgery, recorded from the triceps surae muscle. © ARKANA Forum GmbH 2022. All Rights Reserved

References

1. Ashram YA, Badr-El-Dine MM. Multichannel facial nerve monitoring: value in detection of mechanically elicited electromyographic activity and prediction of postoperative outcome. Otol Neurotol. 2014;35(7):1290–7.
2. Møller AR. Intraoperative neurophysiological monitoring. 2nd ed. Totowa, NJ: Humana Press; 2006. p. 356.
3. Prell J, Rampp S, Romstöck J, Fahlbusch R, Strauss C. Train time as a quantitative electromyographic parameter for facial nerve function in patients undergoing surgery for vestibular schwannoma. J Neurosurg. 2007;106(5):826–32.
4. Prell J, Rachinger J, Scheller C, Alfieri A, Strauss C, Rampp S. A real-time monitoring system for the facial nerve. Neurosurgery. 2010;66(6):1064–73.
5. Romstöck J, Strauss C, Fahlbusch R. Continuous electromyography monitoring of motor cranial nerves during cerebellopontine angle surgery. J Neurosurg. 2000;93(4):586–93.
6. MacDonald DB, Dong C, Quatrale R, Sala F, Skinner S, Soto F, et al. Recommendations of the International Society of Intraoperative Neurophysiology for intraoperative somatosensory evoked potentials. Clin Neurophysiol. 2019;130(1):161–79.
7. Neuloh G, Schramm J. Intraoperative neurophysiological mapping and monitoring for supratentorial procedures. In: Deletis V, Shils JL, editors. Neurophysiology in neurosurgery: a modern intraoperative approach. Amsterdam/Boston, MA: Academic Press; 2002. p. 339–401.
8. Malcharek MJ, Landgraf J, Hennig G, Sorge O, Aschermann J, Sablotzki A. Recordings of long-latency trigeminal somatosensory-evoked potentials in patients under general anaesthesia. Clin Neurophysiol. 2011;122(5):1048–54.
9. Cavalcanti GA, Bruschini H, Manzano GM, Nunes KF, Giuliano LM, Nobrega JA, et al. Pudendal somatosensory evoked potentials in normal women. Int Braz J Urol. 2007;33(6):815–21.
10. Stöhr M, Buettner UW, Dichgans J, Hess CW. Evozierte potenziale: SEP—VEP—AEP—EKP—MEP. Springer Medizin Verlag Heidelberg: Springer e-books; 2005.
11. Khealani B, Husain AM. Neurophysiologic intraoperative monitoring during surgery for tethered cord syndrome. J Clin Neurophysiol. 2009;26(2):76–81.
12. Gonzalez AA, Shilian P, Zada G, Gugino LD. Motor evoked potentials. In: Loftus CM, Biller J, Baron EM, editors. Intraoperative neuromonitoring. New York, NY: McGraw-Hill Education; 2014. p. 389–404.
13. Szelényi A, Langer D, Beck J, Raabe A, Flamm ES, Seifert V, et al. Transcranial and direct cortical stimulation for motor evoked potential monitoring in intracerebral aneurysm surgery. Neurophysiol Clin Neurophysiol. 2007;37(6):391–8.
14. Szelényi A, Kothbauer KF, Deletis V. Transcranial electric stimulation for intraoperative motor evoked potential monitoring: Stimulation parameters and electrode montages. Clin Neurophysiol. 2007;118(7):1586–95.
15. Jones SJ, Harrison R, Koh KF, Mendoza N, Crockard HA. Motor evoked potential monitoring during spinal surgery: responses of distal limb muscles to transcranial cortical stimulation with

pulse trains. Electroencephalogr Clin Neurophysiol. 1996;100:375–83.

16. Sala F, Kothbauer KF. Intraoperative neurophysiological monitoring during surgery for intramedullary spinal cord tumors. In: Nuwer MR, editor. Intraoperative monitoring of neural function. Amsterdam: Elsevier; 2009. p. 235–51.

17. Sala F, Squintani G, Tramontano V. Intraoperative neurophysiologic monitoring during brainstem surgery. In: Loftus CM, Biller J, Baron EM, editors. Intraoperative neuromonitoring. New York, NY: McGraw-Hill Education; 2014. p. 285–97.

18. Sarnthein J, Tomilov M, Baag M, Regli L. Improving intraoperative evoked potentials at short latency by a novel neuro-stimulation technology with delayed return discharge. Clin Neurophysiol. 2021;132(6):1195–9.

19. Szelényi A, Bello L, Duffau H, Fava E, Feigl GC, Galanda M, et al. Intraoperative electrical stimulation in awake craniotomy: methodological aspects of current practice. Neurosurg Focus. 2010;28(2):E7.

20. Matthies C. Monitoring during surgery around the acoustic and vestibular nerves. In: Nuwer MR, editor. Intraoperative monitoring of neural function. Amsterdam: Elsevier; 2009. p. 566–89.

21. Stöhr M, Pfadenhauer K, Scheglmann K, Wagner. Neuromonitoring. Darmstadt: Steinkopff; 1999. p. 386.

22. Krieg SM, Kempf L, Droese D, Rosahl SK, Meyer B, Lehmberg J. Superiority of tympanic ball electrodes over mastoid needle electrodes for intraoperative monitoring of hearing function: clinical article. J Neurosurg. 2014;120(5):1042–7.

23. Møller AR. Intraoperative Neurophysiological Monitoring Techniques for Microvascular Decompression Procedures. In: Loftus CM, Biller J, Baron EM, editors. Intraoperative neuromonitoring. New York: McGraw-Hill Education; 2014. p. 273–84.

24. Luo Y, Regli L, Bozinov O, Sarnthein J. Clinical utility and limitations of intraoperative monitoring of visual evoked potentials. Davies WIL, editor. PLoS One. 2015;10(3):e0120525.

25. Goto T, Kodama K, Hongo K. Monitoring of visual evoked potentials during para- and suprasellar procedures. In: Loftus CM, Biller J, Baron EM, editors. Intraoperative neuromonitoring. New York, NY: McGraw-Hill Education; 2014. p. 243–54.

26. Raabe A, Beck J, Schucht P, Seidel K. Continuous dynamic mapping of the corticospinal tract during surgery of motor eloquent brain tumors: evaluation of a new method: Clinical article. J Neurosurg. 2014;120(5):1015–24.

27. Zentner J. Surgical treatment of epilepsies: diagnosis, surgical strategies, results. Cham: Springer; 2020. p. 404.

28. Deletis V, Sala F. The role of intraoperative neurophysiology in the protection or documentation of surgically induced injury to the spinal cord. Ann N Y Acad Sci. 2001;939:137–44.

29. Deletis V, Seidel K. Neurophysiological identification of long sensory and motor tracts within the spinal cord. In: Neurophysiology in neurosurgery. Elsevier; 2020. p. 163–75. https://linkinghub.elsevier.com/retrieve/pii/B9780128150009000125.

30. Yanni DS, Ulkatan S, Deletis V, Barrenechea IJ, Sen C, Perin NI. Utility of neurophysiological monitoring using dorsal column mapping in intramedullary spinal cord surgery. J Neurosurg Spine. 2010;12:623–8.

31. Quinones-Hinojosa A, Gulati M, Lyon R, Gupta N, Yingling C. Spinal cord mapping as an adjunct for resection of intramedullary tumors: surgical technique with case illustrations. Neurosurgery. 2002;51(5):1199–207.

32. Nair D, Kumaraswamy VM, Braver D, Kilbride RD, Borges LF, Simon MV. Dorsal column mapping via phase reversal method. Neurosurgery. 2014;74(4):437–46.

33. Simon MV, Chiappa KH, Borges LF, Nuwer MR, Deletis V. Phase reversal of somatosensory evoked potentials triggered by gracilis tract stimulation: case report of a new technique for neurophysiologic dorsal column mapping. Neurosurgery. 2012;70(3):783.

34. Deletis V, Bueno De Camargo A. Interventional neurophysiological mapping during spinal cord procedures. Stereotact Funct Neurosurg. 2001;77(1–4):25–8.

35. Minahan RE, Sepkuty JP, Lesser RP, Sponseller PD, Kostuik JP. Anterior spinal cord injury with preserved neurogenic "motor" evoked potentials. Clin Neurophysiol. 2001;112(8):1442–50.

36. Barzilai O, Lidar Z, Constantini S, Salame K, Bitan-Talmor Y, Korn A. Continuous mapping of the corticospinal tracts in intramedullary spinal cord tumor surgery using an electrified ultrasonic aspirator. J Neurosurg Spine. 2017;27(2):161–8.

37. Deletis V, Seidel K, Sala F, Raabe A, Chudy D, Beck J, et al. Intraoperative identification of the corticospinal tract and dorsal column of the spinal cord by electrical stimulation. J Neurol Neurosurg Psychiatry. 2018;89(7):754–61.

38. Randolph GW, Dralle H, with the International Intraoperative Monitoring Study Group, Abdullah H, Barczynski M, Bellantone R, et al. Electrophysiologic recurrent laryngeal nerve monitoring during thyroid and parathyroid surgery: International standards guideline statement. Laryngoscope. 2011;121(S1):S1–16.

39. Raynor BL, Lenke LG, Kim Y, Hanson DS, Wilson-Holden TJ, Bridwell KH, et al. Can triggered electromyograph thresholds predict safe thoracic pedicle screw placement? Spine. 2002;27(18):2030–5.

40. Raynor BL, Lenke LG, Bridwell KH, Taylor BA, Padberg AM. Correlation between low triggered electromyographic thresholds and lumbar pedicle screw malposition: analysis of 4857 screws. Spine. 2007;32(24):2673–8.

41. Deletis V, Urriza J, Ulkatan S, Fernandez-Conejero I, Lesser J, Misita D. The feasibility of recording blink reflexes under general anesthesia. Muscle Nerve. 2009;39(5):642–6.

42. Vogel P. Kursbuch klinische Neurophysiologie: EMG—ENG—Evozierte Potentiale; 35 Tabellen; [mit 100 Video-Clips auf DVD]. 2., aktualisierte Aufl. Stuttgart: Thieme; 2006. p. 230.
43. Vodušek DB, Deletis V. Intraoperative neurophysiological monitoring of the sacral nervous system. In: Deletis V, Shils JL, editors. Neurophysiology in neurosurgery a modern intraoperative approach. Amsterdam/Boston, MA: Academic Press; 2002.
44. Kothbauer KF, Novak K. Intraoperative monitoring for tethered cord surgery: an update. Neurosurg Focus. 2004;16(2):E8.
45. Deletis V, Vodušek DB. Intraoperative recording of the bulbocavernosus reflex. Neurosurgery. 1997;40(1):88–93.
46. Troni W, Benech CA, Perez R, Tealdi S, Berardino M, Benech F. Non-invasive high voltage electrical stimulation as a monitoring tool of nerve root function in lumbosacral surgery. Clin Neurophysiol. 2013;124(4):809–18.
47. Kneist W. Individualisierte Chirurgie bei Rektumkarzinomen. In: Korenkov M, Germer CT, Lang H, editors. Gastrointestinale Operationen und technische Varianten. Berlin, Heidelberg: Springer Berlin Heidelberg; 2013. p. 297–389. https://doi.org/10.1007/978-3-642-32259-4_10.
48. Kauff DW, Wachter N, Bettzieche R, Lang H, Kneist W. Electrophysiology-based quality assurance of nerve-sparing in laparoscopic rectal cancer surgery: Is it worth the effort? Surg Endosc. 2016;30(10):4525–32. https://doi.org/10.1007/s00464-016-4787-z.
49. Kneist W, Kauff DW, Rubenwolf P, Thomas C, Hampel C, Lang H. Intraoperative monitoring of bladder and internal anal sphincter innervation: a predictor of erectile function following low anterior rectal resection for rectal cancer? results of a prospective clinical study. Dig Surg. 2013;30(4–6):459–65.

Perioperative Management

6

Celine Wegner

Contents

C. Wegner (✉)
ARKANA Forum GmbH, Emmendingen, Germany
e-mail: c.wegner@arkana-forum.com

© The Author(s), under exclusive license to Springer Nature Switzerland AG 2024
J. Zentner et al. (eds.), *Intraoperative Neuromonitoring*,
https://doi.org/10.1007/978-3-031-46125-5_6

6.1 Patient Preparation

6.1.1 Positioning the Electrodes

Before placing the electrodes, the **scalp** must be thoroughly **cleaned**. To determine the exact **electrode positions**, the head is measured according to the **10–20 system**. The electrodes are then placed in the pre-marked positions.

Attention should be paid to the position of the anode and cathode when placing **stimulation electrodes**. In transcranial stimulation, anodal stimulation is to be preferred; the stimulation effect takes place mainly under the anode. Therefore, the anode is placed as close as possible to the target area. For the stimulation of peripheral nerves, cathodal stimulation has proven to be effective. This means that the cathode must be placed close to the target area, while the anode is positioned opposite to the desired direction of action potential propagation to prevent an anodal block.

A **ground electrode** must be picked for each recording box and should be located close to the recording electrodes. Depending on the measuring arrangement, the ground electrode can be placed at the hip, leg or shoulder, for example.

When using **monopolar high-frequency (HF) electrosurgery**, it is possible that part of this HF current will flow through the neuromonitoring subdermal needle electrodes(leakage current), which can cause skin burns at the insertion sites if the current density is high. To prevent this, the needle electrodes should not be placed in the direct path between the electrosurgery blade and the dispersive pad electrode of the electrosurgery unit. In addition, only neuromonitoring devices and accessories equipped with HF protection should be used.

6.1.2 Securing the Electrodes

All needle electrodes must be well taped so that they are not accidentally pulled out during patient positioning or other patient manipulations.

6.1.3 Labeling the Electrodes

It is advisable to define a color scheme for the most common and important operations so that it is clear from the electrode color whether the electrode is located at the head, at the lower or upper limbs, or on the left or right side of the patient. This can help to identify an error more easily in the event of any problems.

In addition, clear labeling of the electrode cables is extremely helpful during placement and subsequent connection of the cables. It is recommended to prepare labels and fix them to the corresponding cables. The labeling can include, for example, the needle position (e.g., target muscle), the patient side, and the corresponding channel number.

6.1.4 Connecting the Electrodes

After placement and usually after patient positioning, all electrodes are connected to the respective adapter boxes according to the labeling. Information on electrode assignment and the corresponding plugs can be found in the electrode chart of the software. The adapter boxes are then connected to the stimulator and the amplifier as indicated by the labeling and color code.

Tightly braiding or twisting the electrode cables significantly reduces electrical interference in individual electrodes, which may be important in cortical recordings, for example.

6.2 System Preparation

6.2.1 Starting the Device

Before operating the power switch, make sure that the power plug of the device is connected.

6.2.2 Starting the Software

The monitoring software starts automatically with most manufacturers. Otherwise, the software must be started by double-clicking after booting the PC.

6.2.3 Entering the Patient Data

Before starting the measurement, at least the hospital ID of the patient is entered to ensure clear assignment of the data for easy retrieval and later analysis.

6.2.4 Selecting the Program

An appropriate program is selected from the existing list and, if necessary, adapted to the actual requirements. Alternatively, a new program can be created with the help of the program editor.

When creating new programs, attention should be paid to the order of the recording sites. It is recommended to arrange them from cranial to caudal to aid interpretation and better identify connection errors revealed by unexpectedly short or long response latency in one or more channels.

6.2.5 Measuring the Impedance

Before starting measurements, an impedance test is performed to check whether all electrodes are functional and have optimal contact. Electrodes with excessive impedances should be repositioned or replaced.

It is also very important to make sure that electrodes of one channel have balanced impedances. Again, if there are significant deviations, the respective electrodes should be repositioned or replaced.

6.2.6 Checking the Parameters

Before starting the measurement, all relevant parameters are checked. Particularly important is the control of the stimulation current. The start-

ing and maximum values can be taken from the respective tables in Chap. 5.

6.2.7 Checking and Setting the Artifact Threshold

The artifact threshold is used to reject individual sweeps containing high-amplitude artifacts from averaging. This function reduces a negative influence on averaged evoked potentials caused by interferences such as electrosurgery.

The artifact threshold is checked at the beginning of the measurements and individually adjusted to the respective conditions.

6.3 General Conduct Rules in the Operating Room (OR)

6.3.1 Entering the OR

In the unclean area of the changing room, street clothes, shoes, and all jewelry are removed. Since free lockers are rarely available, it is advisable not to take valuables into the operating unit. Dressed in underwear and socks, one enters the clean side of the changing room. There, on shelves sorted by size, one can find pants and tops, shoes, as well as surgical masks and hoods. One selects the appropriate clothing and gets dressed. The hair must be completely covered by the hood. Before entering the operating room, the surgical mask must be put on, with the mouth, chin, and nose covered (Fig. 6.1). Thereafter, hands and forearms are thoroughly washed and disinfected (Fig. 6.2). During patient contact, e.g., when placing the electrodes, wearing of gloves is strongly recommended.

Artificial fingernails and the carrying of private items (bags, backpacks, etc.) are not permitted in the operating room. Private items must be left in the lockers in the dressing room.

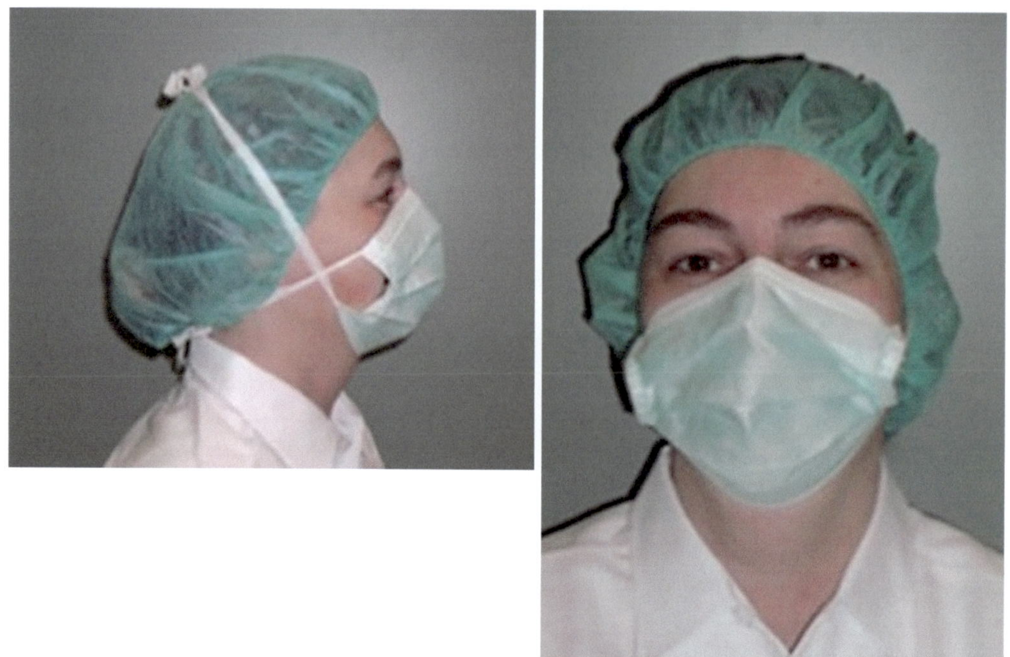

Fig. 6.1 Correctly put on surgical hood and mask. © ARKANA Forum GmbH 2022. All Rights Reserved

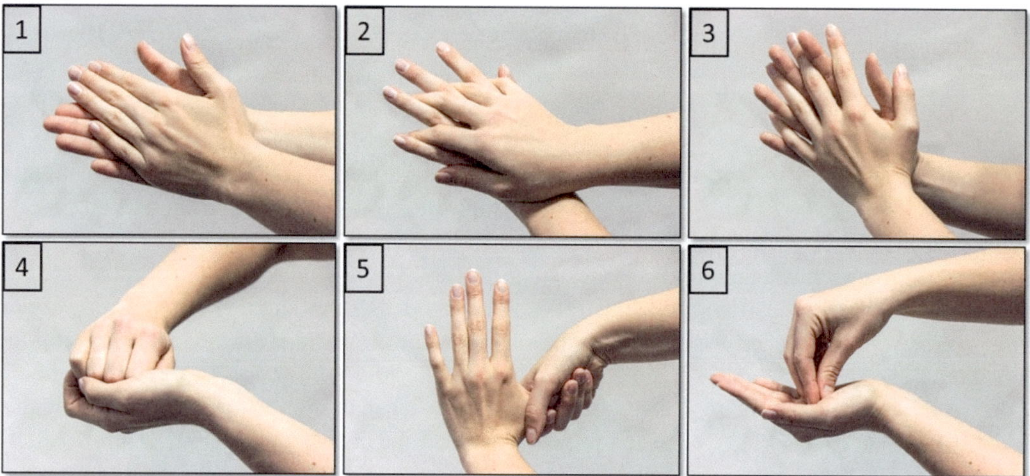

Fig. 6.2 Instructions for hygienic hand disinfection. © ARKANA Forum GmbH 2022. All Rights Reserved

6.3.2 Staying in the OR

If one is new to the OR as an employee, one should first briefly introduce oneself to everyone present and become familiar with the local conditions. As long as neuromonitoring is not yet routine in the hospital, the placement of the monitoring system should be agreed with the surgeon, anesthetist, and OR personell. When preparing the system and the patient, care must also

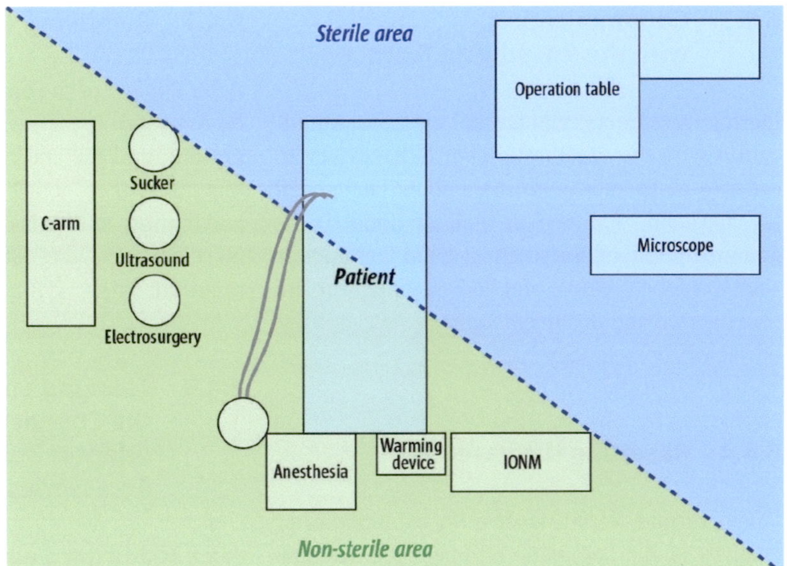

Fig. 6.3 Schematic representation of the structure of an OR. © ARKANA Forum GmbH 2022. All Rights Reserved

be taken not to get too close to the sterile instrument tables and equipment. A minimum distance of one arm's length from sterile areas must be maintained.

The operating room is usually structured in such a way that a virtual line running across the room separates the sterile from the non-sterile part. In the sterile part are prepared operating tables, the surgical team, and, if necessary, the sterile-covered microscope and/or C-arm. The non-sterile part includes the anesthesia team and equipment and surgical supplies. This is also where the neuromonitoring system is placed. When entering the operating room, one should recognize the course of this virtual line and, if possible, stay only in the non-sterile area (Fig. 6.3).

6.3.3   Leaving the OR

At the end of surgery, surgical clothes and shoes are taken off and sorted into the laundry bags and bins provided. Surgical masks and hoods are disposed of in waste containers.

6.4   Measurement Processes

6.4.1   Comparing Results with Preoperative Neurological Status

After the baseline has been defined, the measured results should be compared with the preoperative neurological findings to check the initial intraoperative readings for plausibility.

In general, it makes sense to take note of the medical records as early as the planning stage of the surgery. It may be possible or necessary to adapt or abandon the neuromonitoring plan on the basis of this information.

6.4.2   Checking the Current Flow

After starting the stimulation, the current flow control display is checked to ensure that the set current is actually flowing in full. If this is not the case, the impedance of the stimulation electrodes and the connection lines should be checked again.

6.4.3 Communicating with the Anesthesia Team

During the surgery, regular and close communication with the anesthesia team is necessary in order to be promptly informed about changes in the anesthetic regimen as well as about bolus administration of anesthetics. Vital parameters such as blood pressure and body temperature are also queried and documented, as these can influence electrophysiology.

6.4.4 Resetting the Baseline

Under certain circumstances, for example, after changes of the anesthetic regimen, the baseline must be redefined during surgery. The respective reasons should be noted.

6.4.5 Completing the Measurement Process

The measurement process can only be completed after the surgeon has explicitly confirmed that neuromonitoring is no longer required. All measurement results remain stored under the respective patient ID and can be called up again at any time. A report of the neuromonitoring results can be prepared.

6.4.6 Shutting Down the System

Having completed the measurements, the IONM system must be shut down. Only then the power switch is switched off.

6.4.7 Removing the Electrodes

After the end of the operation, the electrodes can be removed. If the neuromonitoring team is not present until the end of surgery, it is imperative that the staff responsible is informed of the type and number of electrodes used. This ensures that no electrodes are left behind or improperly removed.

6.4.8 Cleaning and Checking the Connection Cables, Adapter Boxes, and Reusable Accessories

After each intervention, the system accessories must be cleaned, disinfected, and checked for any damage. Afterwards, the accessories should be neatly stowed away in the system or in another place. Defective accessories are forwarded to the service department of the manufacturer. Cleaning and sterilization of the accessories is carried out in the sterilization unit of the hospital.

6.4.9 Documenting the Data

After the neuromonitoring has been completed, the data must be documented. This can be accomplished either via the report function of the software or manually. Important items include the modalities and electrodes used, the times of starting and completing the neuromonitoring, the baselines, major events, and possibly a rough course of the patient's blood pressure and temperature during surgery. These data can be supplemented by images and screenshots of the signals.

Anesthesia and IONM

7

Michael Malcharek and Hans-Joachim Priebe

Contents

M. Malcharek (✉)
Praxisklinik, Leipzig, Germany

H. -J. Priebe
Department of Anesthesiology and Critical Care,
University Medical Center, Freiburg, Germany

7.1 Effect of Anesthetics on the Nervous System

The main drugs used for general anesthesia are listed in Table 7.1. Depending on the desired effects of hypnosis, analgesia, and immobilization/muscle relaxation, these drugs exhibit different action profiles at the neuronal or neuromuscular targets.

With regard to anesthesia-induced **unconsciousness**, the primary mechanism of action is

Table 7.1 Most important anesthetics used for general anesthesia (commonly used drugs are printed in bold). TIVA, total intravenous anesthesia; GABA, gamma-amino-butyric acid; NMDA, N-methyl-D-aspartate

Hypnosis	
intravenous substances	• **propofol** • barbiturates • etomidate • ketamine
	• mainly used for induction of anesthesia • propofol also used for maintenance of anesthesia (TIVA) • propofol, thiopental, and etomidate are GABA-agonists • ketamine is a NMDA-antagonist
inhaled substances	• isoflurane • sevoflurane • desflurane
	• usually used for maintenance of anesthesia • sevoflurane may also be used for induction of anesthesia in children • lower allergic potential than propofol • good controllability (especially desflurane, as it is short-acting)
	• nitrous oxide (N_2O)
	• only in combination with other hypnotics • additional analgesic component, good controllability
Analgesia	
opioids	• **remifentanil** • sufentanil • fentanyl
	• morphine-like strong analgesics used during laryngoscopy and intraoperative pain stimuli • remifentanil is ultra-short acting (good controllability) → therefore usually continuous iv. administration • postoperative pain hypersensitivity (especially with remifentanil)
other intravenous substances	• ketamine
	• low potency analgesic, hemodynamic activation • sometimes strong side effects postoperatively (e.g., hallucinations, salivation, disorientation)
inhaled substances	• nitrous oxide (N_2O)
	• potent co-hypnotic with analgesic potential
Immobilization/Relaxation	
depolarizing muscle relaxant	• succinylcholine
	• ultra-short-acting muscle relaxant (approximately 5 min) • noteworthy profile of side effects (e.g., prolonged duration of action in pseudocholinesterase deficiency or after repetitive administration, cardiac arrhythmias, trigger substance for malignant hyperthermia)
non-depolarizing muscle relaxants	• **rocuronium** • mivacurium • (*cis*)-atracurium
	• few side-effects • rapid and effective antagonization of rocuronium by sugammadex • enzyme-independent degradation of (*cis*)-atracurium
other immobilizing/ relaxing substances	• volatile anesthetics • propofol
	• suppressive effect on depolarization of the α-motoneuron at the spinal level → suppression of motorreactions • suppression at the α-motoneuron probably more pronounced with volatile anesthetics than propofol

still unclear. However, three basic working hypotheses are currently discussed:

- Interference with synaptic transmission at the receptor level ("synaptic model").
- Impairment of impulse transmission (e.g., reduction of nerve conduction velocity).
- Inhibitory influence on higher-order control centers in the central nervous system (e.g., the reticular formation).

For the **synaptic model**, a variety of receptors are stimulated or inhibited by various hypnotically active drugs [1]. In a simplified view, the functionally inhibitory gamma-amino-butyric acid (GABA) and glycine receptors, and the excitatory glutaminergic N-methyl-D-aspartate (NMDA) receptors play a crucial role for anesthetic drug interactions. Most hypnotics (e.g., propofol, barbiturates, volatile anesthetics) act by agonistically enhancing the inhibitory effect of the GABA receptors. In contrast, drugs such as ketamine, nitrous oxide, and xenon antagonistically reduce the excitatory effect at the NMDA receptors.

The **hypnotic effect** of various anesthetics is thought to occur via the thalamus, cortex, and higher-level structures in the brainstem (e.g., reticular formation). In addition, there is evidence that different brain regions are affected in a dose-dependent manner [2, 3]. Both, the different mechanisms of action at the molecular level and the different sites of action underscore the complexity of the issue.

Opioids are almost exclusively used for adequate **analgesia** during surgical procedures. They act directly at specific opioid receptors and exhibit electrophysiologically measurable effects only at extremely high doses [4].

With regard to the **immobilizing/relaxing** component of general anesthesia, the reduction in reflex movements does not necessarily argue for direct relaxation of the muscles. Agents acting at GABA receptors and glycine receptors (e.g., propofol and volatile anesthetics) enhance spinal inhibitory effects at the synaptic level, usually resulting in effective immobilization. However, muscle relaxants obviously act directly at the terminal portion of the motor pathway, the motor end plate, while other pathways like the sensory are not affected at all.

In the following, the interactions of various anesthetics used for general anesthesia on the different neuromonitoring modalities will be described.

7.2 Effects of Anesthetics on Electrophysiology

7.2.1 Electroencephalogram

The spontaneous brain electrical activity recorded by the electroencephalogram (EEG) is more sensitive to centrally acting anesthetics than the stimulus-related activity recorded with evoked potentials. This is due to the higher number of synapses within the cortical network that is required to generate the typical EEG patterns. As a result, the EEG reacts sensitively to anesthetics. Thus, **specific EEG changes** occur during the induction of general anesthesia using GABA-ergic substances such as propofol, barbiturates, or volatile anesthetics (synaptic block) (Fig. 7.1).

In order to describe the relationships between these EEG patterns and the corresponding cerebral states of activity, the EEG is divided into different **frequency bands** (delta, <4 Hz; theta, 4–<8 Hz; alpha, 8–13 Hz; beta, >13 Hz). In the awake individual with the eyes open, predominantly beta or "fast" activity is found. If the eyes are closed during relaxation, the brain generates the slower occipital alpha rhythm (relaxed awake state). When general anesthesia is induced with a GABA-ergic substance such as propofol, a short excitatory phase with beta sequences is followed by slow "rhythmic" theta and delta activity with high amplitudes. In the further course, complex patterns appear (e.g., delta waves with alpha or beta spindles). After further deepening of anesthesia, a burst–suppression pattern may occur. This consists of alternating mixed-frequency components of an excitatory character (burst) with an isoelectric line (suppression) (Fig. 7.2). Finally, extremely deep anesthesia can produce persistent EEG suppression.

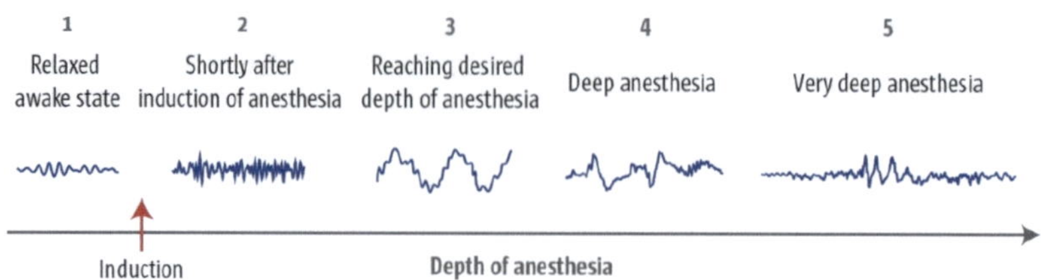

Fig. 7.1 Illustration of EEG patterns during increasing depth of anesthesia by GABA-ergic substances. © ARKANA Forum GmbH 2022. All Rights Reserved

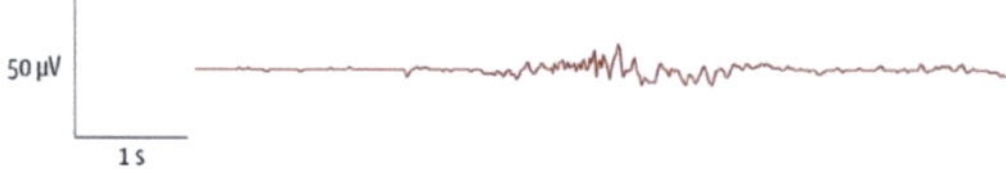

Fig. 7.2 Drug-induced burst–suppression pattern with bursts of fast and slow EEG components separated by segments of suppression. © ARKANA Forum GmbH 2022. All Rights Reserved

The EEG course as described serves as an electrophysiologic basis for estimating the **depth of anesthesia**. This can be done visually to some extent, but it can also be quantified by computerized frequency analysis. This allows various indices to be generated such as the bispectral, narcotrend, entropy, or cerebral state index. All these methods display the estimated depth of anesthesia using a scale of 0–100 (0 = extremely deep anesthesia; 100 = awake patient). The target range for adequate general anesthesia is defined as 40–60.

7.2.2 Somatosensory Evoked Potentials

Despite a similar action mechanism, anesthetic effects on somatosensory evoked potentials (SEPs) are less pronounced than on EEG. Therefore, SEPs have been successfully used for decades in IONM. The major effects of anesthetics on SEPs are listed in Table 7.2.

The GABA agonist **etomidate** and the NMDA antagonist **ketamine** show specific action profiles. At high doses, both drugs cause signal suppression, but at low doses an excitatory component predominates which can increase cortical SEP amplitude (Fig. 7.3). However, continuous administration of etomidate carries the risk

of adrenocortical suppression with subsequently decreased cortisol production [11, 12], so this anesthetic regimen is rarely used in clinical practice.

During both, total intravenous anesthesia (TIVA) based on **propofol** and **inhalation anesthesia**, SEPs can usually be reliably obtained in patients without preexisting neurological deficits and initially stable signal quality. Inhalation anesthetics exhibit a dose-dependent effect [13, 14]. Additional administration of nitrous oxide can cause considerable amplitude suppression [15]. This is especially true for SEPs with low baseline amplitudes, such as tibial nerve SEPs in elderly patients (Fig. 7.4). In patients with unstable SEPs, the use of TIVA appears to be advantageous [16–19]. However, even in these cases, boluses or higher doses of propofol can lead to signal suppression, which is usually not problematic because of the short half-life.

7.2.3 Motor Evoked Potentials

Intraoperative recording of motor evoked potentials (MEPs) during anesthesia is challenging, regardless of whether transcranial or direct cortical stimulation is used. An illustration of the **motor pathways** helps to understand the effects of anesthetics on MEPs (Fig. 7.5).

The **motor cortex** represents the primary target area for transcranial and direct cortical triggering of MEPs (**level I**). Thereby, pyramidal cell axons can be directly depolarized, or pyramidal cells can be indirectly activated by inter-neuronal excitatory synaptic propagation. After direct activation of the pyramidal cell axons, impulse propagation is almost independent of anesthetic

Table 7.2 Influence of anesthetics on SEPs

Anesthetic	A	L	Comments
Hypnotics with specific effects at GABA$_A$ receptors			
Propofol	⇩	⇧	Bolus administration can significantly reduce amplitude [5]
Etomidate	⬆	(−)	• at low doses, increases amplitudes • at high doses, suppresses SEP (and MEP) amplitudes
GABA-ergic substances with other effects			
Barbiturates	(⇩)	(⇧)	Suppressive effect more pronounced on MEPs than on SEPs
Benzodiazepines	⇩	(−)	Dose-dependent mild amplitude suppression [6]
Isoflurane	⬇	⇧	• cortical SEPs basically follow synaptic model (like EEG)
Sevoflurane	⬇	⇧	• no significant influence on asynaptic peripheral (e.g., cubital fossa, Erb' point), or cervical potentials [7]
Desflurane	⬇	⇧	• comparable effects of sevoflurane and desflurane on SEPs [8]
NMDA-receptor-antagonists			
Ketamine	⬆	(−)	Effects similar to etomidate
Nitrous oxide (N$_2$O)	⬇	(⇧)	Higher suppressive effect on amplitudes in combination with isoflurane than isoflurane alone [9]
Xenon	⇩	(−)	
Other drugs			
Opioids	(−)	(−)	Mild effect on SEPs because action is opioid receptor-mediated, minor effect on GABA and NMDA [7]
Muscle relaxants	(−)	(−)	SEPs may be of better quality due to reduced or absent muscle artifact [7]
Dexmedetomidine (α2-agonist)	⇩	(−)	Successful intraoperative use to reduce propofol dose during TIVA for scoliosis surgery [10]

A amplitude, *L* latency, *TIVA* total intravenous anesthesia, *GABA* gamma-amino-butyric acid, *NMDA* N-methyl-D-aspartate

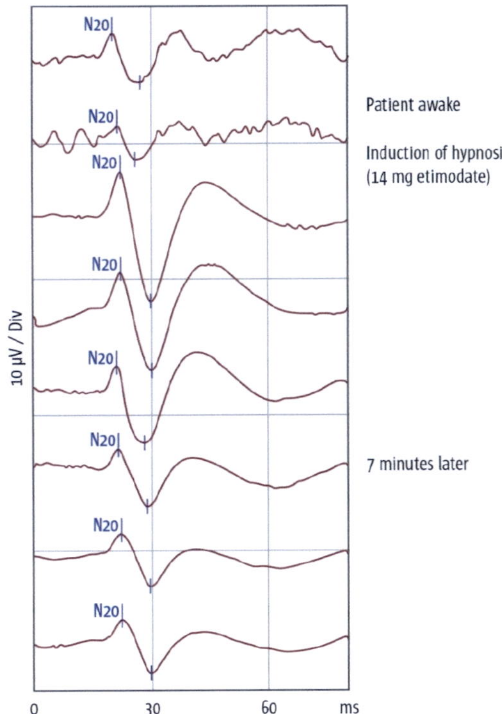

Fig. 7.3 Effect of etomidate on cortical SEPs (Malcharek 2007, unpublished data). © ARKANA Forum GmbH 2022. All Rights Reserved

influences. This is reflected by the epidural recording of **D-waves** (direct waves), which are reliably recordable under general anesthesia because the conduction of the impulse between the stimulation and recording sites is not interrupted by synapses [20, 21]. Consequently, a single stimulation impulse is sufficient to generate a D-wave. In contrast, indirect depolarization, which depends on synaptic transmission, is significantly influenced by anesthetics, comparable to anesthetic-induced EEG changes. Thus, **I-waves** (indirect waves) rarely occur after single pulse stimulation under adequate anesthesia.

In the peripheral recording of MEPs after stimulation of the corticospinal tract, the **α-motoneuron** localized in the anterior horn plays a crucial role (**level II**). Here, in addition to input from the pyramidal cells, other excitatory or inhibitory signals arrive from higher-order centers and from spinal control circuits. The depolarization of the postsynaptic membrane in the α-motoneuron thus represents the result of complex information processing. Anesthetics, especially hypnotics, directly increase the depo-

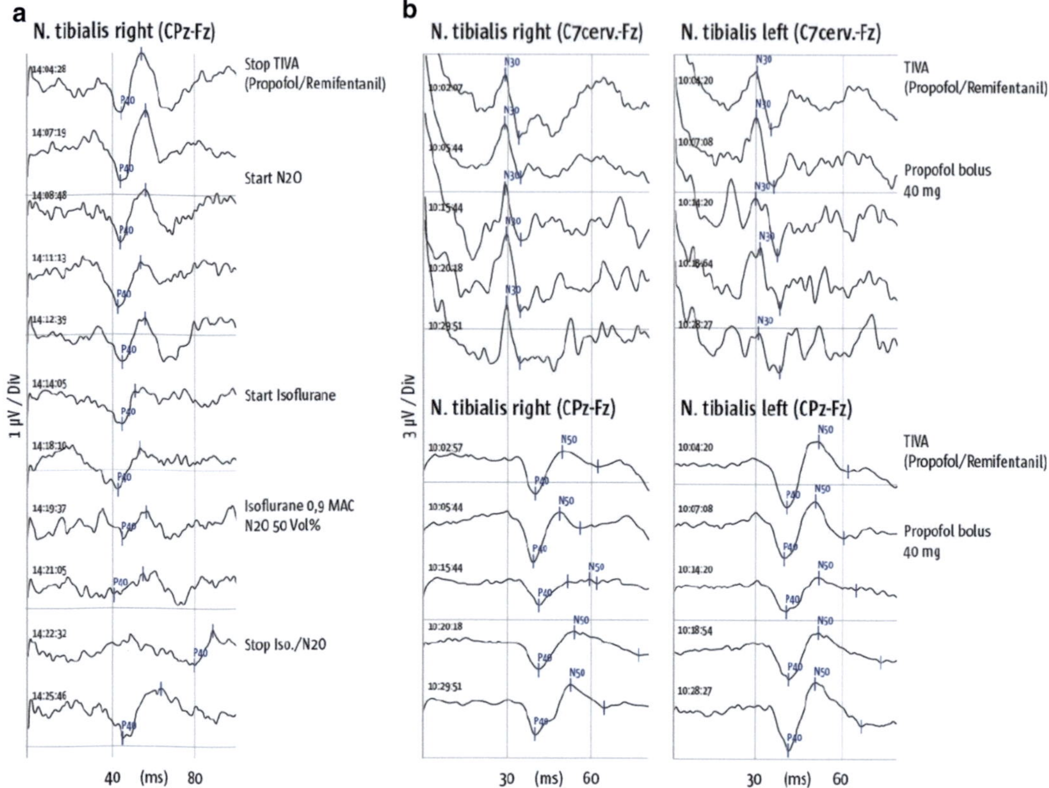

Fig. 7.4 Tibial nerve SEPs during isoflurane/N2O inhalation anesthesia (**a**) and total intravenous anesthesia (TIVA) with propofol and remifentanil (**b**) (Malcharek 2007, unpublished data). © ARKANA Forum GmbH 2022. All Rights Reserved

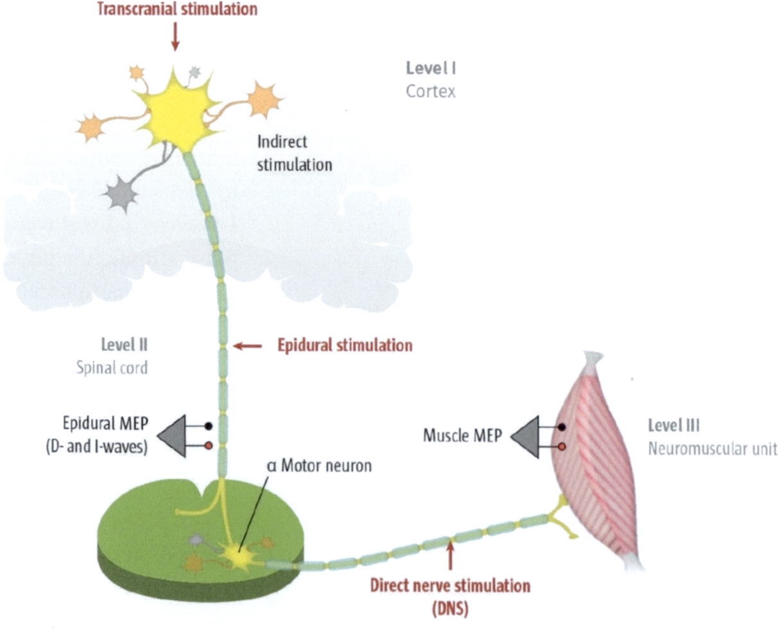

Fig. 7.5 Simplified representation of the different sites for triggering and recording MEPs and compound muscle action potentials in the course of the corticospinal pathway. © ARKANA Forum GmbH 2022. All Rights Reserved

larization threshold acting at GABA, glycine, or NMDA receptors, but simultaneously suppress activating higher-order (e.g., reticular formation) and local (e.g., somatosensory-motor reflex arches) influences. Overall, the depolarization threshold is increased. This increased depolarization threshold can usually only be overcome by a short series of electrical impulses (**multi-pulse or train technique**) [22]. In contrast to the triggering of D-waves, during anesthesia recordings peripheral to the spinal anterior horn require train stimulation.

Another phenomenon associated with an increase in the depolarization threshold of the α-motoneuron is the time-dependent accumulation of anesthetics ("anesthetic fade") (Fig. 7.6). This phenomenon leads to a gradual generalized reduction of MEP amplitudes and an increase in the intensity of stimulation or number of pulses necessary to generate stable MEPs, especially during prolonged surgery [23]. In clinical practice, such gradual changes must be distinguished from abrupt increases in the stimulation intensity associated with bolus administration of anesthetics.

For recordings from the **musculature (level III)** as the third component of the motor system, only the effect of **muscle relaxants** at the motor end plate has to be considered. Hypnotics or analgesics have almost no suppressive effect in this area. If muscle relaxants are being used, they should preferably be administered continuously and dosing monitored by relaxometry aiming at a **train-of-four** (**TOF**) value greater than two. If rocuronium-induced relaxation becomes inappropriately deep, it can quickly be reduced or abolished by the administration of sugammadex, which can quickly reduce or abolish the effects of non-depolarizing muscle relaxants. In particular, it antagonizes the effect of rocuronium by almost 100% in less than 5 min.

Overall, **TIVA** with propofol is most suitable for intraoperative MEP monitoring. After repetitive stimulation, well-defined MEPs can usually be obtained during TIVA in the absence of relaxation. Propofol anesthesia is preferable in patients with a pre-damaged pyramidal tract and associated impaired quality of baseline potentials. The dosage of propofol can be reduced when higher doses of opioids are administered because opioids at higher doses have an additional sedative effect. Reduction of the propofol dosage is also possible during adjuvant administration of ketamine [24, 25]. However, the known side effects of ketamine must be taken into account. Another drug that can be used to reduce the dosage of pro-

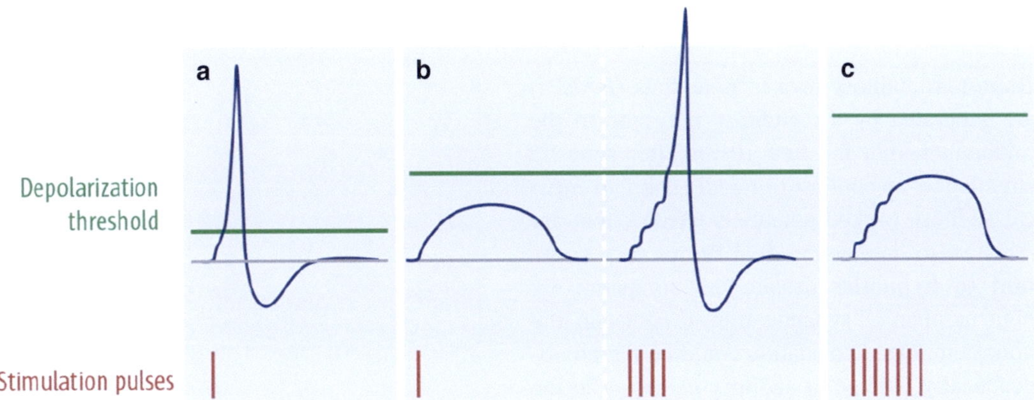

Fig. 7.6 Anesthetic fade: Change in depolarization threshold of the α- motoneuron and duration of anesthesia. Before induction of anesthesia (phase **a**), the α- motoneuron can be depolarized by a single stimulation pulse. After induction and during adequate maintenance of anesthesia (phase **b**), the α-motoneuron can only be depolarized with a pulse train. During deep anesthesia (phase **c**), depolarization of the α-motoneuron is not possible even using a longer pulse train. © ARKANA Forum GmbH 2022. All Rights Reserved

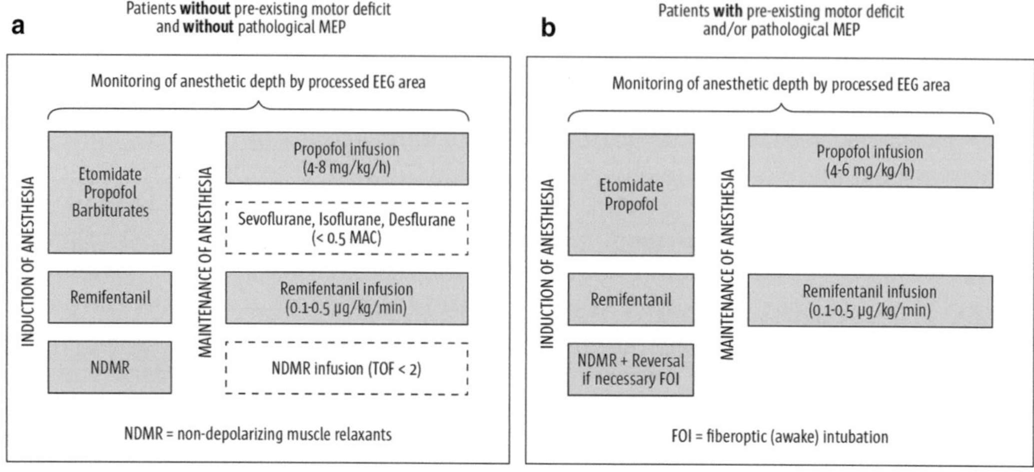

Fig. 7.7 Anesthetic regimen in patients without (**a**) and with (**b**) a pre-damaged pyramidal tract (Malcharek 2006, unpublished data). © ARKANA Forum GmbH 2022. All Rights Reserved

pofol is the selective alpha 2-adrenoceptor agonist dexmedetomidine. Balanced anesthesia with volatile anesthetics and nitrous oxide should be avoided in patients with a pre-damaged pyramidal tract. In neurologically intact patients, volatile anesthetics can safely be used in some, but not all patients. In any case, the minimum alveolar concentration (MAC) should not exceed 0.5–0.6 (Fig. 7.7).

7.2.4 Brainstem Auditory Evoked Potentials

Brainstem auditory evoked potentials (BAEPs) are generated by the auditory nerve up to the midbrain within the first 10 ms after acoustic stimulation. In contrast to middle and late cortical auditory evoked potentials (AEPs), that are sensitive to anesthetics, BAEPs are **very resistant to hypnotics** despite the comparatively high number of synaptic transmissions in the brainstem. One explanation could be the phylogenetically old age of auditory pathways in the brainstem and the importance of acoustic protective reflexes.

The BAEP can be reliably registered during **TIVA** or **inhalational anesthesia**, while subsequent AEPs may be completely suppressed by the same anesthetic regimen (Fig. 7.8).

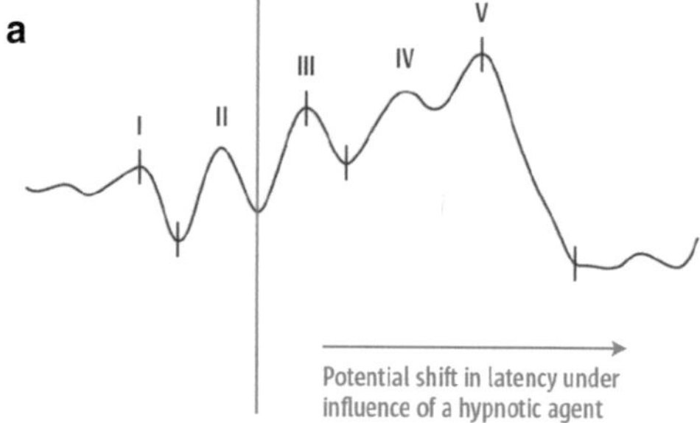

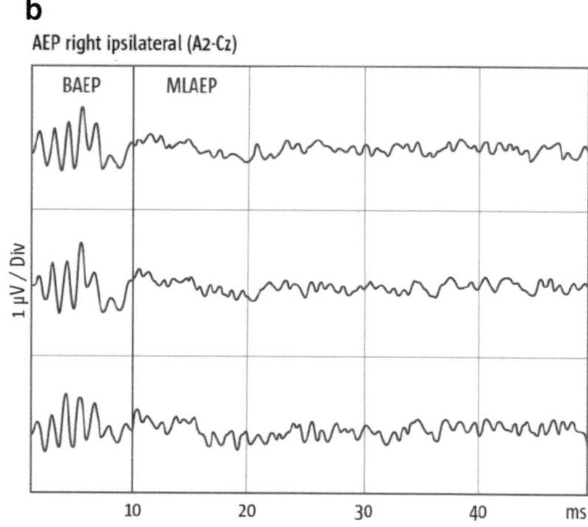

Fig. 7.8 The auditory evoked potential (AEP) and anesthesia. (**a**) Schematic representation of the effect of a volatile anesthetic or propofol on the pontine conduction time of BAEPs (Malcharek 2015, unpublished data); (**b**) Presence of the BAEP and absence of the middle latency AEP (MLAEP) under propofol anesthesia (Malcharek 2009, unpublished data). © ARKANA Forum GmbH 2022. All Rights Reserved

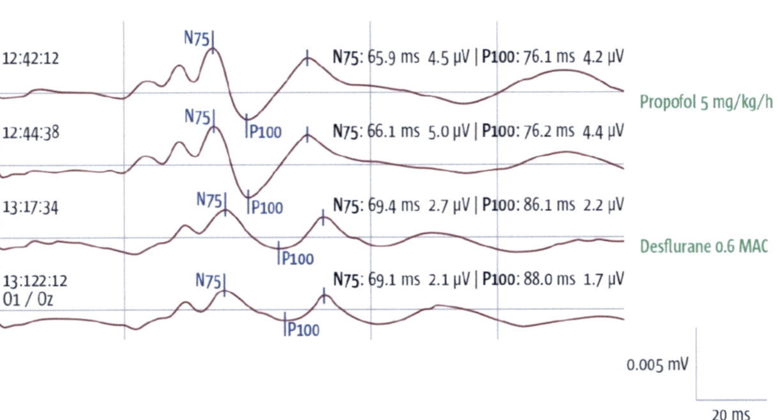

Fig. 7.9 Propofol versus desflurane for VEP monitoring (Malcharek 2015, unpublished data). The N75 and P100 labels used for convenience here do not correspond to pattern reversal VEP peaks in diagnostic laboratory testing. © ARKANA Forum GmbH 2022. All Rights Reserved

7.2.5 Visual Evoked Potentials

Several decades ago, it was assumed that visual evoked potentials (VEPs) are not recordable at all under general anesthesia [26]. However, with the introduction of TIVA based on propofol, intraoperative flash VEP monitoring has become feasible, although significant variations in amplitudes have been described [27].

Figure 7.9 demonstrates VEP amplitude reduction and latency prolongation after switching from propofol/remifentanil to desflurane/remifentanil anesthesia in a single patient without visual deficits. In addition, flash VEPs appear to vary more in terms of morphology, amplitude, and latency under volatile anesthetics compared with TIVA based on propofol. Thus, **TIVA with propofol** seems to be the preferred technique for intraoperative VEP monitoring.

7.3 Awake Craniotomy

Awake craniotomy is an intracranial surgical procedure during which the patient is kept awake and responsive for part of the surgery. It is mostly used for mapping of sensorimotor cortex and language areas, thereby reducing the risk of injuring functional tissue.

Surgical procedures under local anesthesia and sedation were introduced in epilepsy surgery at the beginning of the twentieth century. It was to facilitate localization of the seizure focus by intraoperative electrocorticography (ECoG), elicitation of habitual seizure patterns, and mapping of the sensorimotor cortex and language areas. At that time, electrophysiological and anesthetic techniques did not permit reliable recording of epileptic activity or mapping of eloquent areas under general anesthesia. By today, total intravenous anesthesia (TIVA) with propofol in combination with opioids provides adequate conditions for intraoperative ECoG and functional mapping and monitoring. For preoperative delineation of the language areas, subdural grid electrodes are implanted in a first procedure, and the epileptogenic area is resected in a subsequent procedure. Although current electrophysiologic and anesthetic techniques allow effective ECoG and mapping of the sensorimotor cortex during general anesthesia, awake craniotomy has been re-introduced during the past two decades, because it allows intraoperative localization of the language area without the need for prior placement of grid electrodes. However, awake craniotomy poses several challenges including appropriate selection and preparation of patients and adjustment of surgical and anesthetic management [28].

7.3.1 Patient Selection and Preparation

Optimal preoperative preparation is one of the main factors in determining the short- and long-term outcome of awake craniotomy. It includes appropriate patient selection and comprehensive preoperative patient preparation [29]. Patients eligible for awake surgery must be highly cooperative and motivated, while those with intellectual disability, communication deficits, anxiety, claustrophobia, psychiatric disorders, emotional instability, and age below 10 years are considered unsuitable. Relative contraindications for awake craniotomy include anticipated difficult airway management, obesity, gastroesophageal reflux, chronic cough, and obstructive sleep apnea. However, the only absolute contraindication to awake craniotomy is patient refusal.

Adequate preoperative patient preparation includes detailed explanation of the various aspects of the procedure, including positioning, drill-generated noise during craniotomy, insertion of an indwelling urinary catheter, and mapping-related tasks. The patient must be assured that each surgical intervention will be communicated before it is carried out, and that close communication with the surgeon and the anesthesiologist will be maintained throughout the procedure. This will alleviate the fear of an unanticipated painful event.

7.3.2 Patient Positioning and Monitoring

As the patient has to remain in the same position for several hours, optimal positioning on the operating table providing a comfortable and safe position is important. Most commonly, the supine, half-sitting, or lateral positions are used. To improve patient comfort and reduce the risk of nerve injury, soft pads are placed on the operating table. In particular, hard surfaces that may exert direct pressure to susceptible peripheral nerves are softly padded. Extensive flexion, inclination, or rotation of the head must be avoided because they may provoke airway obstruction and hinder airway intervention. Preferably, the head is fixed in a "sniffing" position. This reduces the risk of airway obstruction during sedation in the spontaneously breathing patient, particularly in the absence of a supraglottic airway device or an endotracheal tube. In addition, this position facilitates airway intervention if needed. Free view of

and access to the patient's face and extremities are important for patient safety, for reliable communication between patient and healthcare team, and for effective sensory, motor, and language testing.

Spontaneous respiration is maintained throughout the procedure and must be continuously monitored by a nasal CO_2 sampling cannula. Supplemental oxygen is provided by face mask or nasal cannula. If electrosurgery is used, care must be taken to limit the oxygen concentration at the operating site to avoid ignition of fire or explosion. Regular control of body temperature is mandatory to prevent cooling of the patient. Warmed blankets or, preferably, a forced air warming blanket are used to avoid a decrease in body temperature.

7.3.3 Scalp Nerve Blocks

Effective elimination of scalp sensation by regional anesthesia is a pivotal part of any awake craniotomy because it is essential for successful performance and patient satisfaction. Local anesthesia is frequently performed under light sedation, mainly with propofol and/or remifentanil. It can be achieved by either direct blockade of each of the six nerves that innervate the scalp (i.e., auriculotemporal, zygomaticotemporal, supraorbital, supratrochlear, greater occipital, and lesser occipital nerves) (Fig. 7.10) or by local anesthetic infiltration at the sites of surgical incision and placement of Mayfield head clamp pins. The direct nerve blocks are technically more demanding, but they require a lower volume of local anesthetic (approximately 40 ml) and provide a longer duration of analgesia. Usually, a mixture of long-acting local anesthetics (0.25% bupivacaine, 0.2% ropivacaine, and 0.25% levobupivacaine) is used and can provide sufficient analgesia for up to 8 h [30]. Additional intraoperative local infiltration of sensitive structures by the surgeon may intermittently be required. Epinephrine 1:200,000 is added to reduce systemic absorption and, thereby, the risk of systemic local anesthetic toxicity. Moreover, epinephrine reduces bleeding during skin incision and prolongs the duration of

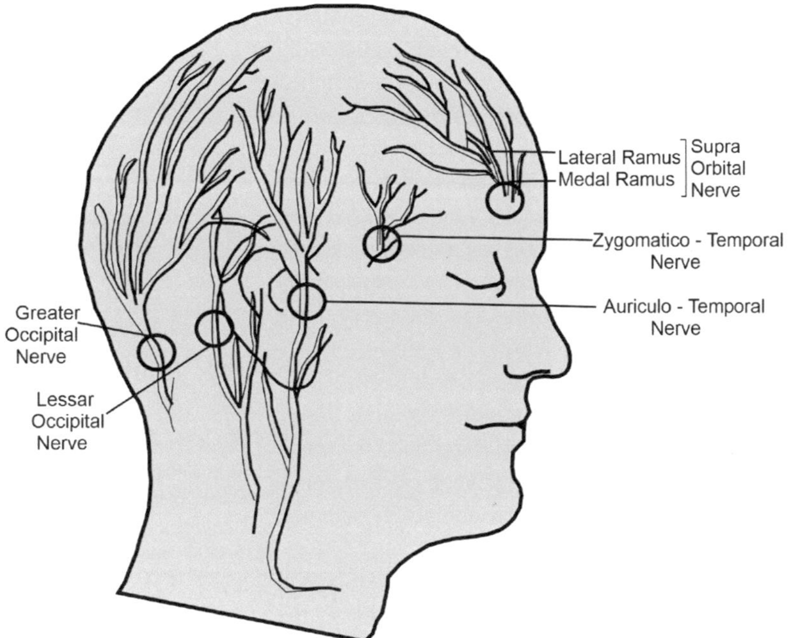

Fig. 7.10 The sites of injection of local anesthetics for block of scalp nerves. From [28], with permission

local anesthesia. To avoid systemic (hypertension, tachycardia) and local (skin necrosis) toxicity, the maximum recommended dose of the epinephrine component must be observed. Despite use of scalp nerve blocks and provision of sedation and analgesia by the anesthesiologist, pain remains the most common complaint during awake craniotomy.

7.3.4 Anesthetic Technique

Various anesthetic protocols for awake craniotomy are available. They can consist of a combination of local anesthesia and moderate sedation, or of a combination of local anesthesia and phases of general anesthesia and moderate sedation. The latter can be managed as asleep-awake-asleep (AAA) or asleep-awake technique. As the term suggests, the AAA technique consists of three phases, with periods of general anesthesia at the beginning and at the end and a period of consciousness in between which allows mapping and monitoring.

During phase 1 of the AAA technique, general anesthesia is administered. Shortly before phase 2, the depth of anesthesia is reduced to a degree of sedation which restores spontaneous respiration and responsiveness to verbal commands. At this time, the commonly used supraglottic airway device (rarely the endotracheal tube) is removed and electrophysiologic mapping and monitoring are started. At all times, the anesthesia team must be prepared to rapidly convert to general anesthesia, if the situation requires it. For phase 3, the patient is re-anesthetized and the airway device re-inserted.

The period of consciousness requires effective local anesthesia. It also requires that all operating room personnel behave with high sensitivity to the patient's awake state. At that time, there must be no casual chatting, and traffic in and out of the operating room should be reduced to prevent disturbing the patient or interfering with essential communication between the patient, surgeon, anesthesiologist, neuropsychologist, and neuromonitoring specialist.

Maintaining an appropriate level of sedation during awake craniotomy is a particular challenge for the anesthesiologist and requires considerable skill and experience. Oversedation may cause respiratory depression, airway obstruction, hypoxemia, and cardiovascular depression, while too little sedation may result in patient movement and anxiety. Sedation must not substantially impair the patient's ability to remain adequately responsive to verbal commands. Most commonly, a combination of propofol and remifentanil is used for sedation as a standard technique which, however, is associated with an increased risk of respiratory depression. Alternatively, sedation with the selective alpha-2-adrenoceptor agonist dexmedetomidine has high efficacy and safety during awake craniotomy and has very little effect on neuronal function. In addition, it provides anxiolysis and analgesia, reduces the sympathetic tone, and saves opioids. At low doses, respiratory and circulatory depression is rather unusual. These favorable characteristics make dexmedetomidine a rational choice for sedation during awake craniotomy.

In the past, the use of an endotracheal tube had been recommended for airway control during the asleep phases. In today's practice, however, the use of a supraglottic airway device is preferred. In experienced hands, the device is easy to insert, remove, and re-insert without the need to change the position of the patient and interrupt surgical activities. In addition, it facilitates transition from the asleep to the awake phase because lighter anesthesia is required. Furthermore, it is associated with a reduced risk of coughing and gagging on awakening.

7.3.5 Mapping

Intraoperative stimulation mapping aims at localizing language areas and the sensorimotor cortex. Cortical stimulation is accomplished by using a low-frequency stimulation pattern consisting of 25–60 Hz pulse trains lasting 1–4 s. The most commonly applied frequencies are 50 Hz (Europe) and 60 Hz (North America). For mapping of language areas, images of simple objects are shown to the patient at regular intervals. Cortical stimulation is applied prior to the presentation of each image and continued until there is a correct response or the next image is presented. Each preselected site is stimulated 3–4 times. Sites where stimulation provokes consistent speech arrest or anomia are considered to be

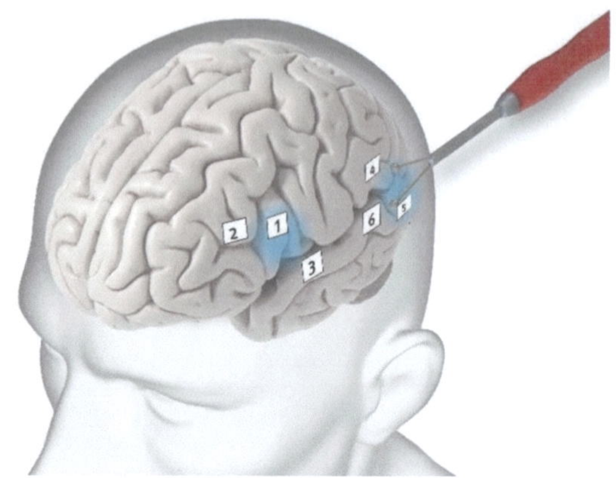

Fig. 7.11 Schematic illustration of intraoperative stimulation mapping of language areas during awake surgery. Using a bipolar fork probe, the area in question is scanned. Language area stimulation blocks speech function. 1–3: Broca's area; 4–6: Wernicke's area. © ARKANA Forum GmbH 2022. All Rights Reserved

essential to language function (Fig. 7.11). As for language areas, the motor and sensory cortex are stimulated using a similar stimulation pattern. Motor responses are observed, and the patient is asked to report sensory sensations. Stimulation of the cortex may cause seizures, particularly in the presence of focal lesions.

7.3.6 Evidence, Benefits, and Complications

Awake craniotomy can be expected to be advantageous when compared to craniotomy under general anesthesia because it should allow a greater extent of tumor resection at lower risk of neurological deficits such as motor and speech function damage [31]. However, randomized controlled trials comparing long-term outcomes following awake craniotomy vs. those following craniotomies under general anesthesia are lacking. The current supportive evidence in favor of awake craniotomy is mainly based on prospective cohort and retrospective chart reviews [32]. In a cohort study of 575 patients, awake craniotomy compared to craniotomy under general anesthesia was associated with a higher tumor resection rate in the eloquent area, lesser permanent neurological deficit, and fewer new-onset postoperative neurological deficits [33]. Additional benefits of awake craniotomy include reduced need of postoperative monitoring thereby shortening or eliminating intensive care unit stay, shorter hospital stays, and reduced postoperative pain, nausea, and vomiting [34].

Although such benefits were not consistently documented by other studies [32], awake craniotomy with brain mapping is considered by some the treatment of choice for resections of brain tumors or lesions in or near eloquent areas of the brain [35–38]. However, even if awake craniotomy is considered the treatment of choice for specific procedures, addressing the lack of randomized controlled trials unequivocally documenting the long-term benefit of awake craniotomy vs. craniotomy under general anesthesia, and explaining the rationale for recommending awake craniotomy, could well be considered an integral part of the preoperative consultation for ethical reasons [39].

Most frequent intraoperative complications of awake craniotomy include seizures (mostly occurring during stimulation for brain mapping), hypertension (mostly caused by pain, agitation, and anxiety, more rarely by hypoxemia and hypercarbia), nausea and vomiting (usually caused by opioids, anxiety, or surgical stimulation), and respiratory problems (e.g., hypoxemia and hypercarbia caused by airway obstruction secondary to oversedation). Seizure activity is effectively treated by irrigation of the brain with sterile cold (4 °C) isotonic saline or Ringer's solution. If ineffective, bolus doses of propofol or midazolam should be administered. Nausea and vomiting are treated by ondansetron, dexamethasone, and low-dose propofol. In the case of hypertension, the underlying cause needs to be taken care of. Relief of airway obstruction may require decrease in the depth of sedation, insertion of an oral or nasopharyngeal airway, or assisted ventilation via a supraglottic airway device. Failed awake craniotomy (defined as need or conversion to general anesthesia or inadequate mapping or monitoring) occurred on average in 2% of awake craniotomies [40].

7.3.7 Summary

In summary, awake craniotomy has experienced a renaissance during the past years and has become an accepted technique for various neurosurgical interventions. This renaissance has been facilitated by remarkable progress in anesthetic techniques. The choice of a specific anesthetic regimen for awake craniotomy largely depends on the preference of the individual anesthesiologist. Special expertise is required to assure patient comfort and successful management. Effective local anesthesia and smooth and predictable transition from unconsciousness to a cooperative state remain major challenges. The importance of a sensitive and experienced multidisciplinary operating room team (i.e., surgeons, anesthesiologists, neuromonitoring specialists, and nurses) for successful awake craniotomy cannot be overemphasized. As the procedural demands are considerable, awake craniotomy should be restricted to centers highly experienced in this technique. Informed patient consent must be based on a thorough preoperative discussion between patient, neurosurgeon, and neuroanesthesiologist addressing in detail benefits, complications, and the stages of awake craniotomy.

7.4 Test Questions

1. What are the three main components goals of general anesthesia?
2. Which of the drugs commonly used to induce and maintain the various components of general anesthesia are best suited during intraoperative use of IONM? What are their respective advantages?
3. What does the term TIVA mean, and what is the relevance of TIVA during IONM?
4. Which anesthetics should not be used during application of IONM, and for what reasons?
5. Which IONM modalities are affected by muscle relaxants and which are not? Provide reasons for your statement.
6. What are three possible mechanisms of action of anesthetics?

7. Which main groups of receptors are important in the differentiation of hypnotics?
8. On which receptors do analgesics act and when do they affect IONM signals?
9. The processed EEG is used to control the depth of anesthesia. What substances show typical EEG patterns after induction and during maintenance of general anesthesia?
10. What EEG frequency bands can be observed during induction of anesthesia (transition from patient awake with the eyes closed to deep anesthesia) and which method can be used to monitor depth of anesthesia?
11. How do the effects on SEPs differ between volatile anesthetics and propofol?
12. What is the effect of etomidate on SEPs?
13. What types of intraoperative MEP stimulation are available?
14. Where can MEP signals be recorded? List specific features/advantages of each method.
15. Why must train (multi-pulse) stimulation be used for MEP recordings from target muscles?
16. What is meant by "anesthetic fade"?
17. Which substance influences EMG recordings after stimulation of a peripheral nerve? In contrast to MEP signals, which substances have no effect on EMG?
18. What effect do anesthetics have on the recording of AEPs?
19. What differences in flash VEP signal quality may exist between different anesthetic regimens (e.g., TIVA with propofol/remifentanil versus inhalation anesthesia with desflurane/remifentanil)?

References

1. Alkire MT, Hudetz AG, Tononi G. Consciousness and anesthesia. Science. 2008;322(5903):876–80.
2. Nelson LE, Lu J, Guo T, Saper CB, Franks NP, Maze M. The alpha2-adrenoceptor agonist dexmedetomidine converges on an endogenous sleep-promoting pathway to exert its sedative effects. Anesthesiology. 2003;98(2):428–36.
3. Veselis RA, Feshchenko VA, Reinsel RA, Dnistrian AM, Beattie B, Akhurst TJ. Thiopental and propofol affect different regions of the brain at similar pharmacologic effects. Anesth Analg. 2004;99(2):399–408.
4. Kalkman CJ, Drummond JC, Ribberink AA, Patel PM, Sano T, Bickford RG. Effects of propofol, etomidate, midazolam, and fentanyl on motor evoked responses to transcranial electrical or magnetic stimulation in humans. Anesthesiology. 1992;76(4):502–9.
5. Laureau E, Marciniak B, Hébrard A, Herbaux B, Guieu JD. Comparative study of propofol and midazolam effects on somatosensory evoked potentials during surgical treatment of scoliosis. Neurosurgery. 1999;45(1):69–75.
6. Sloan TB, Fugina ML, Toleikis JR. Effects of midazolam on median nerve somatosensory evoked potentials. Br J Anaesth. 1990;64(5):590–3.
7. Sloan TB, Jäntti V. Anesthetic effects on evoked potentials. In: Nuwer MR, editor. Intraoperative monitoring of neural function. Amsterdam: Elsevier; 2009. p. 94–126.
8. Freye E, Brückner J, Latasch L. No difference in electroencephalographic power spectra or sensory-evoked potentials in patients anaesthetized with desflurane or sevoflurane. Eur J Anaesthesiol. 2004;21(5):373–8.
9. Thornton C, Creagh-Barry P, Jordan C, Luff NP, Doré CJ, Henley M, et al. Somatosensory and auditory evoked responses recorded simultaneously: differential effects of nitrous oxide and isoflurane. Br J Anaesth. 1992;68(5):508–14.
10. Anschel DJ, Aherne A, Soto RG, Carrion W, Hoegerl C, Nori P, et al. Successful intraoperative spinal cord monitoring during scoliosis surgery using a total intravenous anesthetic regimen including dexmedetomidine. J Clin Neurophysiol. 2008;25(1):56–61.
11. Wagner RL, White PF. Etomidate inhibits adrenocortical function in surgical patients. Anesthesiology. 1984;61(6):647–51.
12. Wagner RL, White PF, Kan PB, Rosenthal MH, Feldman D. Inhibition of adrenal steroidogenesis by the anesthetic etomidate. N Engl J Med. 1984;310(22):1415–21.
13. Boisseau N, Madany M, Staccini P, Armando G, Martin F, Grimaud D, et al. Comparison of the effects of sevoflurane and propofol on cortical somatosensory evoked potentials. Br J Anaesth. 2002;88(6):785–9.
14. Ku ASW, Hu Y, Irwin MG, Chow B, Gunawardene S, Tan EE, et al. Effect of sevoflurane/nitrous oxide versus propofol anaesthesia on somatosensory evoked potential monitoring of the spinal cord during surgery to correct scoliosis. Br J Anaesth. 2002;88(4):502–7.
15. Schaney CR, Sanders J, Kuhn P, LaJohn S, Heard C. Nitrous oxide with propofol reduces somatosensory-evoked potential amplitude in children and adolescents. Spine. 2005;30(6):689–93.
16. Chen Z. The effects of isoflurane and propofol on intraoperative neurophysiological monitoring during spinal surgery. J Clin Monit Comput. 2004;18(4):303–8.
17. Clapcich AJ, Emerson RG, Roye DP, Xie H, Gallo EJ, Dowling KC, et al. The effects of propofol, small-dose isoflurane, and nitrous oxide on cortical somatosensory evoked potential and bispectral index monitoring in adolescents undergoing spinal fusion. Anesth Analg. 2004:1334–40.

18. Fletcher J, Clarke C, Bailey A, Georges L. The effect of desflurane and propofol, at a BIS of 60, on the somatosensory evoked potential. In: Anesthesiology® Annual Meeting; 2005 Oct 22 [cited 2017 Jul 25]. Available from: http://w.asaabstracts.com/strands/asaabstracts/abstract.htm?year=2005&index=4&absnum=356

19. Liu EHC. Effects of isoflurane and propofol on cortical somatosensory evoked potentials during comparable depth of anaesthesia as guided by bispectral index. Br J Anaesth. 2005;94(2):193–7.

20. Hicks RG, Woodforth IJ, Crawford MR, Stephen JP, Burke DJ. Some effects of isoflurane on I waves of the motor evoked potential. Br J Anaesth. 1992;69(2):130–6.

21. Woodforth IJ, Hicks RG, Crawford MR, Stephen JPH, Burke D. Depression of I waves in corticospinal volleys by sevoflurane, thiopental, and propofol. Anesth Analg. 1999;89(5):1182–7.

22. Pechstein U, Ceclzich C, Nadstawek J, Schramm J. Transcranial high-frequency repetitive electrical stimulation for recording myogenic motor evoked potentials with the patient under general anesthesia. Neurosurgery. 1996;39(2):335–44.

23. Lyon R, Feiner J, Lieberman JA. Progressive suppression of motor evoked potentials during general anesthesia: the phenomenon of "anesthetic fade". J Neurosurg Anesthesiol. 2005;17(1):13–9.

24. Erb TO, Ryhult SE, Duitmann E, Hasler C, Luetschg J, Frei FJ. Improvement of motor-evoked potentials by ketamine and spatial facilitation during spinal surgery in a young child. Anesth Analg. 2005;100(6):1634–6.

25. Inoue S, Kawaguchi M, Kakimoto M, Sakamoto T, Kitaguchi K, Furuya H, et al. Amplitudes and intrapatient variability of myogenic motor evoked potentials to transcranial electrical stimulation during ketamine/N$_2$O- and propofol/N$_2$O-based anesthesia. J Neurosurg Anesthesiol. 2002;14(3):213–7.

26. Cedzich C, Schramm J, Mengedoht CF, Fahlbusch R. Factors that limit the use of flash visual evoked potentials for surgical monitoring. Electroencephalogr Clin Neurophysiol Potentials Sect. 1988;71(2):142–5.

27. Halliday AM. The visual evoked potential in healthy subjects. In: Halliday AM, editor. Evoked potentials in clinical testing. 2nd ed. Edinburgh: Churchill Livingstone; 1993. (Clinical neurology and neurosurgery monographs).

28. Girvin JP. Operative techniques in epilepsy. Cham: Springer International Publishing; 2015. https://doi.org/10.1007/978-3-319-10921-3.

29. Potters J-W, Klimek M. Awake craniotomy: improving the patient's experience. Curr Opin Anaesthesiol. 2015;28(5):511–6.

30. Osborn I, Sebeo J. "Scalp block" during craniotomy: a classic technique revisited. J Neurosurg Anesthesiol. 2010;22(3):187–94.

31. Kim SH, Choi SH. Anesthetic considerations for awake craniotomy. Anesth Pain Med. 2020;15:269–74.

32. Brown T, Shah AH, Bregy A, Shah NH, Thambuswamy M, Barbarite E, et al. Awake craniotomy for brain tumor resection: the rule rather than the exception? J Neurosurg Anesthesiol. 2013;25:240–7.

33. Sacko O, Lauwers-Cances V, Brauge D, Sesay M, Brenner A, Roux FE. Awake craniotomy vs surgery under general anesthesia for resection of supratentorial lesions. Neurosurgery. 2011;68:1192–8. discussion 1198–9

34. Manninen PH, Tan TK. Postoperative nausea and vomiting after craniotomy for tumor surgery: a comparison between awake craniotomy and general anesthesia. J Clin Anesth. 2002;14(4):279–83.

35. Kayama T. Guidelines committee of the Japan awake surgery conference : the guidelines for awake craniotomy guidelines committee of the Japan awake surgery conference. Neurol Med Chir (Tokyo). 2012;52:119–41.

36. Eseonu CI, Rincon-Torroella J, ReFaey K, Lee YM, Nangiana J, Vivas-Buitrago T, et al. Awake craniotomy vs craniotomy under general anesthesia for perirolandic gliomas: evaluating perioperative complications and extent of resection. Neurosurgery. 2017;81:481–9.

37. Gerritsen JKW, Arends L, Klimek M, Dirven CMF, Vincent AJE. Impact of intraoperative stimulation mapping on high-grade glioma surgery outcome: a meta-analysis. Acta Neurochir. 2019;161:99–107.

38. Singh K, Dua A. Anesthesia for awake craniotomy. In: StatPearls. Treasure Island, FL: StatPearls Publishing; 2023.

39. Kirsch B, Bernstein M. Ethical challenges with awake craniotomy for tumor. Can J Neurol Sci J Can Sci Neurol. 2012;39(1):78–82.

40. Nossek E, Matot I, Shahar T, Barzilai O, Rapoport Y, Gonen T, Sela G, Korn A, Hayat D, Ram Z. Failed awake craniotomy: a retrospective analysis in 424 patients undergoing craniotomy for brain tumor. J Neurosurg. 2013;118(2):243–9.

Application of Intraoperative Neuromonitoring

8

David MacDonald, Barbara Bischoff, and Josef Zentner

Contents

D. MacDonald (✉)
ARKANA Forum GmbH, Emmendingen, Germany

B. Bischoff
Department of Neurosurgery, Sozialstiftung Bamberg, Bamberg, Germany

J. Zentner
Department of Neurosurgery, University Medical Center, Freiburg, Germany

8.1 Interpretation of the Potential Findings

The response signals generated during IONM are mainly assessed on the basis of their **amplitude** and **latency**. There are no normal control values for the anesthetic state, but typical intraoperative values in patients undergoing surgery can be found in Chap. 5. The following paragraphs concern basic aspects of interpreting the signals in the context of non-surgical and surgical influences. More detailed information is available in the respective specialist literature.

With respect to non-surgical influences on potentials, it should first be noted that signal

© The Author(s), under exclusive license to Springer Nature Switzerland AG 2024
J. Zentner et al. (eds.), *Intraoperative Neuromonitoring*,
https://doi.org/10.1007/978-3-031-46125-5_8

latency can depend on **body size**. Thus, somatosensory evoked potential (SEP) and motor evoked potential (MEP) latencies increase with patient height and limb length. Also, brainstem auditory evoked potential (BAEP) and visual evoked potential (VEP) mean latencies are somewhat longer in men than in women due to larger average head circumference. Second, systemic factors such as **anesthesia**, **body temperature**, and **blood pressure** must be considered. Some anesthetics have a significant influence on potentials, even bolus application of agents that exert only a little effect per se. As body temperature decreases, axonal conduction velocity decreases by 1–2 m/s per °C, thus latency increases. Hypotension below a patient's lower limit of autoregulation can reduce evoked potential amplitudes due to nervous system ischemia, and even modest blood pressure reduction can cause evoked potential deterioration in patients with impaired autoregulation. Third, changes in potentials may be due to **technical influences**, such as in adequate electrode contact, high impedance, or displacement of the monitored structures after surgical debulking.

After stabilization of anesthesia and before surgery begins, the **initial baseline values** are registered. Thereafter, the evolution of the potentials over time is observed during the operation, especially during the decisive surgical steps. It may be necessary to **reset baselines** after surgical opening or after encountering generalized "baseline drift." One then looks for signal deterioration that might signify a risk of neurologic injury due to surgical influences. Here, it is necessary to decide which alterations of the potentials are considered acceptable and which are attributed a pathological significance. It seems obvious that **irreversible disappearance** of a previously stable potential is important and predictive of a serious neurological deficit. Conversely, **reversible disappearance or deterioration** with signal restoration after intervention can suggest but not prove injury prevention or mitigation. Less obvious, on the other hand, is the significance of **irreversible deterioration** of a still-present signal that persists to the end of the surgery.

In order to interpret surgery-related signal deterioration, **critical limit values** must be defined, i.e., values for amplitude reduction or latency prolongation that allow a statement to be made as to whether the monitored structures are at risk or not. Since absolute limits do not exist, they have to be defined empirically relative to the patient's most recent baselines. According to general experience, signal alterations within the limits should be associated with an uneventful neurological outcome, whereas additional neurological deficits must be expected with signal deterioration beyond the critical limits.

In **clinical practice**, 50% **amplitude reduction** is a generally accepted limit for BAEPs and VEPs, as well as D-waves when applied to spinal cord monitoring. It is also a traditional limit for SEPs, but it is advisable to adjust the SEP amplitude reduction limit according to observed reproducibility [1]. Muscle MEP limit values are controversial due to the intrinsically high variability and sensitivity of these potentials. Certainly, MEP disappearance is always a major limit and is often the first pathological sign. However, 50% MEP amplitude reduction is an appropriate critical limit for brain, brainstem, and cranial nerve monitoring, while an 80% reduction limit is applicable to spinal cord monitoring. Note that the reduction must exceed trial-to-trial amplitude variability to be relevant. In addition, various stimulation **threshold elevation** limits have been proposed for muscle MEPs [2].

Latency prolongation often accompanies amplitude reduction and can be another limit value, but is generally less important. This is because an intraoperative damage causes acute neuronal or axonal failure that mainly reduces amplitude, while demyelination that mainly prolongs latency is a subacute or chronic process that does not develop during surgery. Still, ≥ 1 ms latency delay is relevant for BAEPs, and $\geq 10\%$ latency prolongation is a traditional limit for SEPs, but only with concurrent amplitude reduction.

Signal deterioration beyond the empirical limits must generally be considered critical. However, the interpretation also depends on the modality used, the signal quality, and the examination conditions. It is not so much the absolute values that are important, but rather the dynamics of signal alterations during the course of surgery. In principle, the more rapidly a well-defined potential deteriorates, the greater the significance with regard to the expected postoperative neurological status.

The empirically defined limit values serve as **warning** or **intervention criteria** for the surgeon. At the latest when the limit values are exceeded, the surgeon must be warned with regard to impending neurological deficits. As a consequence, the surgeon must try to intervene in an adequate way to reverse both the signal deterioration and the associated functional impairment. Appropriate measures may include undoing recent surgical maneuvers, changing the dissection site, reducing the spatula traction, or simply pausing the dissection.

Definition of the warning criteria is important to the reliability and value of monitoring. Excessively sensitive limits will cause numerous **false positives**. Here, the surgeon is inappropriately warned of minor signal alteration irrelevant to neurological outcome. Consequently, a surgeon confused by the monitoring may terminate the procedure too early, leaving the patient with suboptimal surgical treatment. Furthermore, as in Aesop's fable about crying wolf, a surgeon jaded by too many false positives may eventually fail to intervene for truly pathologic deterioration, with disastrous consequences for the patient.

On the other hand, overly specific limits risk **false negatives**. Here, the signal deterioration is inappropriately considered acceptable, while a neurological deficit is present postoperatively. False negatives are dangerous because the surgeon believes the patient to be in a state of supposed safety and assumes that the surgical steps to this point have been harmless. In principle, the choice of limit values and the interpretation of signal deterioration should be done in such a way that false negatives are extremely rare, while false positives are more acceptable but must not become excessive.

Understanding that warning criteria represent empirical values that are ultimately arbitrarily determined and that it is not the absolute values, but rather the dynamics of signal alterations in the course of surgery that matter, **communication** between the monitoring team and the surgeon is of particular importance. The surgeon must inform the monitoring team about the essential surgical steps to ensure rapid monitoring feedback during critical phases of the operation. Conversely, the monitoring team must keep the surgeon informed about critical signal deterioration and its response to intervention.

Overall, various aspects must be taken into account when interpreting the monitoring results. The efficacy of IONM depends on the qualification of the monitoring team and effective communication with the surgical and anesthesia staff.

8.2 IONM in Neurosurgery

8.2.1 Brain Tumors

Brain tumors originate from the brain tissue or meninges (**primary brain tumors**) or arise outside the brain and grow as metastases in the brain (**secondary brain tumors**). Depending on their pathologic characteristics and growth behavior, brain tumors are usually classified into World Health Organization (WHO) grades of I to IV, with WHO grade I tumors (e.g., pilocytic astrocytoma) showing a benign course, while WHO grade IV tumors (e.g., glioblastoma) are malignant and grow rapidly. Brain tumors can become symptomatic by causing focal neurological deficits and/or signs of increased intracranial pressure. In principle, the complete removal of the tumor represents the best prerequisite for a favorable course of the disease. The major obstacle in surgical treatment is that tumors often involve functionally important areas (motor cortex, language areas, etc.). These areas, however, must be spared to avoid postoperative neurological deficits.

The aim of electrophysiological techniques in tumor surgery is the identification (**mapping**) and the control (**monitoring**) of functionally relevant areas. Impairment of potentials and function can result from direct surgical manipulation and indirectly from pressure or spatula traction. The choice of IONM modalities and methods depends on the location of the tumor and the planned surgical approach. For example, the median nerve **SEP phase reversal** is useful for localizing the central sulcus, **MEPs** can be elicited by both transcranial and direct cortical stimulation, and use of the monopolar stimulation through the tip of the surgical suction device during resection facilitates continuous (dynamic) mapping and monitoring of the pyramidal tract (see also Sect. 8.2.3).

During transcranial stimulation, care must be taken to ensure that patient movements from triggered muscle contractions do not interfere with the surgical procedure. Furthermore, it should be kept in mind that monitoring may be disturbed during the use of certain surgical devices, such as the electrosurgery unit or the cavitron ultrasonic surgical aspirator. In addition, during motor stimulation, the monitoring team should be alert to the appearance of prolonged muscle responses, which may be indicative of an epileptic seizure. Usually, seizures can be quickly resolved by irrigation of the cortex with cold (4 °C) saline or Ringer's solution.

Case Example: Astrocytoma
Clinical Setting:

The patient presented with medically intractable epilepsy after incomplete resection of a left frontodorsal WHO grade II astrocytoma in a previous surgery. Brain magnetic resonance imaging (MRI) showed tumor recurrence (Fig. 8.1). The follow-up surgery aimed at complete removal of the tumor with IONM guidance.

Procedure and Monitoring:

After opening the dura mater, the **median nerve SEP phase reversal** was examined with a subdural strip electrode to localize the central sulcus and by deduction the precentral motor gyrus (Fig. 8.2). The same electrode was then applied for direct cortical triggering of **muscle MEPs** that remained stable during surgery (Fig. 8.3) [4–8]. The patient had a postoperative supplementary motor area syndrome that eventually resolved completely. Figure 8.4 shows the result of reoperation on postoperative MRI.

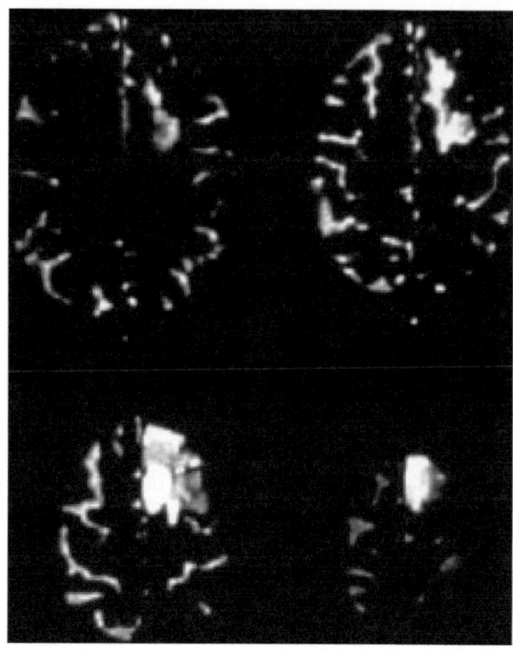

Fig. 8.1 Preoperative MRI showing a recurrent left frontodorsal astrocytoma. From [3], with permission

Case Example: Right Frontal Brain Tumor
Clinical Setting:

The patient presented with medically controlled seizures and no neurologic deficit. Neuroimaging showed a right frontal tumor encroaching on the suspected motor gyrus. The surgical plan was total lesion removal with IONM guidance.

Procedure and Monitoring:

After craniotomy and dural opening, left median nerve cortical SEPs were recorded from a 6-contact subdural strip electrode placed at a right angle across the putative central sulcus. This showed a phase reversal suggesting that the central sulcus was between electrodes 4 (negative, presumably postcentral) and 5 (positive, presumably precentral). By inference, electrode 5 should have been nearest to the primary motor gyrus. However, direct cortical stimulation through the same contacts produced lowest thenar MEP threshold at electrode 4, showing that it was closest to primary motor cortex instead (Fig. 8.5). This enabled the surgeon to proceed with complete tumor removal, which would have been compromised had the SEP result been accepted. Thus, it is advisable to follow cortical SEP map-

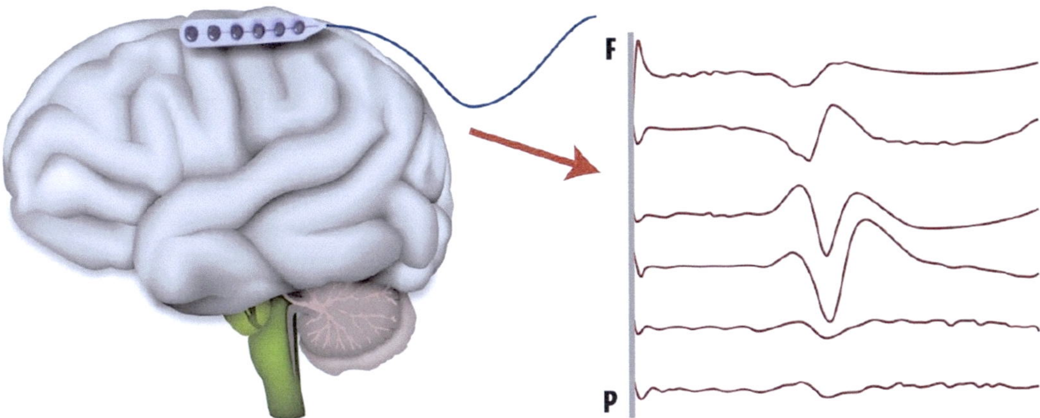

Fig. 8.2 Schematic representation of the median nerve SEP phase reversal. After stimulation of the right median nerve, SEPs were recorded from all contacts of the strip electrode. The site of phase reversal (arrow) corresponds to the central sulcus. By inference, this also suggests the precentral motor gyrus. F, frontal; P, parietal.© ARKANA Forum GmbH 2022. All Rights Reserved

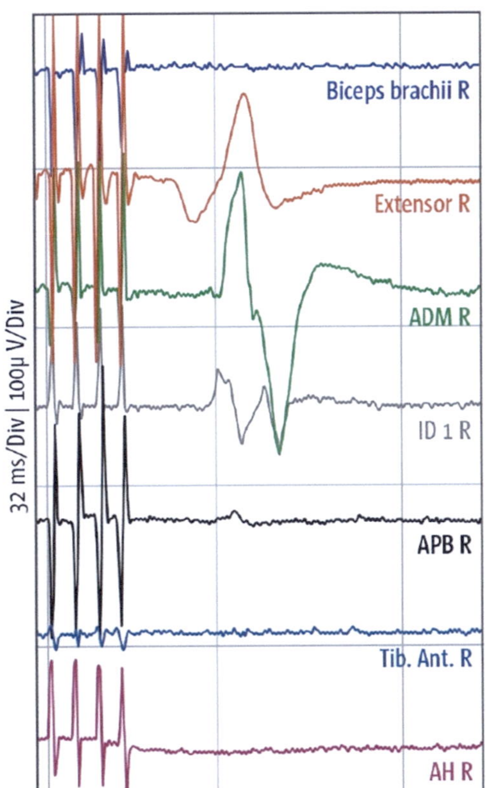

Fig. 8.3 Muscle MEP monitoring during the removal of the recurrent tumor shown in Fig. 8.1. Stimulation was performed via the appropriate contact of the strip electrode used to determine the median nerve SEP phase reversal. Extensor, extensor digitorum muscle; ADM, abductor digiti minimi muscle; ID1, first dorsal interosseus muscle; APB, abductor pollicis brevis muscle; Tib. Ant., tibialis anterior muscle; AH, abductor hallucis muscle; R, right. © ARKANA Forum GmbH 2022. All Rights Reserved

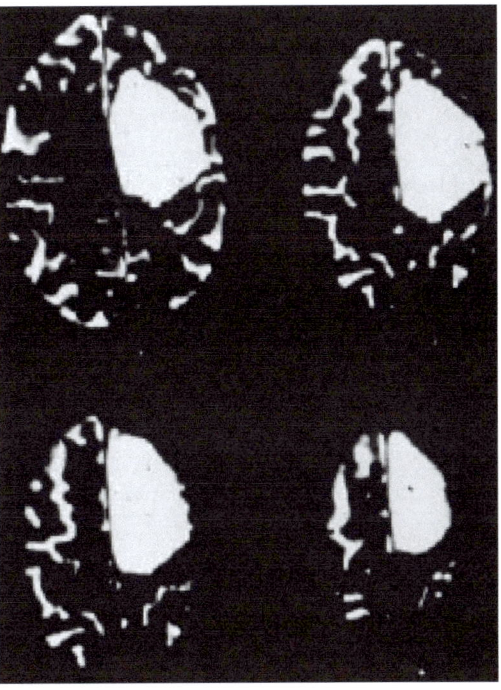

Fig. 8.4 Postoperative MRI. The tumor had been completely removed up to the precentral sulcus. From [3], with permission

ping with MEP mapping whenever primary motor cortex localization is critical. Monitoring of left arm and leg MEPs by interleaved 0.5 Hz cortical stimulation at the site of electrode 4 and at the leg area of the same gyrus produced stable potentials throughout surgery (Fig. 8.6). The patient had no postoperative motor deficit.

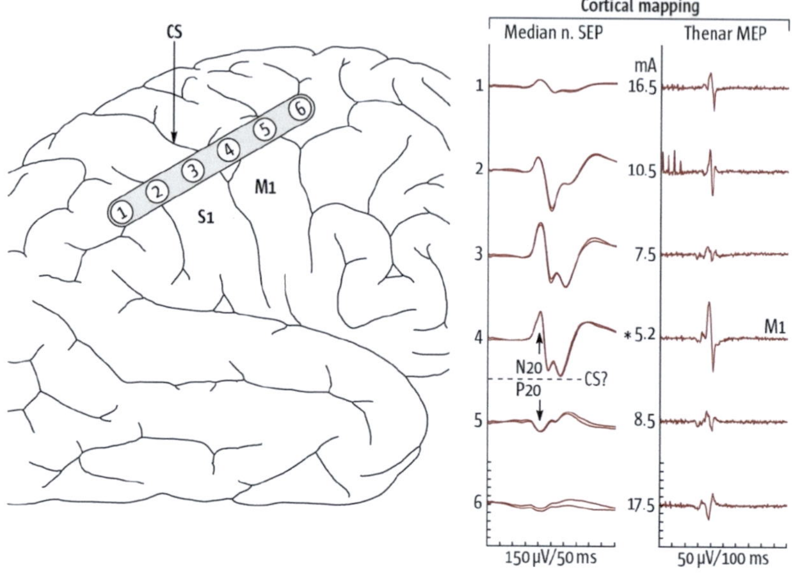

Fig. 8.5 Discrepant cortical mapping. Median nerve (n.) cortical SEPs implied that electrode 5 was on the primary motor gyrus (M1), but lowest thenar MEP threshold (*) in mA showed that electrode 4 was actually closest to M1. CS, central sulcus; S1, primary sensory gyrus. Modified from [1], with permission

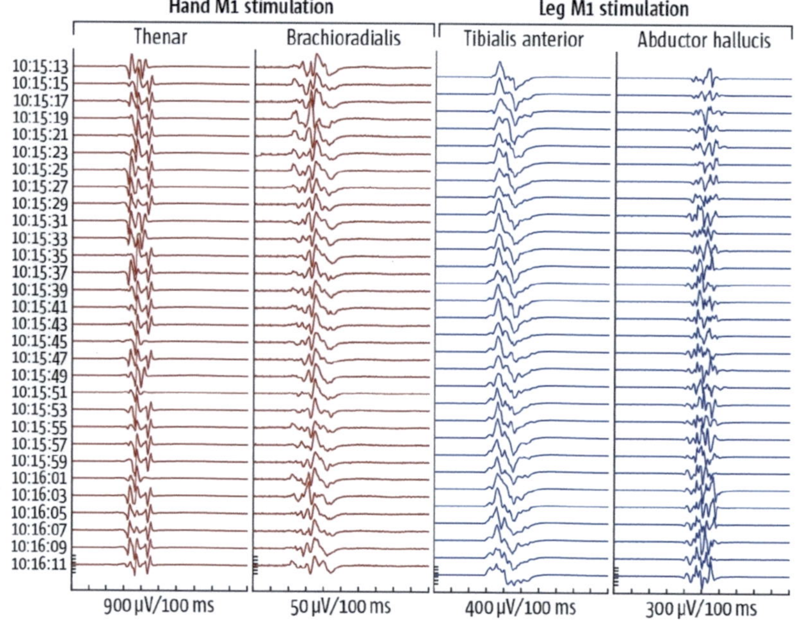

Fig. 8.6 A segment of interleaved left arm and leg direct cortical stimulation MEP monitoring during right frontal tumor resection. Hand area stimulation was done at the site of electrode 4 in Fig. 8.5. M1, primary motor gyrus.© ARKANA Forum GmbH 2022. All Rights Reserved

8.2.2 Vascular Diseases

Intracranial **aneurysms** and **arteriovenous malformations** are of particular importance in vascular neurosurgery. They are congenital malformations that enlarge over the course of years due to the constant blood flow and can eventually rupture to cause life-threatening **intracranial hemorrhage**. Aneurysms arise from a weakness of the muscular layer in the vessel wall; they are usually localized at the branching of large cerebral arteries at the brain base. Rupture of an aneurysm results in subarachnoid hemorrhage, which manifests in sudden-onset headache and neck stiffness (meningism). Arteriovenous malformations are pathologic short circuits between arteries and veins. They are fed by one or more arteries and drain into superficial and/or deep veins. Their rupture leads to intracerebral hemorrhage.

Treatment options include neuroradiological intervention (e.g., endovascular coiling) and microsurgery (e.g., clipping, resection). However, either approach may inadvertently result in occlusion of a vessel important for the supply of an eloquent brain area.

Electrophysiological techniques aim to monitor sensory and motor pathways with **SEPs** and **MEPs** of the upper and/or lower extremities, depending on the vascular territory involved. Of particular importance for the monitoring team in the context of vascular procedures is the quick detection of evoked potential deterioration, especially after the placement of a temporary or permanent clip. Only this gives the surgeon adequate time to react (e.g., by removing and repositioning the clip) before infarction ensues and thus to prevent a postoperative neurological deficit (Fig. 8.7) [9–12]. After placement of the permanent clip for definitive elimination of the vascular malformation, close attention must be paid to the further signal course for at least 8–10 minutes.

Case Example: Aneurysm
Clinical Setting:

The patient presented with **subarachnoid hemorrhage** confirmed by brain CT (Fig. 8.8). Cerebral angiography demonstrated an aneurysm at the bifurcation of the left middle cerebral artery. Surgical treatment aimed at the elimination of the aneurysm by clipping, with IONM guidance.

Procedure and Monitoring:

The surgery proceeded in a standard fashion while monitoring bilateral median and tibial nerve **SEPs** (Fig. 8.9) and upper and lower limb **MEPs** (Fig. 8.10). The contralateral potentials were monitors, while ipsilateral potentials served as controls. Stable potentials throughout the procedure indicated an uneventful outcome. Considering the affected middle cerebral artery territory, it would have been sufficient to monitor only upper limb evoked potentials in this case.

8.2.3 Skull Base Surgery

Skull base surgery is particularly concerned with **tumors** and **vascular processes** involving the cranial nerves. In the **anterior** and **middle cra-**

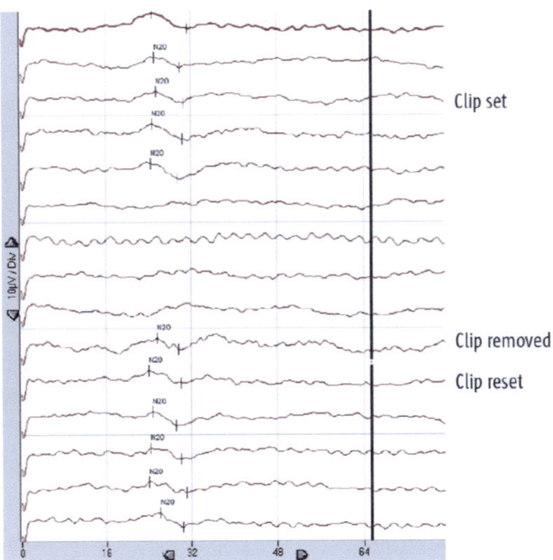

Fig. 8.7 Median nerve SEP disappearance after clip placement, with signal restoration after removing and repositioning the clip. © ARKANA Forum GmbH 2022. All Rights Reserved

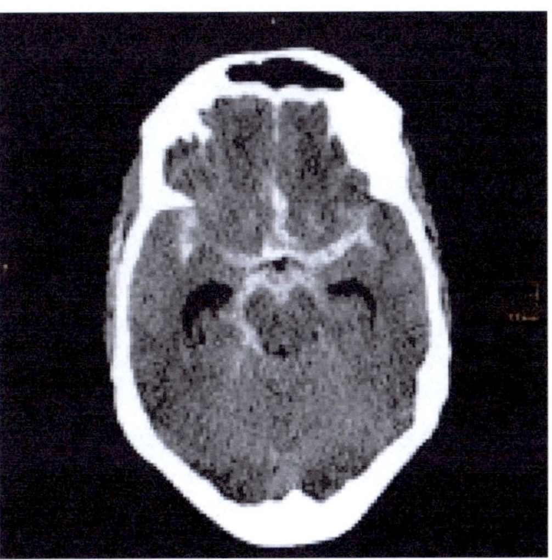

Fig. 8.8 Preoperative CT showed extensive subarachnoid hemorrhage. © ARKANA Forum GmbH 2022. All Rights Reserved

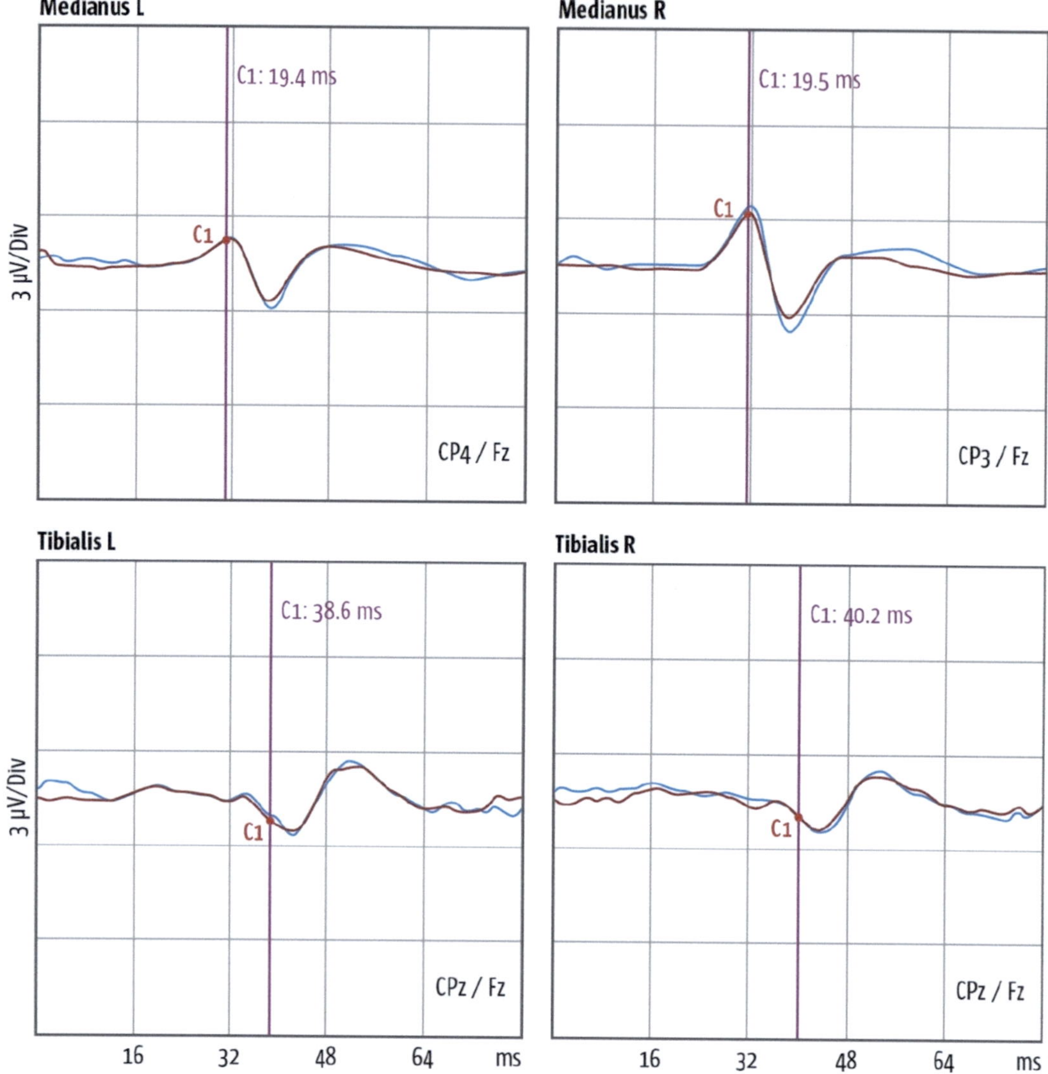

Fig. 8.9 Bilateral median and tibial nerve SEPs recorded during aneurysm clipping. © ARKANA Forum GmbH 2022. All Rights Reserved

nial fossae, the most common pathologies are perisellar, cavernous sinus, or trigeminal ganglion tumors. In the **posterior cranial fossa,** tumors of the cerebellopontine angle predominate. The most common pathology to be operated on in this area is the **vestibular schwannoma.** It is a benign tumor originating from the vestibular part of the vestibulocochlear nerve. For historical reasons, the term acoustic neuroma is still used for this tumor, which, however, rarely originates from the cochlear part of the nerve. Vestibular schwannomas become symptomatic with vertigo, tinnitus, and hearing loss. They can get very large and lead to compression of the brainstem with disturbance of cerebrospinal fluid circulation.

Of further importance in the cerebellopontine angle are **vascular-nerve conflicts** characterized by compression of a cranial nerve by an aberrant vascular loop, causing **trigeminal neuralgia,** glossopharyngeal neuralgia, or **hemifacial spasm.** The operative principle in vascular-nerve conflict is to detach the vessel from the nerve and then permanently separate them with an implant such as a Teflon pad.

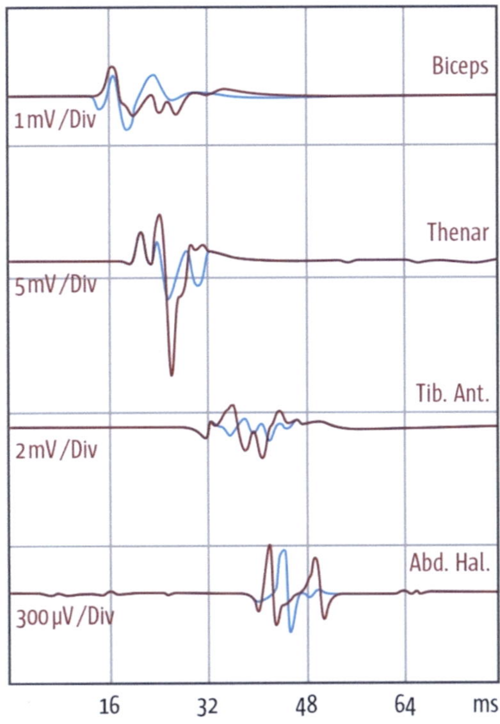

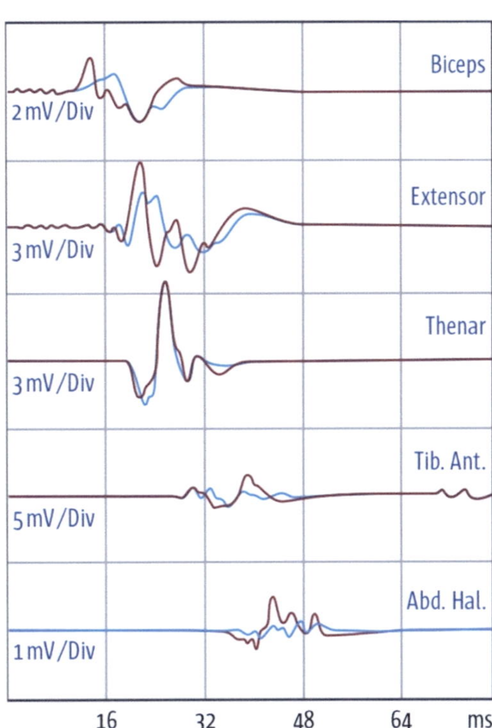

Fig. 8.10 Bilateral upper and lower limb MEPs recorded during aneurysm clipping. Extensor, extensor digitorum muscle; Tib. Ant., tibialis anterior muscle; Abd. Hal., abductor hallucis muscle. © ARKANA Forum GmbH 2022. All Rights Reserved

During skull base and cerebellopontine angle surgeries, neuromonitoring focuses on the cranial nerves that are particularly at risk. Common methods include **BAEPs**, free-running electromyography (**EMG**), **triggered EMG** with compound muscle action potentials (**CMAPs**), and **corticobulbar MEPs**. Less common techniques include auditory nerve action potentials (NAPs), electrocochleography (ECochG), and brainstem reflexes. In processes affecting the brainstem, it is advisable to additionally monitor the long ascending and descending pathways with **MEPs** and **SEPs**.

In principle, BAEPs should be tried in every case (Figs. 8.11 and 8.12). However, this is often unsuccessful in large vestibular schwannomas due to preexisting hearing loss with pathological BAEP absence. Preoperative testing is always recommended. If hearing is preserved, one may consider adding auditory NAPs or ECochG as complementary methods to aid signal interpretation.

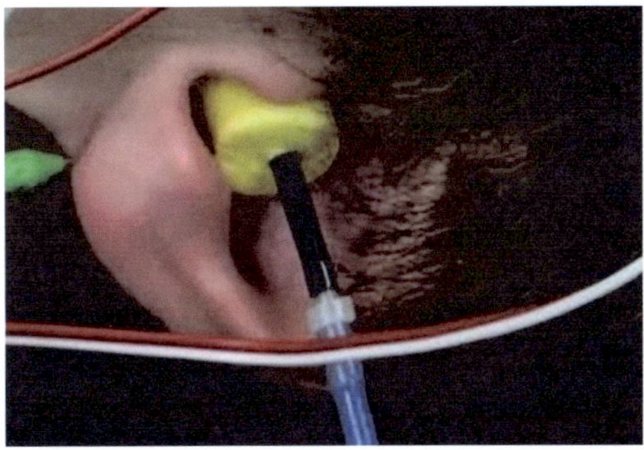

Fig. 8.11 Placement of the earplugs for BAEP monitoring. © ARKANA Forum GmbH 2022. All Rights Reserved

Corticobulbar MEPs are triggered contralaterally by anodal stimulation at C3 or C4 versus a Cz cathode (see also Sect. 5.4.2). Recording may be possible with standard filter settings, but opening the software high-pass filter to 0.2–2 Hz or constraining it to 50–100 Hz can help to separate these short-latency responses from stimulus artifact. The onset latency of the response is impor-

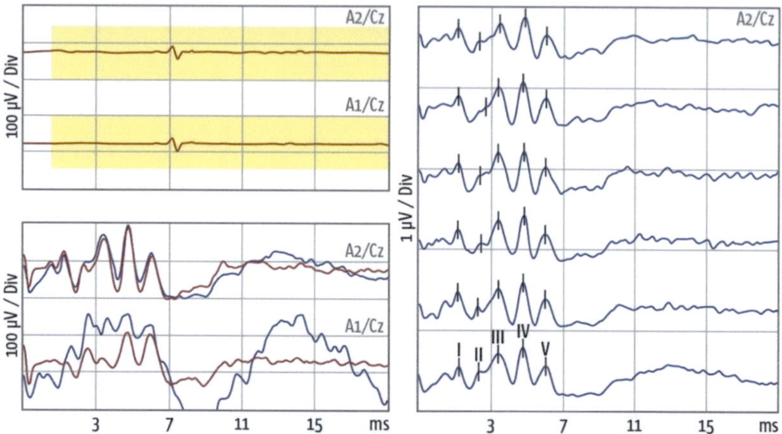

Fig. 8.12 BAEPs with waves I–V. Analysis emphasizes wave V amplitude and latency. © ARKANA Forum GmbH 2022. All Rights Reserved

tant because too-short latency implies direct nerve activation. For example, facial MEP onset latency should be>10 ms to exclude direct nerve excitation and thereby confirm a central MEP origin [13, 14]. Similarly, it is important to exclude single-pulse responses that imply direct nerve activation. This is done by preceding or following the pulse train stimulus with a single pulse.

Intermittent **mapping** is used to localize the nerves. This can be accomplished with a monopolar or bipolar-concentric stimulation probe using 1–3 Hz frequency, 0.2–0.5 ms pulse duration, and 0.01–2 mA intensity while recording cranial CMAPs. For direct excitation of a functionally intact nerve, 0.01–0.1 mA is normally sufficient. However, higher intensities of 1–2 mA may be required if there is tumor tissue on the nerve. Analysis includes CMAP amplitude and latency. In order to avoid providing a false sense of security, it is important to understand that distal nerve stimulation at the porus acusticus still produces a CMAP even in case the nerve is proximally damaged or transected [15, 16]. Thus proximal stimulation near the brainstem is essential for assessing facial nerve functional integrity during these surgeries.

Continuous (dynamic) mapping by monopolar cathodal stimulation through the tip of the surgical suction device is an alternative [17] (Fig. 8.13). The major advantage of this technique is that the surgeon does not have to change instruments for dissection and mapping, thus facilitating continuous mapping during the resec-

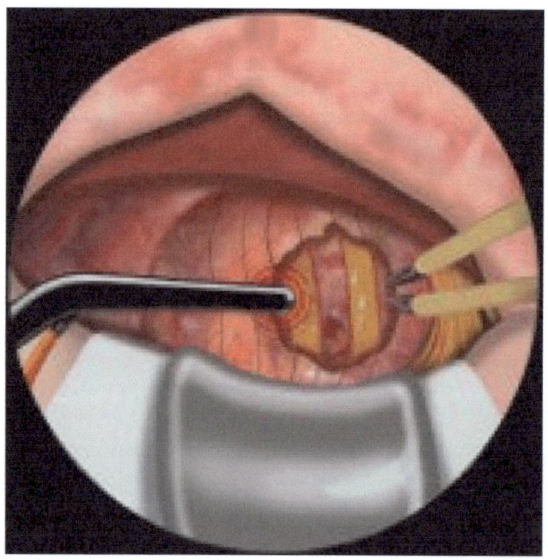

Fig. 8.13 Schematic illustration of continuous (dynamic) mapping with monopolar stimulation through the tip of the surgical suction device (left). © Inselspital, Bern University Hospital, Dept. of Neurosurgery 2022. All Rights Reserved

tion. In addition, some neuromonitoring systems offer the possibility to set an alarm tone that sounds as soon as a predefined stimulation threshold is reached [18, 19].

Free-running EMG can be assessed either by qualitative visual or quantitative computer analysis. Visual interpretation provides rapid detection of nerve irritation which, however, is relatively nonspecific. Quantitative assessment employs train-time analysis, an automated algorithm that sums up the duration of A-trains that are considered pathological, and generates a visible and audible alarm when a certain threshold is reached. Train-time analysis improves the sensitivity and specificity of facial nerve EMG monitoring, but the algorithm currently is not generally available [18–20].

Case Example: Vestibular Schwannoma
Clinical Setting:

The patient presented with right hearing loss. Right BAEPs were absent, and MRI demonstrated a large right **vestibular schwannoma** Koss Grade IV compressing the brainstem (Fig. 8.14). Surgery aimed at gross total resection with IONM guidance to preserve facial nerve function [17].

Procedure and monitoring: The surgery proceeded with the patient in the Fukushima position. Monitoring included free-running EMG, CMAPs, and corticobulbar MEPs from muscles innervated by cranial nerves **V–VII** and **IX–XII**; the facial nerve (**VII**) muscles were the orbicularis oculi, nasalis, orbicularis oris, and mentalis (Figs. 8.15, 8.16 and 8.17). There were also monitored bilateral median nerve SEPs and MEPs of

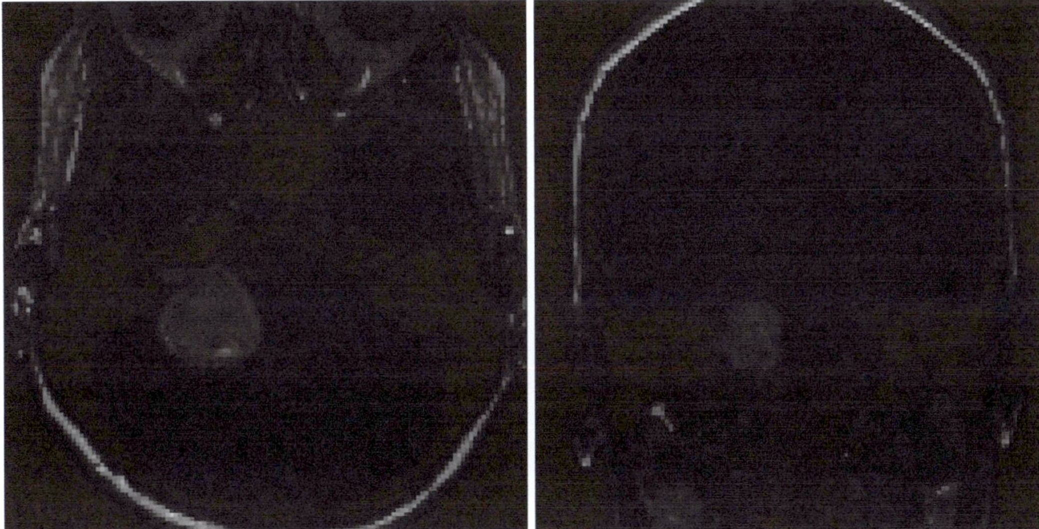

Fig. 8.14 Preoperative MRI showed a large right vestibular schwannoma with compression of the brainstem. © Inselspital, Bern University Hospital, Dept. of Neurosurgery 2022. All Rights Reserved

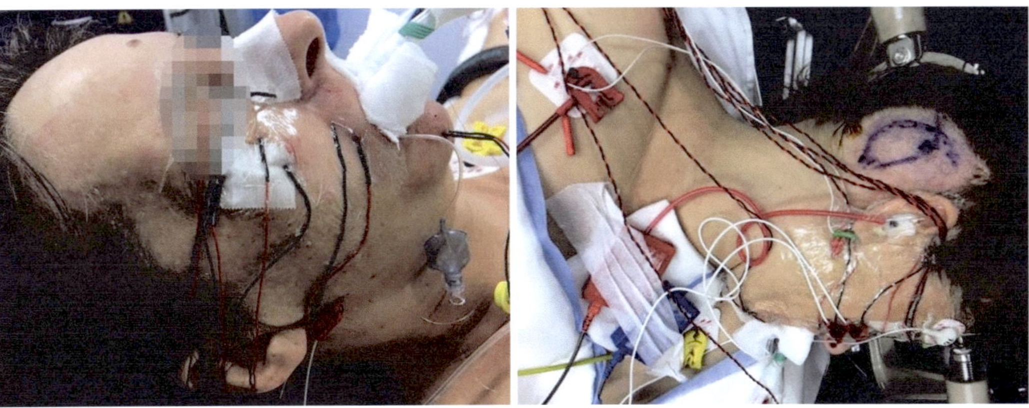

Fig. 8.15 Electrode placements before (left) and after (right) positioning of the patient with a large vestibular schwannoma shown in Fig. 8.14. © Inselspital, Bern University Hospital, Dept. of Neurosurgery 2022. All Rights Reserved

the upper extremities. None of the monitored potentials showed significant deterioration during surgery although facial MEP duration

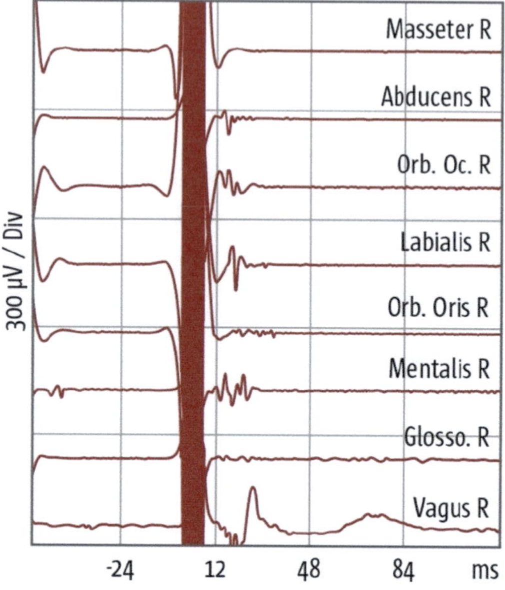

Fig. 8.16 Corticobulbar MEPs before (left) and after (right) resection of the right vestibular schwannoma shown in Fig. 8.14. Abducens, abducens nerve, lateral rectus muscle; Orb. Oc., orbicularis oculi; Orb. Oris, orbicularis oris; Glosso., glossopharyngeal nerve, soft palate muscle. © Inselspital, Bern University Hospital, Dept. of Neurosurgery 2022. All Rights Reserved

increased, suggesting dispersion of facial nerve motor axon conduction. The patient had no postoperative facial weakness or other neurologic deficits.

Case Example: Hearing Loss during Large Vestibular Schwannoma Resection
Clinical Setting:

The patient presented with progressive right hearing impairment. Neuroimaging revealed a 4 cm right vestibular schwannoma. The surgical plan was gross total lesion removal with IONM.

Procedure and Monitoring:

The surgery proceeded with the patient in the park bench position. Monitoring include bilateral BAEPs, median nerve SEPs, and facial and thenar MEPs, as well as right masseter, frontalis, and orbicularis oris EMG and CMAPs. The right BAEP showed irreversible wave V and then wave I disappearance during tumor resection before the cochlear nerve had been found (Fig. 8.18). Attempted interventions including surgical pause, irrigation, and raising blood pressure were ineffective. The patient had postoperative right ear deafness. This case exemplifies the low chance of hearing preservation during large (>2 cm) vestibular schwannoma resection.

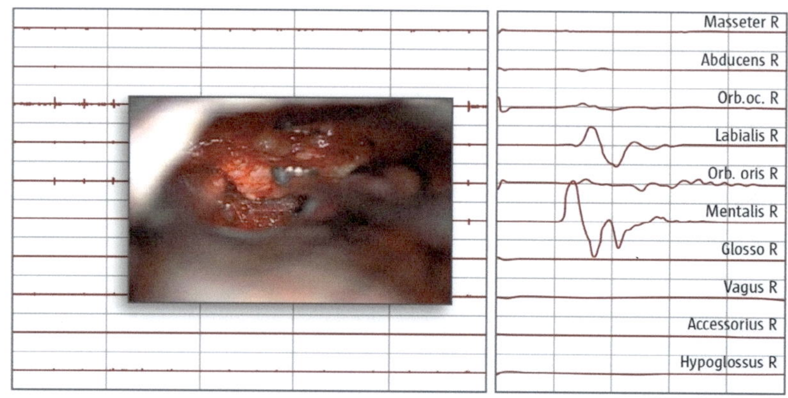

Fig. 8.17 Free-running EMG with overlayed operative microscope video (left) and CMAPs (right) of facial and other cranial muscles during resection of the right vestibular schwannoma shown in Fig. 8.14. Abducens, abducens nerve, lateral rectus muscle; Orb. Oc., orbicularis oculi muscle; Orb. Oris, orbicularis oris muscle; Glosso, glossopharyngeal nerve, soft palate muscle; Vagus, vagus nerve, vocalis muscle; Accessorius, accessory nerve, trapezius muscle; Hypoglossus, hypoglossal nerve, tongue muscle. © Inselspital, Bern University Hospital, Dept. of Neurosurgery 2022. All Rights Reserved

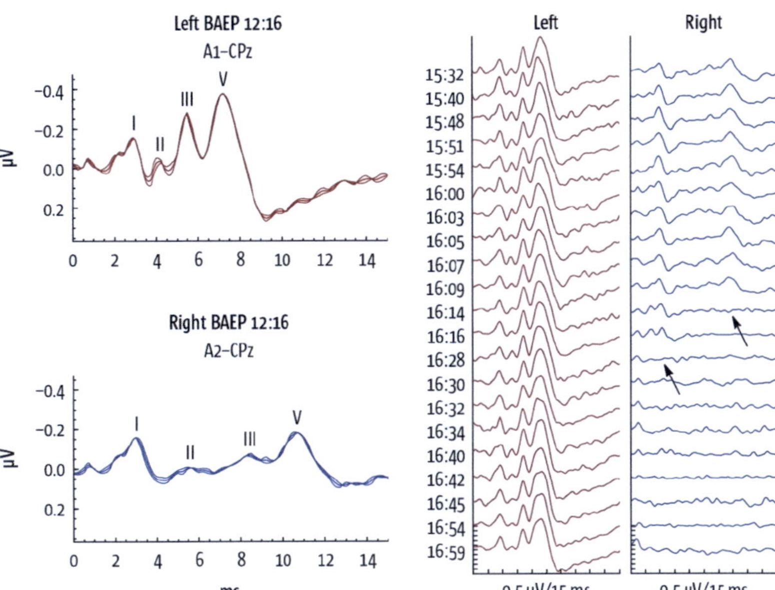

Fig. 8.18 BAEP in large vestibular schwannoma surgery. Baselines at 12:16 showed abnormal right BAEPs with prolonged interpeak intervals and reduced wave V amplitude. Irreversible wave V and then wave I disappearance during resection (arrows) did not respond to attempted intervention. From [21], with permission. © ARKANA Forum GmbH 2022. All Rights Reserved

Case Example: Hearing Preservation during Small Vestibular Schwannoma Resection

Clinical Setting:

The patient presented with tinnitus and mild left hearing impairment. Neuroimaging showed a 1 cm vestibular schwannoma, and preoperative BAEPs were normal. The patient strongly desired hearing preservation. The surgical plan was total or sub-total resection aiming for hearing preservation with IONM guidance.

Procedure and Monitoring:

The surgery proceeded with the patient in the sitting position. Monitoring included bilateral BAEPs and median nerve SEPs, as well as left masseter, frontalis, and orbicularis oris EMG and CMAPs; muscle MEP techniques had not yet been developed. During resection, there was reversible left BAEP deterioration and disappearance that responded to intervention (Fig. 8.19). Postoperative BAEPs were normal, and the patient had no additional hearing impairment. This case exemplifies BAEP-guided hearing preservation during small (<2 cm) vestibular schwannoma resection.

Case Example: Brainstem Metastasis

Clinical Setting:

The patient presented with four-limb motor and sensory deficits and MRI revealed a space-occupying **metastasis** in the ventral pons (Fig. 8.20). The nuclei of most cranial nerves as well as the ascending sensory and descending motor pathways were likely in close vicinity to the tumor. Resection of the metastasis was planned using the transnasal-transsphenoidal route with IONM.

Procedure and Monitoring:

The surgery proceeded in a transnasal-transsphenoidal approach. Monitoring included bilateral median and tibial nerve **SEPs** and bilateral abductor digiti minimi and abductor hallucis muscle **MEPs** to assess long sensory and motor pathways. In addition, **cranial nerves V–IX** were monitored using free-running EMG, corticobulbar MEPs, and BAEPs.

Monitorable BAEPs, SEPs, limb MEPs, and cranial nerve V, VI, VII, and IX corticobulbar MEPs were present at the beginning of the operation. The initial MEP stimulus intensity was

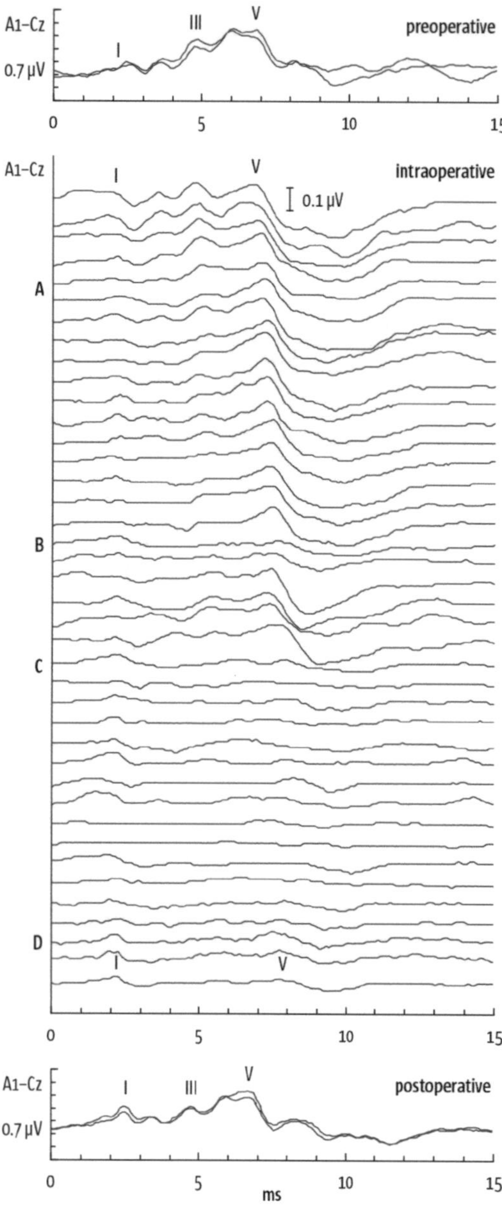

Fig. 8.19 BAEP in small vestibular schwannoma surgery. Preoperative BAEPs were normal. There was intraoperative wave V latency delay (**A**), subsequent >50% amplitude reduction (**B**) that responded to a surgical pause, and then disappearance when the surgeon tried to remove the last small portion of tumor capsule from the nerve (**C**). After a long pause and irrigation, wave V began to recover (**D**). The surgeon left the residual capsule and postoperative BAEPs were normal, with unchanged hearing function. © ARKANA Forum GmbH 2022. All Rights Reserved

90 mA. After coagulation of some small arteries branching from the basilar artery to the metastasis, there was irreversible four-limb SEP and MEP deterioration and then disappearance (Figs. 8.21 and 8.22). These potentials were absent at the end of the operation, except for small intermittent right abductor hallucis MEPs at 230 mA stimulus intensity. Corticobulbar MEPs showed partial deterioration but remained present, while BAEPs were unaffected. Consistent with monitoring results, the patient had additional postoperative motor and sensory deficits in the upper and lower extremities.

Case Example: Trigeminal Neuralgia
Clinical Setting:

The patient presented with chronic left trigeminal neuralgia that was resistant to medical treatment with carbamazepine. Preoperative MRI demonstrated a **vascular-nerve conflict** with compression of the left trigeminal nerve by the inferior cerebellar artery. Decompression of the nerve with IONM guidance according to the approach described by **Jannetta** was planned.

Procedure and Monitoring:

A left lateral suboccipital trephination was done. After opening the dura, the trigeminal nerve and the aberrant loop of the inferior cerebellar artery were exposed. Thereafter, the vascular loop was detached from the nerve, and a Teflon pad was placed between them (Fig. 8.23).

Monitoring included assessment of the vestibulocochlear nerve (**VIII**) using **BAEPs** (Fig. 8.24) and the facial nerve (**VII**) by free-running EMG and corticobulbar MEPs. In more complex cases, mapping may be used to identify cranial nerves V and VII. In addition, SEP and MEP monitoring may be advisable if the brainstem is affected [22, 23].

8.2.4   Spinal Neurosurgery

Neurosurgical spinal procedures that have a significant risk of neurological complications involve **tumors**, **dysraphic malformations** and,

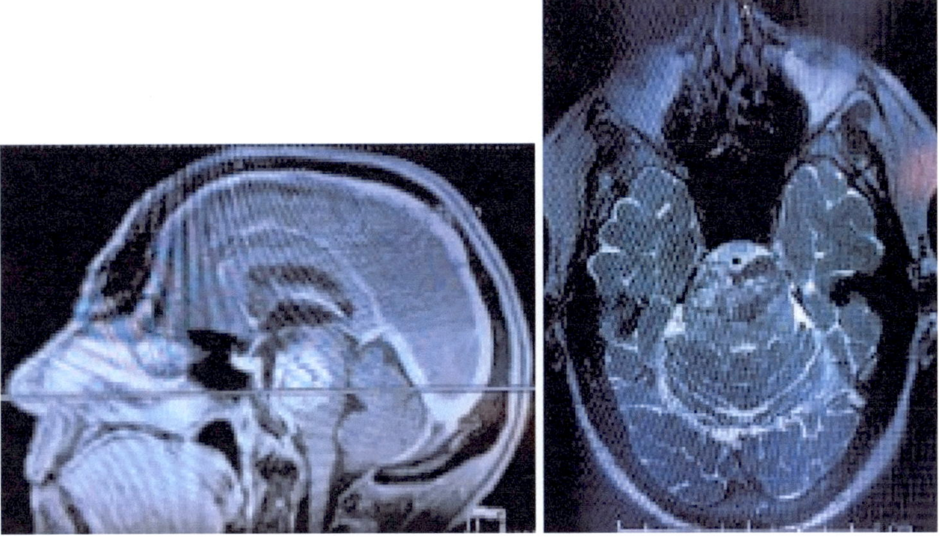

Fig. 8.20 MRI of a large metastasis in the ventral pons © ARKANA Forum GmbH 2022. All Rights Reserved

Fig. 8.21 Left and right median nerve SEPs in the case shown in Fig. 8.20. At the beginning of surgery (top), SEPs were well-defined, but deteriorated after starting tumor resection (middle, blue line) and disappeared before the end of surgery (bottom, blue line). © ARKANA Forum GmbH 2022. All Rights Reserved

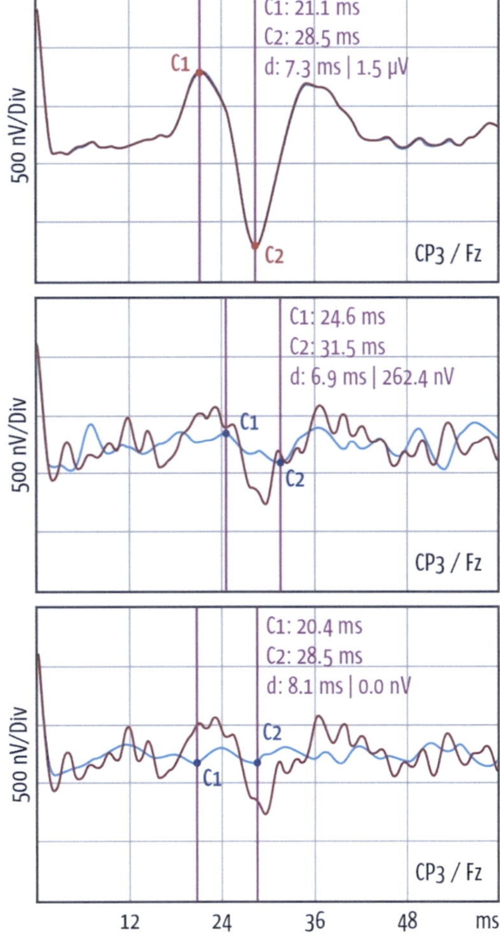

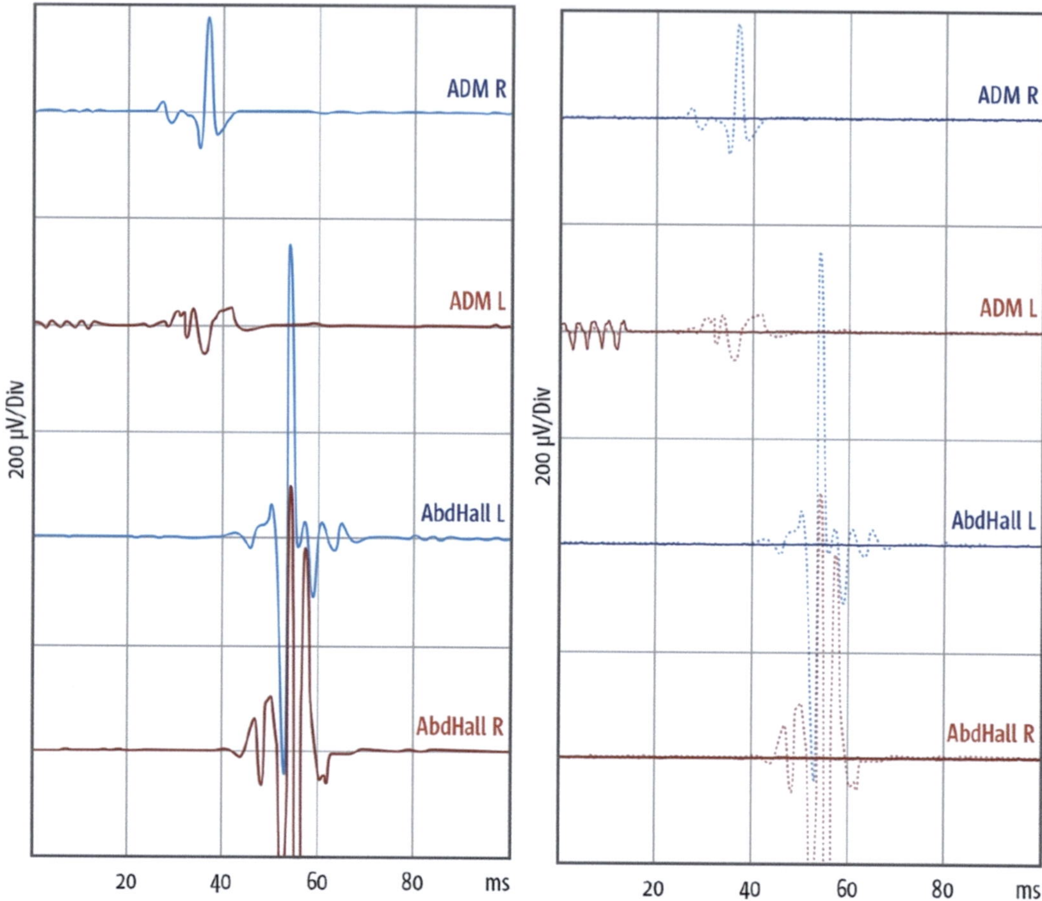

Fig. 8.22 Left and right MEPs of the abductor digiti minimi (ADM) and the abductor hallucis longus (AbdHall) muscles in the case shown in Fig. 8.20. Well-defined baseline MEPs from all muscles were obtained (left). At the end of surgery, MEPs were completely lost at all recording sites (right). © ARKANA Forum GmbH 2022. All Rights Reserved

to a lesser extent, interventions for the treatment of **spasticity** or **pain**. Spinal tumors are classified as extradural, intradural-extramedullary, and intramedullary depending on their spatial relationship to the spinal cord and the meninges. In particular, intramedullary tumor resections have a high risk of additional postoperative neurologic deficits. The aim of IONM in spinal neurosurgery is to assess the function of the spinal cord and to identify and control the emerging nerve roots.

For spinal cord monitoring, **SEPs** are used to study the ascending and **MEPs** to assess the descending pathways. In the case of severe pre-existing cervical myelopathy, it may be useful to start monitoring before positioning the patient in order to detect any position-related risk to spinal cord function. Additional spinal epidural or subdural **D-wave** monitoring is indicated for intramedullary tumor resections because preservation above 50% of baseline amplitude predicts good long-term motor outcome. This can enable gross total removal even when muscle MEP disappearance predicts early postoperative weakness, since temporary weakness is an acceptable outcome for these specific procedures.

The functionality of nerve roots emerging from the spinal cord can be assessed by **direct**

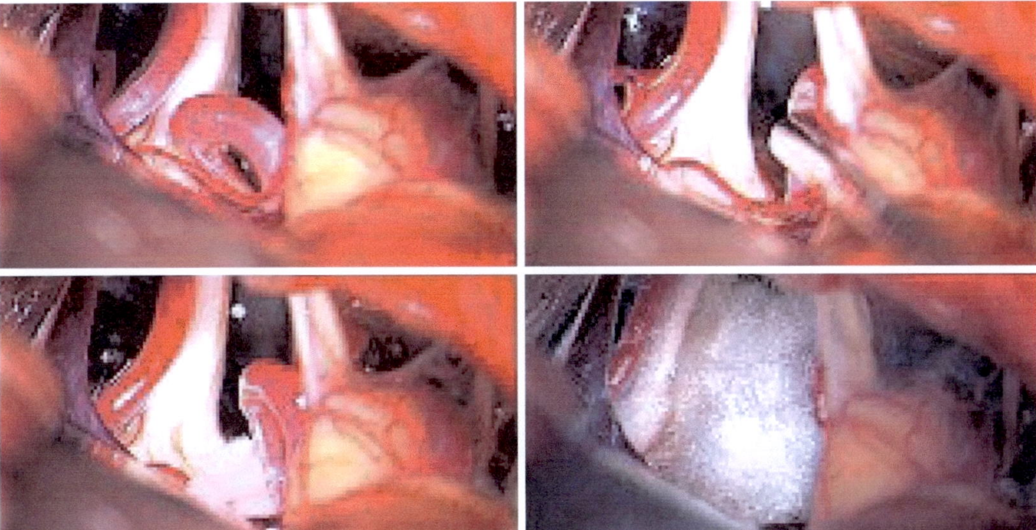

Fig. 8.23 Intraoperative view of surgical treatment of trigeminal neuralgia according to Jannetta. Compression of the left trigeminal nerve by the inferior cerebellar artery (top left). The inferior cerebellar artery is detached from the nerve (top right). A Teflon pad is placed between nerve and artery (bottom left) and fixed with fibrin glue (bottom right). © ARKANA Forum GmbH 2022. All Rights Reserved

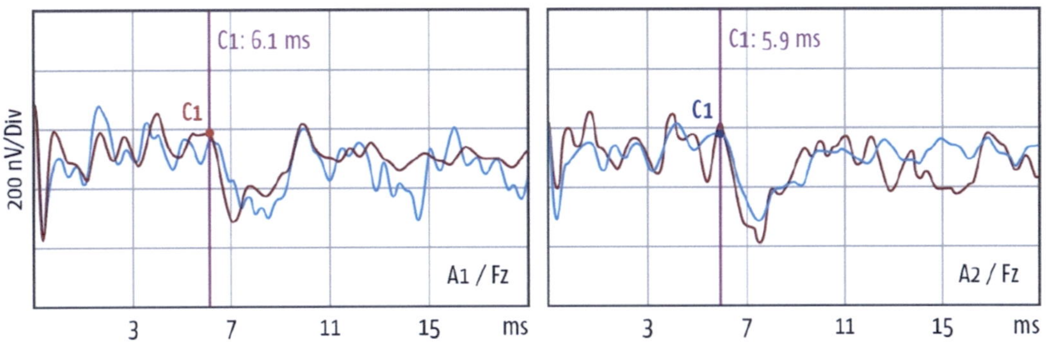

Fig. 8.24 Recording of bilateral BAEPs during surgery for trigeminal neuralgia as shown in Fig. 8.23. Stable potentials indicated preservation of hearing function. © ARKANA Forum GmbH 2022. All Rights Reserved

stimulation. This applies, for example, to neurinomas. The surgically exposed nerve fiber is stimulated by means of a probe, and the response is recorded from the target muscle. If it becomes intraoperatively apparent that the nerve root involved in the tumor is no longer functional, complete tumor resection can be performed without compromising function. Direct intraoperative stimulation can also be used to identify the dorsal root entry zone (DREZ) in selective dorsal rhizotomy for the treatment of spasticity and pain. **Spinal cord mapping** can help to identify the dorsal columns and corticospinal tracts.

Case Report: Ependymoma
Clinical Setting:

The patient presented with motor and sensory deficits in the upper and lower extremities. Preoperative MRI showed an **intramedullary tumor** in the cervical medulla with multiple cysts, typical of an ependymoma (Fig. 8.25). The surgical plan was gross total tumor removal with IONM guidance.

Procedure and Monitoring:

First, surgical exposure of the dura mater was performed by laminotomy. After opening the dura, the spinal cord was incised in its dorsal midline. Thereafter, the tumor was hollowed. Finally, complete resection of the tumor was achieved (Fig. 8.26).

Monitoring included **SEPs** and **MEPs** of all extremities (Fig. 8.27). Stable potentials throughout surgery indicated an uneventful outcome. Facultatively, D-waves from the spinal cord can also be recorded. In addition, mapping and monitoring of the affected nerve roots by stimulation with a hand-held probe and registering the free-running EMG may be advisable in selected cases [24–27].

Case Report: Thoracic Intramedullary Spinal Cord Tumor
Clinical Setting:

The patient presented with mild bilateral leg sensory disturbance and weakness without spasticity, hyperreflexia, or Babinski signs. Neuroimaging disclosed a T4–6 intramedullary tumor, probably an ependymoma. The surgical plan was gross total removal with IONM guidance.

Procedure and Monitoring:

The surgery proceeded like the previous case, except the surgeon inserted spinal epidural electrodes for D-wave recording after laminectomy. Monitoring included bilateral optimized periph-

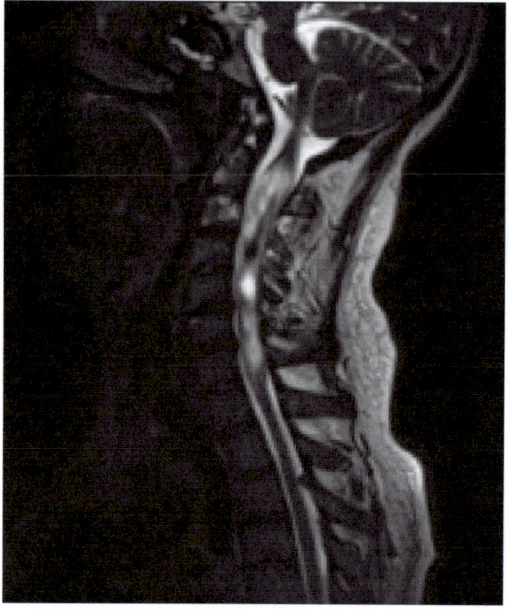

Fig. 8.25 MRI demonstrating a cystic intramedullary tumor of the cervical medulla. © ARKANA Forum GmbH 2022. All Rights Reserved

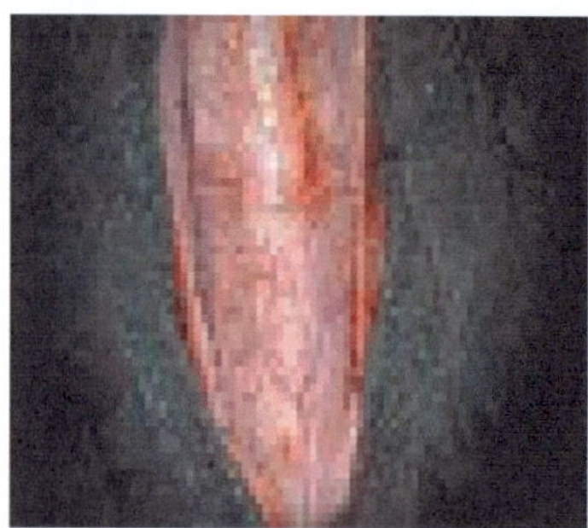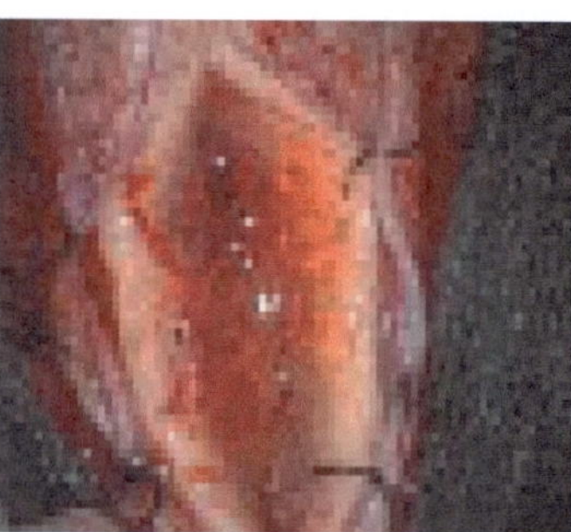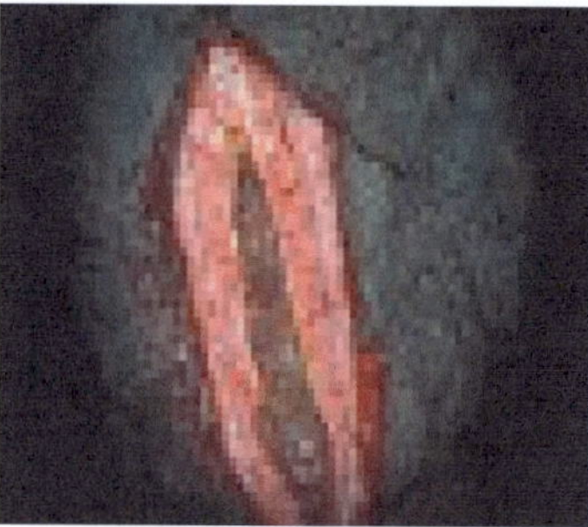

Fig. 8.26 Intraoperative view of the removal of the ependymoma of the cervical medulla shown in Fig. 8.25. Bulging spinal cord after opening of the dura (left); visualization of the tumor after incision of the spinal cord (middle); appearance after complete removal of the tumor (right). © ARKANA Forum GmbH 2022. All Rights Reserved

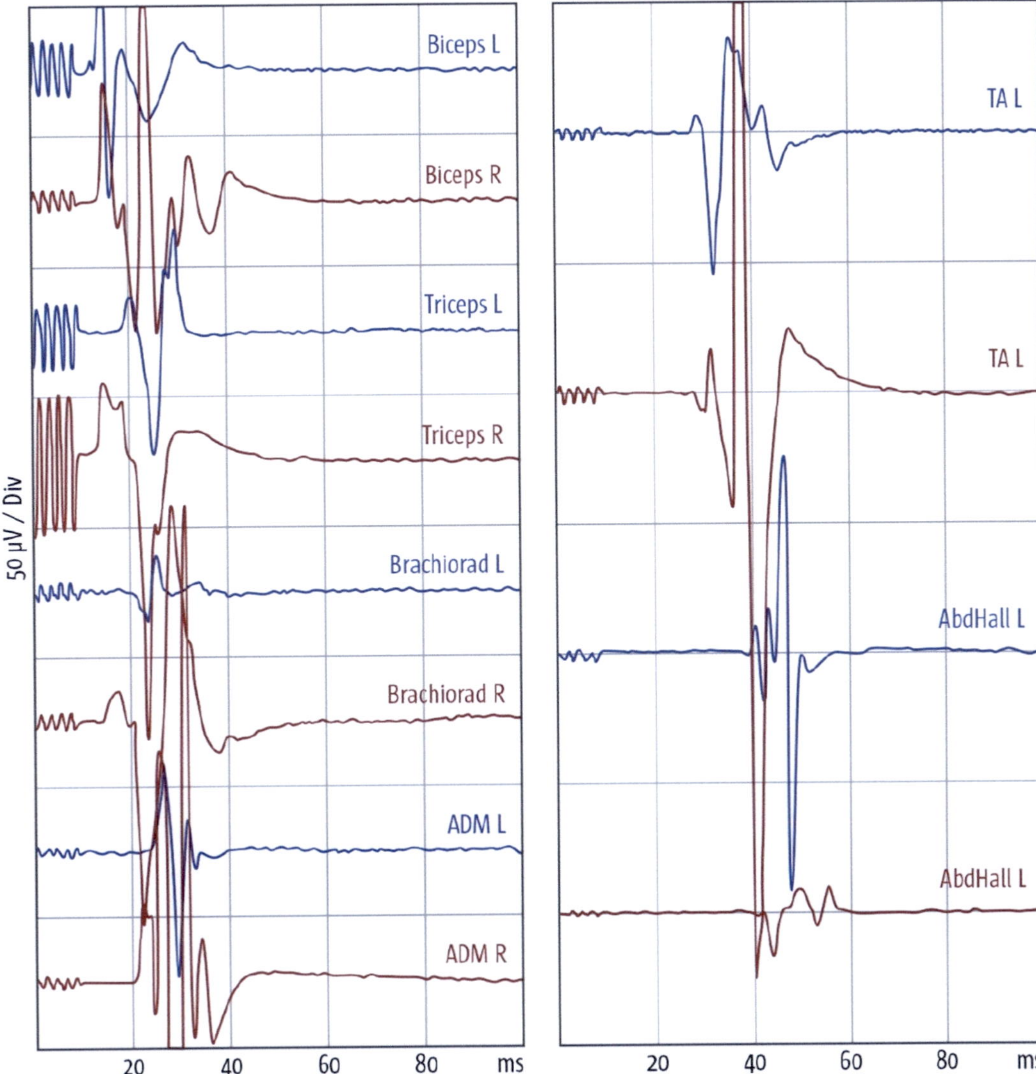

Fig. 8.27 Recording of MEPs from the upper (left) and lower (right) extremities during resection of the intramedullary tumor of the of the cervical medulla. Brachiorad, brachioradialis muscle; ADM abductor digiti minimi muscle, TA, tibialis anterior muscle, AbdHall abductor hallucis muscle; R, right; L, left. © ARKANA Forum GmbH 2022. All Rights Reserved

eral–cortical median and tibial nerve SEPs, four-limb muscle MEPs, and rostral and caudal D-waves. The upper limb potentials and rostral D-wave served as controls. The spinal cord MEP warning criterion was disappearance unexplained by confounding factors. The cortical SEP limit was visually obvious amplitude reduction from recent pre-change values and clearly exceeding spontaneous variability, with no confounding factor explanation. All potentials were stable during dorsal midline myelotomy and tumor resection (Fig. 8.28). There were no new postoperative deficits.

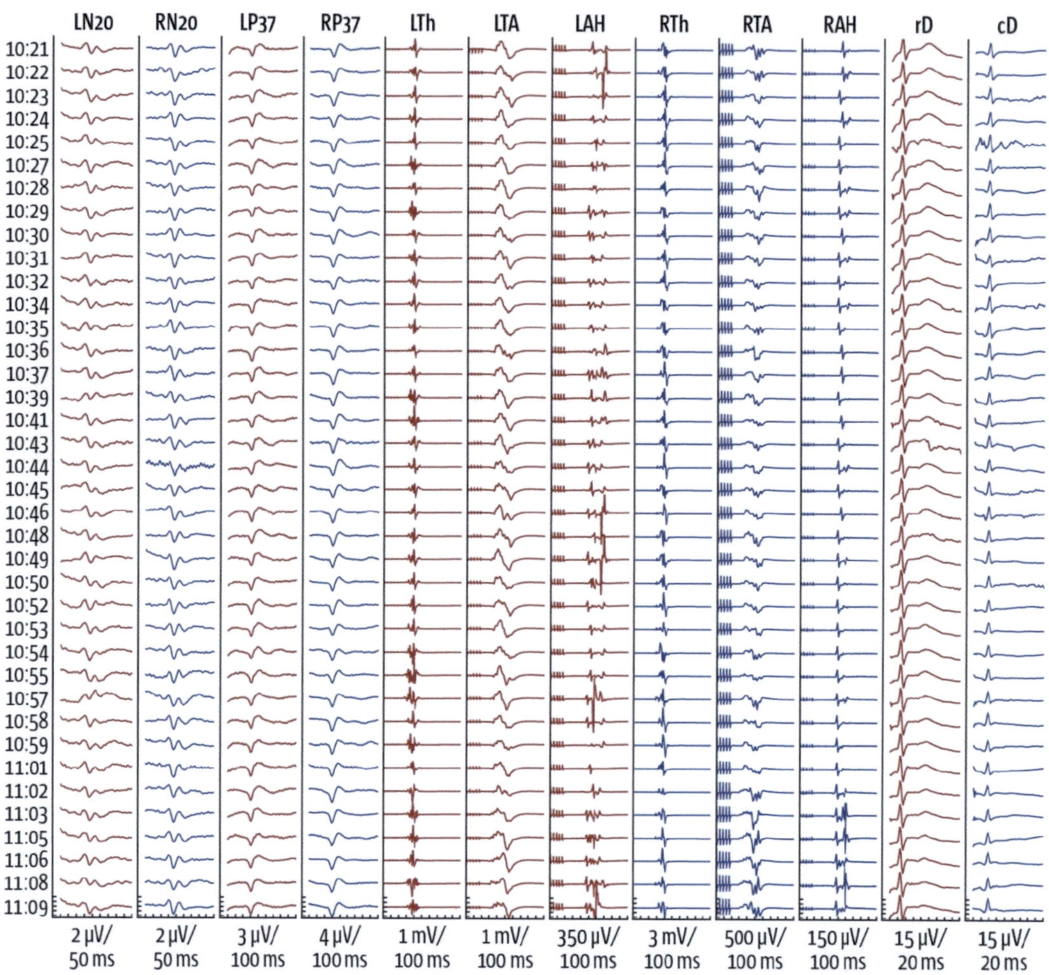

Fig. 8.28 Stable four-limb cortical SEPs, muscle MEPs, and rostral and caudal D-waves during T4–6 intramedullary spinal cord tumor resection. Peripheral cubital and popliteal fossa SEPs recorded as technical controls were also stable (not shown). Note that SEP optimization enabled rapid surgical feedback every 1–2 min without compromising reproducibility. L, left; R ,right; N20 and P37, median and tibial nerve cortical SEPs; Th, thenar muscle; TA, tibialis anterior muscle; AH, abductor hallucis muscle; rD and cD, rostral and caudal D-wave. © ARKANA Forum GmbH 2022. All Rights Reserved

8.3 IONM in Orthopedic Surgery

Of particular importance for IONM in orthopedics are interventions to correct **scoliosis**. This is an idiopathic, congenital, or acquired deviation of the spine with a sideways curve and rotation that may be caused by neuromuscular problems and/or asymmetry of some vertebrae. Surgical procedures to correct scoliosis are associated with a significant risk of paraplegia due to spinal cord compression, traction, or ischemia. Furthermore, spinal orthopedic surgery involves the implantation of **pedicle screws** as part of stabilization procedures. Misdirected screws breaching the pedicle wall can damage nerve roots that run in close spatial relationship, or even the spinal cord. In addition, some procedures involve the insertion of **sublaminar hooks** or **wires** that can injure the spinal cord by entering the spinal canal.

Traditionally, **SEPs** have been used for intraoperative assessment of spinal cord function in scoliosis surgery. They are particularly successful for this application, since the patients usually have intact preoperative neurological function, so that well-defined potentials are obtained even under anesthesia. In recent years, **MEP** monitoring is widely employed to directly assess motor pathways. Indeed, some centers monitor only MEPs, although their combination with SEP monitoring is widely recommended. With spinal cord monitoring, the otherwise necessary wake-up test during surgical correction of scoliosis can be avoided.

When placing pedicle screws, the risk of perforation of the pedicle can be assessed by means of stimulation of the nerve root either at the medial pedicle wall within the pedicle borehole (Fig. 8.29), via the pedicle screw (Fig. 8.30) or by the Kirschner wire inserted prior to screw implantation (Figs. 8.31 and 8.32). An excessively low threshold for triggering CMAPs in the target muscles of the roots at risk may indicate a pedicle breach. The surgeon can then inspect the screw and redirect it if necessary. Free-running EMG may also be helpful.

Case Example: Scoliosis
Clinical Setting:

The patient presented with back pain and intact neurological function. Preoperative CT demonstrated **congenital scoliosis** caused by

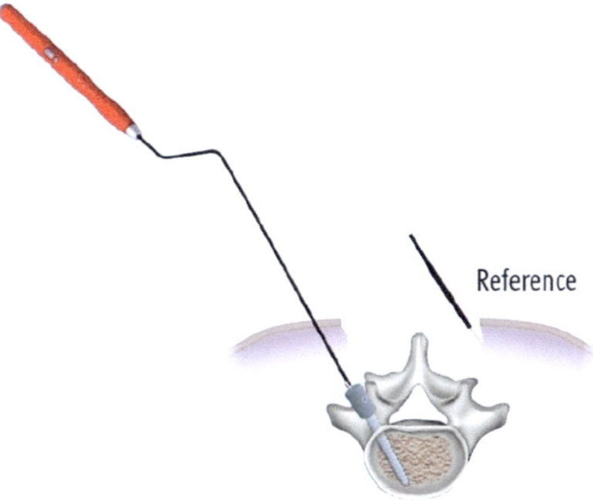

Fig. 8.30 Stimulation of the pedicle screw. © ARKANA Forum GmbH 2022. All Rights Reserved

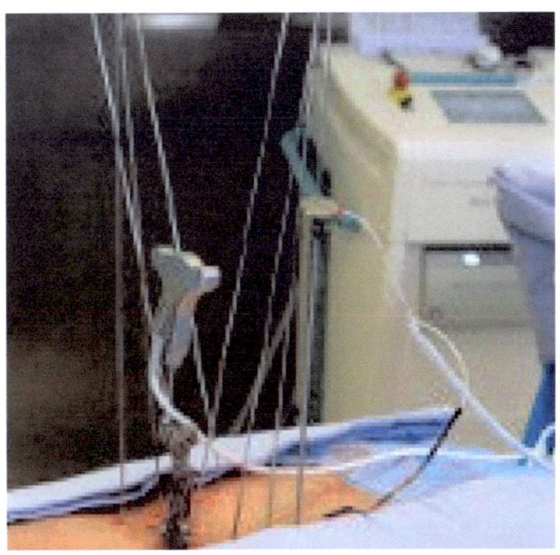

Fig. 8.31 Pedicle stimulation via Kirschner wires. © ARKANA Forum GmbH 2022. All Rights Reserved

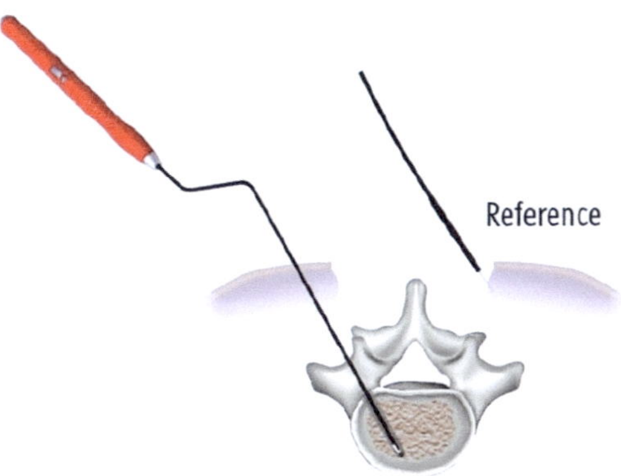

Fig. 8.29 Stimulation in the pedicle borehole. © ARKANA Forum GmbH 2022. All Rights Reserved

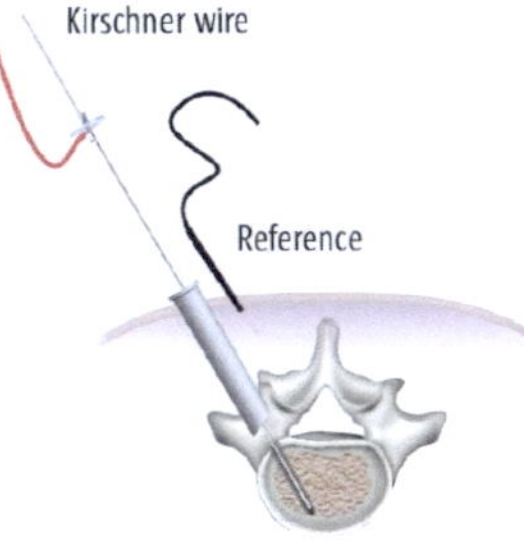

Fig. 8.32 Schematic representation of monopolar pedicle stimulation via a Kirschner wire. © ARKANA Forum GmbH 2022. All Rights Reserved

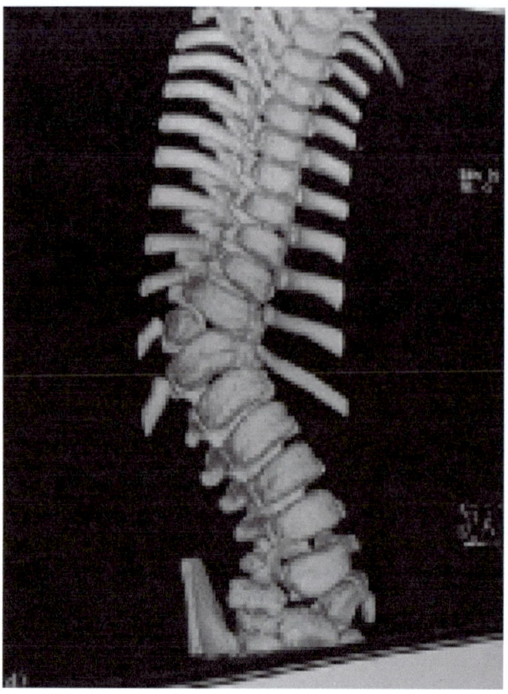

Fig. 8.33 Preoperative CT showed scoliosis due to thoracic and lumbar hemivertebrae. © ARKANA Forum GmbH 2022. All Rights Reserved

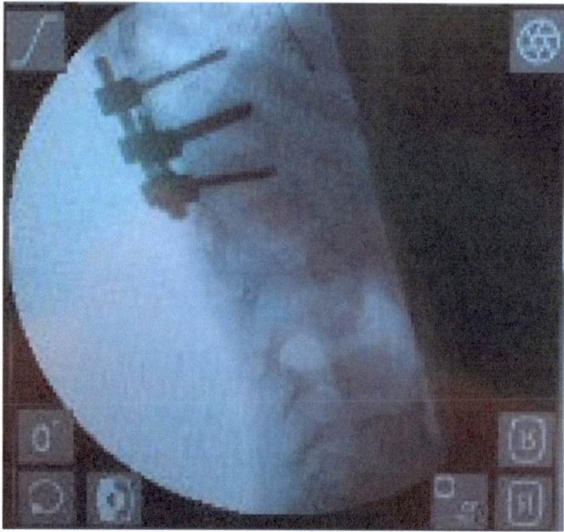

Fig. 8.34 Intraoperative x-ray of the thoracolumbar spine after correction of the scoliosis. © ARKANA Forum GmbH 2022. All Rights Reserved

hemivertebrae at the lower thoracic and upper lumbar spine (Fig. 8.33). Surgical correction of scoliosis with IONM was planned.

Procedure and Monitoring:

During surgery, the hemivertebrae were resected, the scoliosis was corrected, and the thoracic and lumbar spine were fixed in the new position using pedicle screws and rods (Fig. 8.34).

Monitoring included **MEPs** from the upper and lower limbs (Fig. 8.35). Stable potentials throughout surgery indicated an uneventful neurological outcome. More often, SEPs and free-running EMG are also monitored [28, 29].

Case Example: Congenital Kyphoscoliosis Clinical Setting:

The patient presented with thoracolumbar kyphoscoliosis and no neurologic deficits. Imaging revealed multiple vertebral anomalies and hemivertebrae. The surgical plan was posterior spinal fusion and instrumentation with hemivertebrectomies and full curve correction under IONM control.

Procedure and Monitoring:

The surgery proceeded in standard fashion with the patient prone. Monitoring included bilateral peripheral–cortical optimized median and tibial nerve SEPs, MEPs from the thenar, tibialis anterior, and abductor hallucis muscles, and leg EMG. The upper limb potentials served as systemic controls and brachial plexus monitors. The spinal cord MEP warning criterion was disappearance unexplained by confounding factors. The cortical SEP limit was visually obvious amplitude reduction from recent pre-change values and clearly exceeding spontaneous variability, with no confounding factor explanation.

Right after inserting a left high-thoracic sublaminar hook, there was abrupt left leg MEP disappearance and 30% tibial nerve SEP amplitude reduction (Fig. 8.36). Rapid signal restoration followed immediate hook removal. Full curve correction was achieved with omission of this hook, and the patient had no postoperative deficits.

This case exemplifies reversible signal decrements that are typical of scoliosis surgery monitoring events. This is because the pathophysiology is usually spinal cord compression, traction, or ischemia that are potentially reversible with quick intervention. Thus, reversing these pro-

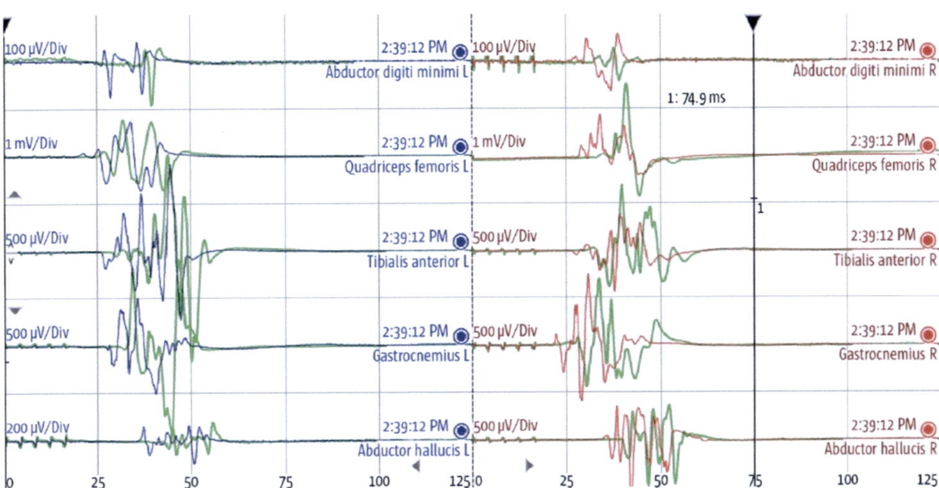

Fig. 8.35 Bilateral MEP monitoring during surgery for thoracolumbar scoliosis shown in Figs. 8.33 and 8.34. The MEPs were recorded from the abductor digit minimi muscles as controls and several muscles of the lower extremities as monitors. *L* left, *R* Right. © ARKANA Forum GmbH 2022. All Rights Reserved

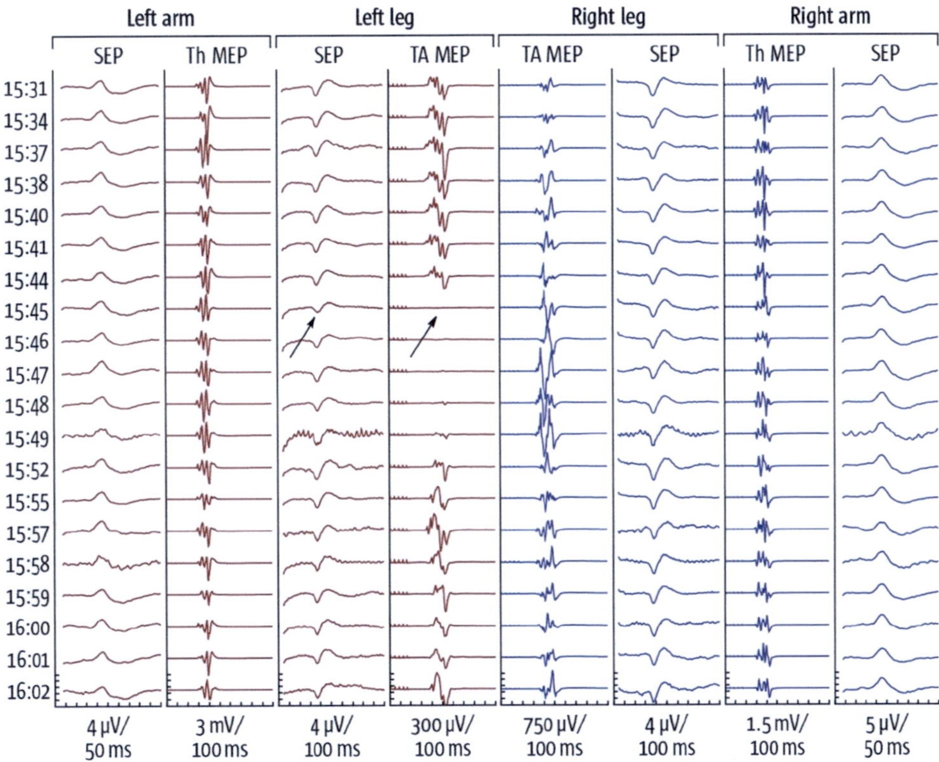

Fig. 8.36 Quickly reversible focal evoked potential decrements during scoliosis surgery. The surgeon inserted a high-thoracic left sublaminar hook at 15:44. One minute later, there was abrupt left tibialis anterior (TA) MEP disappearance and 30% tibial nerve cortical SEP reduction (arrows). To simplify, the figure omits abductor hallucis MEPs that also disappeared, as well as cubital and popliteal fossa SEPs that were stable. Quick signal recovery followed immediate hook removal to relieve suspected acute spinal cord compression. Note that SEP optimization enabled rapid surgical feedback every 1–3 min without compromising reproducibility. Th, thenar. From [21], with permission

cesses depends on rapid surgical feedback to pick up deterioration at an early stage, thereby enabling the surgeon to intervene before structural neural damage begins to set in.

8.4 IONM in Vascular Surgery

Procedures in vascular surgery for which neuromonitoring is relevant relate in particular to **thoracoabdominal aneurysms** of the aorta and **carotid stenosis.** Aneurysms arise from a weakness of the aortic wall and can cause massive life-threatening hemorrhage from rupture. Carotid stenosis is a narrowing of the carotid artery that reduces cerebral blood flow and can cause transient ischemic attacks or stroke.

The aim of neuromonitoring in the surgical treatment of thoracoabdominal aneurysms is the early detection of spinal cord ischemia that risks infarction with paraplegia. The ischemia centers in and may be limited to the lumbosacral gray matter, especially the anterior horns that contain lower motor neurons. Therefore, spinal cord monitoring with muscle **MEPs** is essential for this application. The addition of **SEPs** enhances interpretation of the results, but SEPs alone are insufficient. The critical phase for monitoring begins with the clamping of the aorta. From this moment on, the monitored potentials must be continuously observed until the vessel is unclamped [30].

In the surgical treatment of carotid stenosis, called carotid endarterectomy, the goal is to detect any critical reduction of cerebral blood flow at an early stage. Monitoring for this application is usually accomplished by median and sometimes also tibial nerve **SEPs,** and/or by multichannel **EEG**. The addition of **MEPs** may further improve sensitivity. Again, special attention is paid to the evoked potential course during the clamp time. In case of signal deterioration, the surgeon must be informed immediately in order to facilitate appropriate measures to maintain cerebral blood flow, such as inserting a shunt to bypass the clamped segment [31–34].

Case Example: Thoracoabdominal Aneurysm
Clinical Setting:

The patient presented with abdominal pain and no neurologic deficits. Investigations revealed an extensive atherosclerotic thoracoabdominal aneurysm. The surgical plan was open repair with IONM.

Procedure and Monitoring:

The surgery proceeded with left atrio-femoral bypass. Instead of cannulating the left femoral artery, which blocks left leg blood flow, the surgeon cannulated a femoral artery side graft in order to include the limb in the bypass flow circuit. This strategy preserves left leg evoked potentials that otherwise disappear due to limb ischemia. Monitoring included bilateral thenar, tibialis anterior, and abductor hallucis MEPs and four-limb peripheral–cortical optimized SEPs. Upper limb potentials provided systemic control, and peripheral SEPs controlled for limb ischemia. The MEP warning limit was disappearance unexplained by confounding factors.

There was gradual generalized evoked potential baseline drift related to systemic factors throughout the surgery, and leg MEPs showed substantial trial-to-trial amplitude variability. More importantly, leg MEPs abruptly disappeared 2 min after the first proximal aortic cross-clamp (Fig. 8.37). Quick MEP restoration followed immediate clamp release for probable cord ischemia. Clamping a slightly lower aortic level produced no MEP deterioration. The surgeon thought that the first aortic segment contained segmental arteries critical for spinal cord blood supply. There were no further pathological decrements, and the patient had no postoperative neurologic deficits, but, unfortunately, later died of cardiac complications.

Case Example: Carotid Stenosis
Clinical Setting:

The patient presented with symptoms of left cerebral ischemia. Investigations revealed critical left carotid stenosis. Thus, **carotid endarterectomy** with IONM was planned.

Procedure and Monitoring:

After exposure, the carotid artery was clamped above and below the affected segment. The ves-

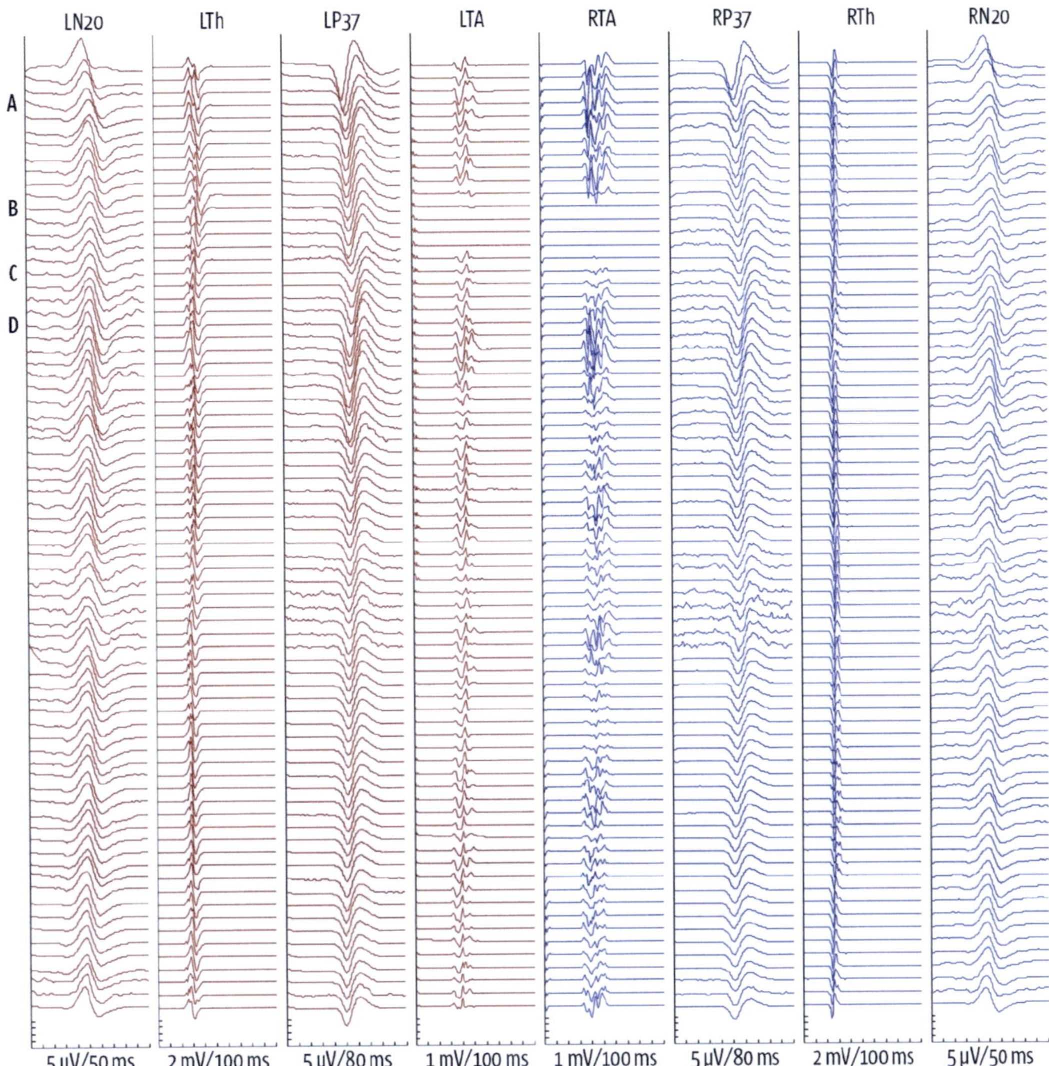

Fig. 8.37 Open thoracoabdominal aneurysm repair. (**A**) Left femoral side graft cannulation. (**B**) Bilateral leg MEP disappearance after proximal aortic clamping. (**C**) Restoration after clamp release. (**D**) Clamping a lower aortic level. To simplify, the figure omits abductor hallucis MEPs that also showed reversible disappearance, as well as cubital and popliteal fossa SEPs that were stable. L, left; R, right; N20 and P37, median and tibial nerve cortical SEPs; Th, thenar; TA, tibialis anterior. Modified from [30], with permission

sel was opened, and the plaques causing stenosis were removed. Thereafter, the artery was repaired and unclamped, thus restoring the blood flow.

Monitoring consisted of bilateral median nerve **SEPs**, with left median nerve responses as a control (Fig. 8.38). The SEPs remained stable throughout the procedure, and the neurological outcome was uneventful. Facultatively, tibial nerve SEPs, EEG, and/or MEPs can be registered in addition.

Case Example: Carotid Stenosis
Clinical Setting:

The patient presented with symptoms of left cerebral ischemia. Investigations revealed critical left carotid stenosis. The surgical plan was **carotid endarterectomy** with EEG monitoring.

Procedure and Monitoring:

The surgery proceeded like the previous case. Monitoring consisted of 16-channel EEG. The

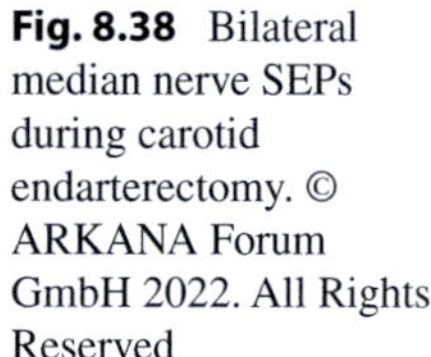

Fig. 8.38 Bilateral median nerve SEPs during carotid endarterectomy. © ARKANA Forum GmbH 2022. All Rights Reserved

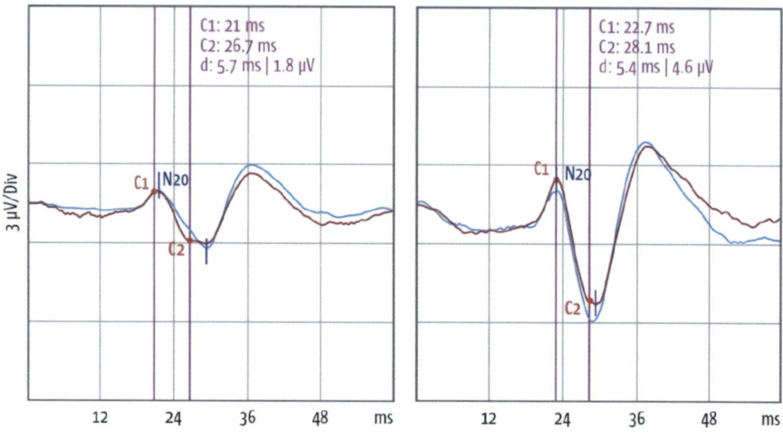

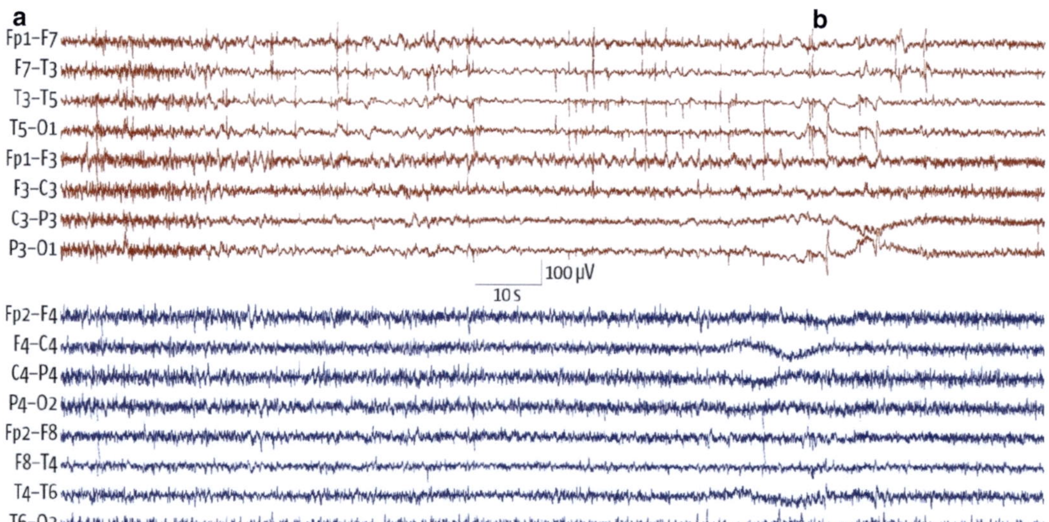

Fig. 8.39 Carotid endarterectomy with EEG monitoring. (**a**) Clamp left carotid artery. (**b**) Shunt established. Note the compressed time base to visualize evolving EEG patterns. The brief high-amplitude deflections are dissimilar metal artifacts from the metallic clamps. © ARKANA Forum GmbH 2022. All Rights Reserved

pre-clamp EEG baseline showed an approximately symmetric mixed-frequency anesthesia pattern. Within 20 s of left carotid artery clamping, there was left temporo-centro-parietal fast activity amplitude reduction, followed by increased slow activity amplitude, and then suppression of all frequencies (Fig. 8.39). The surgeon inserted a shunt and the EEG began to return to baseline within 20 s. There were no further EEG events, and the patient had no postoperative deficit.

This case exemplifies typical EEG alterations due to focal cerebral ischemia. Because EEG requires expertise and multiple scalp electrodes, many IONM programs use evoked potentials instead. Nevertheless, EEG was the first technique applied to endarterectomy and is very effective when properly deployed. It is also possible to quantify the results with computerized compressed spectral displays, but one must still observe the raw signals to differentiate between true EEG and artifact.

8.5 IONM in General Surgery

8.5.1 Thyroid Surgery

The thyroid gland is located in the neck below the larynx in front of the trachea. It has left and right lobes that are connected by an isthmus (Fig. 8.40). Goiter, an enlargement of the thyroid gland, represents worldwide the most common endocrine gland disease (endocrinopathy). The enlarged thyroid gland may function normally, may be underactive (hypothyroidism), or may be overactive (hyperthyroidism). During operations on the thyroid gland, the **recurrent laryngeal nerve** is particularly at risk. This nerve runs behind the thyroid gland and supplies the laryngeal muscles. Injury to the recurrent laryngeal nerve leads to vocal cord paralysis. Unilateral paralysis results in hoarseness, while bilateral paralysis may cause respiratory distress.

The **recurrent laryngeal recurrent nerve** is monitored by recording the **CMAPs** from its target vocalis muscle. Recording is performed either invasively via needle electrodes or, more often, non-invasively via an electrode attached to the endotracheal tube, which is in contact with the vocalis muscle. For intermittent stimulation of the recurrent laryngeal nerve, a hand-held probe is used.

Alternatively, the **vagus nerve** can be stimulated directly by an electrode wrapped around it, thus facilitating continuous CMAP recording. The first vagus nerve stimulation (V1) serves to test the pre-resection functional status of the recurrent laryngeal nerve in its entire course. This is followed by stimulation of the recurrent laryngeal nerve (R1) which is used to identify the nerve, thus supporting its visualization. After completion of the resection, a further functional check of both nerves is performed. The post-resection response signal of the vagus nerve is used to demonstrate the function of the complete pathway from the vagus nerve via the recurrent laryngeal nerve to the vocal cords. This step (V2) is essential because mere post-surgical stimulation of the recurrent laryngeal nerve can result in a positive response signal despite a cut or damaged nerve if the stimulation is distal to the lesion [35–38].

During resection of the cranial poles of the thyroid gland, the external branch of the **superior laryngeal nerve** must be spared. This branch innervates the cricothyroid muscle. Functional control can be achieved by direct electrical stimulation. Contraction of the cricothyroid muscle, which can be observed visually during surgery or recorded via needle electrodes, clearly indicates preservation of nerve function. In approx. 70–80% of patients, a connection (ramus communicans) between the external branch of the superior laryngeal nerve and the recurrent laryngeal nerve is present. In these cases, a signal can also be recorded from the vocalis muscle, which may be visually and acoustically displayed by the IONM device.

Case Example: Goiter
Clinical Setting:

The patient presented with a goiter that was not seen in normal posture, but could be found by palpation. Endocrine and metabolic functions were within the normal ranges. Excision of the goiter with IONM was planned.

Procedure and Monitoring:

First, the **vagus nerve** was exposed, and a stimulation electrode was wrapped around the nerve. Vocalis CMAPs were recorded from needle electrodes (Fig. 8.41). During tumor resection, the **recurrent laryngeal nerve** was identified by stimulation (Fig. 8.42). After com-

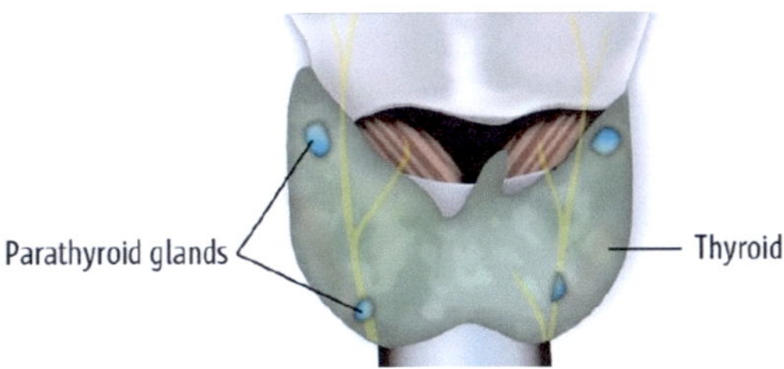

Fig. 8.40 Schematic illustration of the anatomy and location of the thyroid gland. © ARKANA Forum GmbH 2022. All Rights Reserved

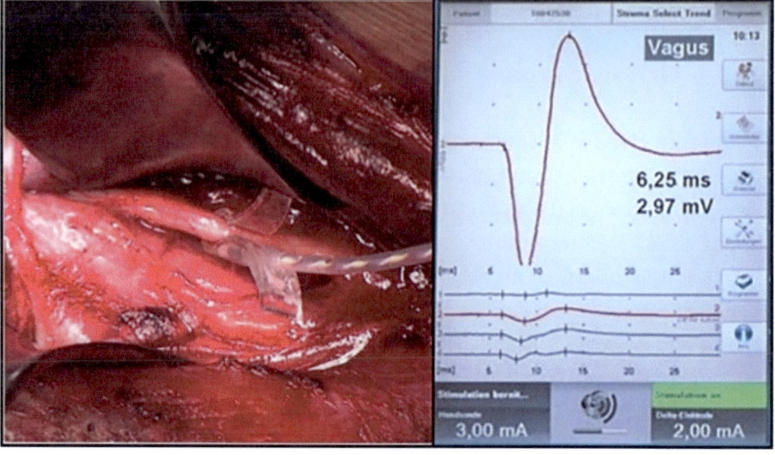

Fig. 8.41 Vocalis CMAPs recorded during continuous stimulation of the vagus nerve. © ARKANA Forum GmbH 2022. All Rights Reserved

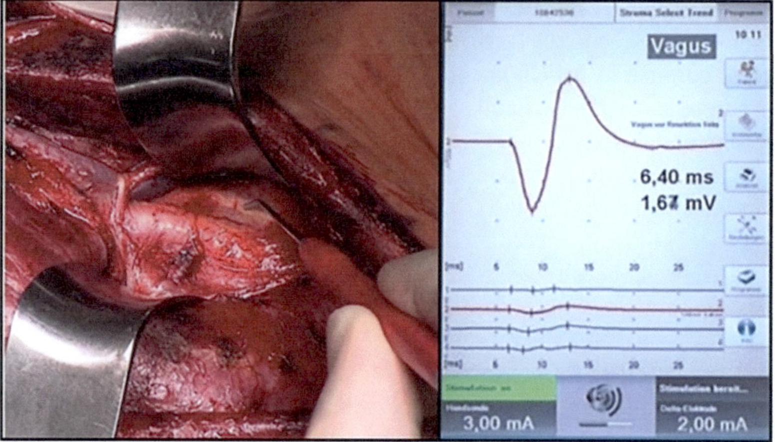

Fig. 8.42 Vocalis CMAPs recorded during intermittent stimulation of the recurrent laryngeal nerve. © ARKANA Forum GmbH 2022. All Rights Reserved

plete resection of the goiter, the recurrent laryngeal nerve was stimulated again. Preserved post-resection response signals both after stimulation of the vagus nerve and the recurrent laryngeal nerve were indicative of an intact function of the complete pathway.

8.5.2 Colorectal Surgery

Colorectal carcinoma is a tumor of the rectum with the inferior margin at a maximum distance of 16 cm from the anocutaneous line. It represents the second most common malignant tumor. Tumor resection can be performed conventionally or by laparoscopy. After dissection, the rectum is detached from the pelvis minor. Dissection in the pelvis minor is strictly oriented to the anatomy of the marginal layers. This approach allows removal of the affected part of the rectum together with the mesorectum, which contains possible lymph node metastases. Particular care must be taken during this procedure to protect the nerves at the pelvic floor and wall.

Colorectal surgery risks impairment of **anal sphincter**, **bladder**, and **sexual** function. The reason for this is that the respective fine nerve structures (inferior hypogastric plexus and splanchnic pelvic nerves) often cannot be visually identified and thus cannot always be preserved if the tumor is radically removed. Pelvic IONM uses the techniques of autonomic nervous system monitoring and allows identification and monitoring of these fine nerve structures. Stimulation is accomplished with a hand-held probe which is applied to the pelvic wall while **bladder pressure** and **internal anal sphincter EMG** are observed. These signals must be

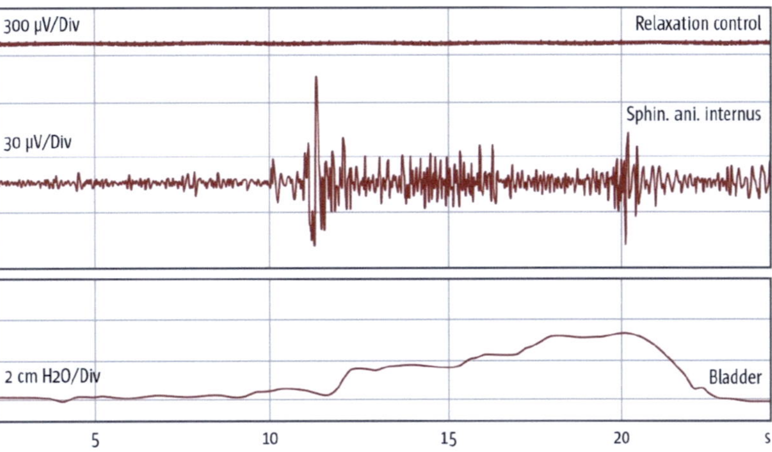

Fig. 8.43 Relaxation control recorded from the external sphincter ani muscle (top), and responses of the internal sphincter ani muscle (middle) and bladder pressure (bottom) during resection of a rectal carcinoma. Preserved responses indicated an uneventful outcome. © ARKANA Forum GmbH 2022. All Rights Reserved

closely monitored when the rectum is detached from the lesser pelvis, during which the inferior hypogastric plexus and the splanchnic pelvic nerves are particularly at risk [39, 40]. When interpreting the signals, special care must be taken not to mistake mechanical or electrical disturbances as positive responses.

Case Example: Rectal Carcinoma
Clinical Setting:

The male patient presented with rectal symptoms, weight loss, and anorexia. Investigations revealed a rectal carcinoma. Radical tumor removal with pelvic IONM was planned.

Procedure and Monitoring:

After extensive dissection and exposure, stimulation of the pelvic wall was performed with a hand-held probe. Monitoring included the **internal sphincter ani** and the **detrusor vesicae muscles**. Immediately before measurement was commenced, the bladder was filled with 200 ml of Ringer's solution. As a control of muscle relaxation, additional recording was done from the external sphincter ani muscle (Fig. 8.43).

8.6 IONM in Otolaryngology

The **parotid gland** is located in front of and slightly below the ear between the skin and the masseter muscle. It is divided into two lobes by connective tissue. When removing tumors of the parotid gland, the facial nerve, which runs between the two lobes, is at risk.

Monitoring of the **facial nerve** during parotid surgery in otolaryngology has been used for decades. The facial nerve was stimulated with a hand-held probe, and contraction of facial muscles was observed. Later, facial nerve monitoring was extended to middle ear and inner ear procedures. Intermittent stimulation with a monopolar probe during drilling at the mastoid allows estimation of the distance to the nerve. In addition to monitoring by intermittent stimulation, continuous observation of the free-running EMG has proven helpful. Here, particular attention should be paid to A-trains [41, 42] (see also Sect. 5.2.1).

Case Example: Removal of the Parotid Gland (Parotidectomy)
Clinical Setting:

The patient presented with a parotid mass that proved to be a **pleomorphic adenoma.** Complete parotidectomy with facial nerve monitoring was planned.

Procedure and Monitoring:

The patient's head was turned slightly so that the parotid gland was easily accessible (Fig. 8.44). After exposure, the facial nerve was identified by direct stimulation with a monopolar hand-held probe while recording orbicularis oris and orbicularis oculi CMAPs (Fig. 8.45). Particular attention was paid to spontaneous A-trains. Preserved CMAPs at the end of surgery were associated with intact postoperative facial nerve function. As an alternative, bipolar stimulation can be used, and recording can be extended to the fron-

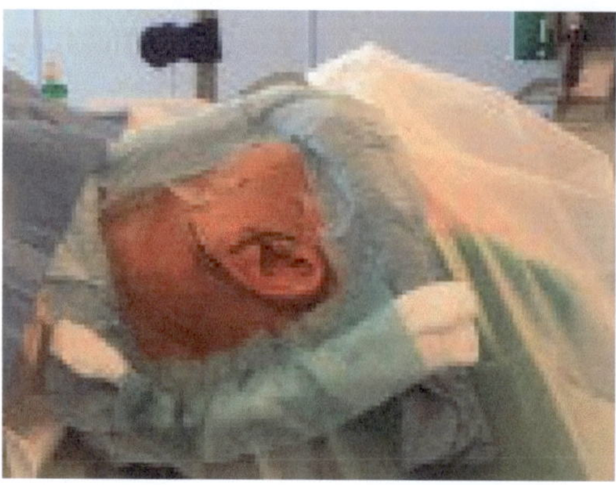

Fig. 8.44 Positioning of the patient for parotidectomy (skin incision is marked). © ARKANA Forum GmbH 2022. All Rights Reserved

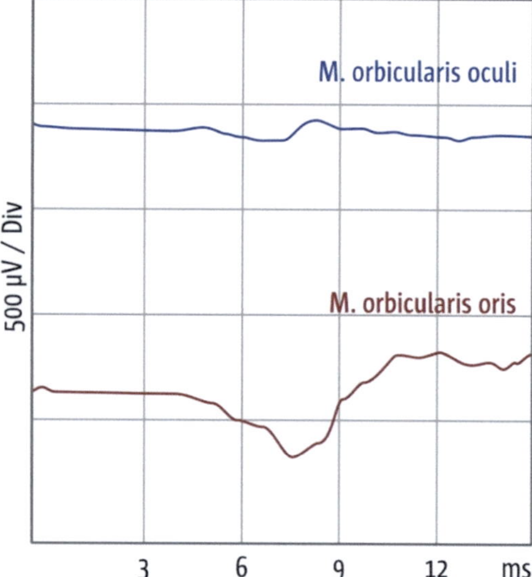

Fig. 8.45 Orbicularis oculi and orbicularis oris CMAPs after stimulation of the facial nerve. © ARKANA Forum GmbH 2022. All Rights Reserved

talis and mentalis muscles using a four-channel technique in order to better differentiate the individual branches of the facial nerve.`.

References

1. MacDonald DB, Dong C, Quatrale R, Sala F, Skinner S, Soto F, et al. Recommendations of the International Society of Intraoperative Neurophysiology for intraoperative somatosensory evoked potentials. Clin Neurophysiol. 2019;130(1):161–79.

2. MacDonald DB, Skinner S, Shils J, Yingling C. Intraoperative motor evoked potential monitoring—a position statement by the American Society of Neurophysiological Monitoring. Clin Neurophysiol. 2013;124(12):2291–316.

3. Zentner J, Hufnagel A, Pechstein U, Wolf HK, Schramm J. Functional results after resective procedures involving the supplementary motor area. J Neurosurg. 1996;85(4):542–9.

4. Cedzich C, Taniguchi M, Schäfer S, Schramm J. Somatosensory evoked potenial phase reversal and direct motor cortex stimulation during surgery in and around the central region. Neurosurgery. 1996;38:962–70.

5. Fujii M, Maesawa S, Motomura K, Futamura M, Hayashi Y, Koba I, et al. Intraoperative subcortical mapping of a language-associated deep frontal tract connecting the superior frontal gyrus to Broca's area in the dominant hemisphere of patients with glioma. J Neurosurg. 2015;122(6):1390–6.

6. Kim K, Cho C, Bang M, Shin HI, Phi JH, Kim SK. Intraoperative neurophysiological monitoring: a review of techniques used for brain tumor surgery in children. J Korean Neurosurg Soc. 2018;61(3):363–75.

7. Kombos T, Süss O, Kern BC, Funk T, Hoell T, Kopetsch O, et al. Comparison between monopolar and bipolar electrical stimulation of the motor cortex. Acta Neurochir. 1999;141:1295–301.

8. Suess O, Suess S, Brock M, Kombos T. Intraoperative electrocortical stimulation of Brodman area 4: a 10-year analysis of 255 cases. Head Face Med. 2006;2(1) https://doi.org/10.1186/1746-160X-2-20.

9. Kang D, Yao P, Wu Z, Yu L. Ischemia changes and tolerance ratio of evoked potential monitoring in intracranial aneurysm surgery. Clin Neurol Neurosurg. 2013;115(5):552–6.

10. Motoyama Y, Kawaguchi M, Yamada S, Nakagawa I, Nishimura F, Hironaka Y, et al. Evaluation of combined use of transcranial and direct cortical motor evoked potential monitoring during unruptured aneurysm surgery. Neurol Med Chir (Tokyo). 2011;51(1):15–22.

11. Szelényi A, Bueno de Camargo A, Flamm ES, Deletis V. Neurophysiological criteria for intraoperative prediction of pure motor hemiplegia during aneurysm surgery. J Neurosurg. 2003;99:575–8.

12. Szelényi A, Langer D, Beck J, Raabe A, Flamm ES, Seifert V, et al. Transcranial and direct cortical stimulation for motor evoked potential monitoring in intracerebral aneurysm surgery. Neurophysiol Clin Neurophysiol. 2007;37(6):391–8.

13. Deletis V, Fernández-Conejero I. Intraoperative monitoring and mapping of the functional integrity of the brainstem. J Clin Neurol. 2016;12(3):262.

14. Ulkatan S, Deletis V, Fernandez-Conejero I. Central or peripheral activations of the facial nerve? J Neurosurg. 2007;106(3):519–20.

15. Amano M, Kohno M, Nagata O, Taniguchi M, Sora S, Sato H. Intraoperative continuous monitoring of

evoked facial nerve electromyograms in acoustic neuroma surgery. Acta Neurochir. 2011;153(5):1059–67.

16. Morota N, Ihara S, Deletis V. Intraoperative neurophysiology for surgery in and around the brainstem: role of brainstem mapping and corticobulbar tract motor-evoked potential monitoring. Childs Nerv Syst. 2010;26(4):513–21.

17. Seidel K, Biner MS, Zubak I, Rychen J, Beck J, Raabe A. Continuous dynamic mapping to avoid accidental injury of the facial nerve during surgery for large vestibular schwannomas. Neurosurg Rev. 2020;43(1):241–8.

18. Prell J, Strauss C, Rachinger J, Alfieri A, Scheller C, Herfurth K, et al. Facial nerve palsy after vestibular schwannoma surgery: dynamic risk-stratification based on continuous EMG-monitoring. Clin Neurophysiol. 2013;125:415.

19. Romstöck J, Strauss C, Fahlbusch R. Continuous electromyography monitoring of motor cranial nerves during cerebellopontine angle surgery. J Neurosurg. 2000;93(4):586–93.

20. Sala F. Take the a train. Clin Neurophysiol. 2015;126(9):1647–9.

21. MacDonald DB, Dong C. Evoked potentials and intraoperative monitoring. In: Greenfield LJ, Geyer JD, Carney PR, editors. Reading EEGs: a practical approach. 2nd ed. Philadelphia: Wolters Kluwer; 2020.

22. Malcharek MJ, Landgraf J, Hennig G, Sorge O, Aschermann J, Sablotzki A. Recordings of long-latency trigeminal somatosensory-evoked potentials in patients under general anaesthesia. Clin Neurophysiol. 2011 May;122(5):1048–54.

23. Minahan RE, Mandir AS. Neurophysiologic intraoperative monitoring of trigeminal and facial nerves. J Clin Neurophysiol. 2011;28(6):551–65.

24. Ito Z, Matsuyama Y, Ando M, Kawabata S, Kanchiku T, Kida K, et al. What is the best multimodality combination for intraoperative spinal cord monitoring of motor function? A multicenter study by the monitoring Committee of the Japanese Society for spine surgery and related research. Glob Spine J. 2016;6(3):234–41.

25. Kothbauer KF. Intraoperatives neurophysiologic monitoring for intramedullary spinal cord tumor surgery. Oper Tech Neurosurg. 2003;6(1):2–8.

26. Kothbauer KF. The interpretation of muscle motor evoked potentials for spinal cord monitoring. J Clin Neurophysiol. 2017;34(1):32–7.

27. Yanni DS, Ulkatan S, Deletis V, Barrenechea IJ, Sen C, Perin NI. Utility of neurophysiological monitoring using dorsal column mapping in intramedullary spinal cord surgery. J Neurosurg Spine. 2010;12:623–8.

28. Schwartz DM. Neurophysiological detection of impending spinal cord injury during scoliosis surgery. J Bone Jt Surg Am. 2007;89(11):2440.

29. Shiban E, Meyer B, Stoffel M, Weinzierl M. Intraoperatives neurophysiologisches monitoring (IOM) in der Wirbelsäulenchirurgie. Wirbels. 2017;01(03):203–18.

30. MacDonald DB, Janusz M. An approach to intraoperative neurophysiologic monitoring of thoracoabdominal aneurysm surgery. J Clin Neurophysiol. 2002;19(1):43–54.

31. Fielmuth S, Uhlig T. The role of somatosensory evoked potentials in detecting cerebral ischaemia during carotid endarterectomy: an assessment of its validity under regional anaesthesia. Eur J Anaesthesiol. 2008;25(8):648–56.

32. Malcharek MJ, Herbst V, Bartz GJ, Manceur AM, Gille J, Hennig G, et al. Multimodal evoked potential monitoring in asleep patients versus neurological evaluation in awake patients during carotid endarterectomy: a single-Centre retrospective trial of 651 patients. Minerva Anestesiol. 2015;81(10):1070–8.

33. So VC, Poon CCM. Intraoperative neuromonitoring in major vascular surgery. Br J Anaesth. 2016;117:ii13–25.

34. Thirumala PD, Natarajan P, Thiagarajan K, Crammond DJ, Habeych ME, Chaer RA, et al. Diagnostic accuracy of somatosensory evoked potential and electroencephalography during carotid endarterectomy. Neurol Res. 2016;38(8):698–705.

35. Angeletti F, Musholt PB, Musholt TJ. Continuous intraoperative neuromonitoring in thyroid surgery. Surg Technol Int. 2015;27:79–85.

36. De la Quintana BA, Iglesias Martínez A, Salutregui I, Agirre Etxabe L, Arana González A, Yurrebaso SI. Continuous monitoring of the recurrent laryngeal nerve. Langenbeck's Arch Surg. 2018;403(3):333–9.

37. Dionigi G, Kim HY, Wu CW, Lavazza M, Ferrari C, Leotta A, et al. Vagus nerve stimulation for standardized monitoring: technical notes for conventional and endoscopic thyroidectomy. Surg Technol Int. 2013;23:95–103.

38. Randolph GW, Dralle H, With the International Intraoperative Monitoring Study Group, Abdullah H, Barczynski M, Bellantone R, et al. Electrophysiologic recurrent laryngeal nerve monitoring during thyroid and parathyroid surgery: international standards guideline statement. Laryngoscope. 2011;121(S1):S1–16.

39. Kauff DW, Lang H, Kneist W. Risk factor analysis for newly developed urogenital dysfunction after total mesorectal excision and impact of pelvic intraoperative neuromonitoring? A prospective 2-year follow-up study. J Gastrointest Surg. 2017;21(6):1038–47.

40. Schiemer JF, Zimniak L, Grimminger P, Lang H, Kneist W. Robot-guided neuromapping during nerve-sparing taTME for low rectal cancer. Int J Color Dis. 2018;33:1803.

41. Marchesi M, Biffoni M, Trinchi S, Turriziani V, Campana FP. Facial nerve function after parotidectomy for neoplasms with deep localization. Surg Today. 2006;36(4):308–11.

42. Ozturk K, Akyildiz S, Gode S, Turhal G, Gursan G, Kirazli T. The effect of partial superficial parotidectomy on amplitude, latency and threshold of facial nerve stimulation. Eur Arch Otorrinolaringol. 2016;273(6):1527–31.

Efficiency and Safety of Intraoperative Neuromonitoring

9

David MacDonald and Josef Zentner

Contents

D. MacDonald (✉)
ARKANA Forum GmbH, Emmendingen, Germany

J. Zentner
Department of Neurosurgery, University Medical
Center, Freiburg, Germany

Efficiency

It has been shown during the last decades that the different **modalities** used in intraoperative neuromonitoring (IONM) **fulfill the requirements of the monitoring concept**. All methods presented here are able to indicate impending neurological

impairment at the stage of reversibility and can thus in principle be used in everyday clinical practice. However, the question arises as to which **application areas** IONM has proven particularly successful, which **patients** should be monitored and which modalities should be used if any. In this context, it is also important to consider the **limitations** of IONM. Finally, the question arises whether and to what extent the expenses associated with IONM are justified from an **economic point of view**.

As early as 1991, a consensus paper from the United States **National Institutes of Health** stated that intraoperative monitoring of **cranial nerves VII and VIII** is useful during neurosurgical procedures in the cerebellopontine angle. Similarly, monitoring of the facial nerve has proven to be beneficial in otolaryngology for surgical procedures at the parotid gland and petrous bone. The value of monitoring cranial nerves VII and VIII in reducing neurological deficits has been demonstrated with statistical significance [1]. In addition, in 2004, the **American Academy of Neurology** recommended the use of electroencephalography to monitor cerebral blood flow during carotid endarterectomy, recording of brainstem auditory evoked potentials in procedures at the brainstem, and the application of somatosensory evoked potentials for spinal procedures [2].

From **today's view**, the range of IONM applications can be expanded with the currently available technical facilities. Monitoring of **cranial nerves** should be considered in complex interventions at the skull base as well as in thyroid and parotid surgery. In brain tumor and vascular surgery, assessment of **motor and sensory pathways**, including **functional topographic mapping**, has proven to be helpful. In addition, monitoring of spinal cord function has gained general acceptance, particularly for the removal of intramedullary tumors, the correction of scoliosis, and the surgical treatment of thoracoabdominal aneurysms. Finally, monitoring of **peripheral nerves** and **nerve roots** during tumor resection and pedicle screw implantation has proven useful.

In addition to the main goal of reducing neurological morbidity, monitoring has proven to be a **didactic tool**: Surgeons have not only learned on which occasions potentials and function can be lost, but have also learned to avoid these situations by modifying surgical strategy and dissection techniques. By providing surgeons with constant feedback on the functional impact of surgical steps, monitoring focuses their attention and motivation to preserve important structures. If the surgeon is willing and able to incorporate the information gained through monitoring into the surgical strategy, one can speak of **functionally guided surgery**.

Obviously, it makes little sense to monitor the auditory nerve in a patient who is already deaf preoperatively, or brainstem function during removal of a frontal tumor. However, IONM should be applied whenever functionally relevant neural structures are at risk during surgery and when these structures are amenable to adequate intraoperative electrophysiological surveillance. Thus, a major **limitation** becomes apparent: Only **circumscribed neural structures or pathways** are amenable to IONM. Therefore, the choice of the appropriate modality to assess structures and pathways at risk is of essential importance. Further limitations are **technical problems** that may occur despite the availability of modern techniques and that are not always resolvable. Finally, the **clinical relevance** of potential findings is not always clear.

Economic constraints in health care raise questions about the **cost-benefit ratio** of IONM. To date, only sparse data are available on this issue, and most of them are hardly reliable. It is relatively easy to calculate the costs incurred by IONM. Much more difficult, however, is the calculation of costs resulting from health impairment caused by postoperative neurological deficits that could have been avoided with a certain probability by monitoring. Corresponding calculations usually only take the primary costs in medical care into account. Secondary costs due to loss of work, performance restrictions, etc., are even more difficult to evaluate, while the subjective reduction in the quality of life of patients suffering postoperative neurological deficits largely escapes calculation.

It is difficult to assess objective **health-care costs with and without IONM**. Standard blinded randomized studies cannot be used. The frequently used comparison with historical data in which IONM was not applied is only of limited value. This is particularly true since more favorable neurological outcomes may rather result from improved surgical techniques than from monitoring, so that the influence of the IONM can only be concluded with reservations.

Despite these limitations, for some IONM applications **robust data** with regard to the cost-benefit ratio are available. For example, not only a medical but also an economic added value could be demonstrated for monitoring of the **facial nerve** in middle ear surgery [3]. The same applies to monitoring of **cranial nerves VII and VIII** during neurosurgical interventions in the **cerebellopontine angle** [4].

Furthermore, there are convincing considerations for the use of IONM in orthopedic operations for the **correction of scoliosis**. Although neurological deficits are rare in these procedures, they can be extremely serious when they occur, including permanent paraplegia or even quadriplegia. A reduction of such severe deficits from 1% without IONM to 0.5% with IONM, which should be achievable even with a conservative estimate, not only would bring an enormous improvement in the quality of treatment for the patients concerned but also would be advantageous from an economic point of view [1].

Similar considerations of the cost-benefit ratio are available for the use of the IONM in **pedicle screw implantation**. For example, experience with monitoring has been reported in the implantation of 5000 pedicle screws in 1000 patients, with additional postoperative neurologic deficits noted in only one patient (0.1%) [5]. Notably, corresponding complications without IONM were documented in 2–10% of patients in comparable series. Even assuming a complication rate of only 2% without IONM, cost calculations demonstrate an economic gain from monitoring [5].

Due to the abovementioned limitations, demonstration of the significance of IONM from an economic point of view cannot be expected in all application fields in the future either. The justification for the use of the IONM must not be based primarily on a cost-benefit analysis. Rather, the main factors are the **improvement in medical care** to be achieved with IONM and the **increase in the quality of life** of the patients concerned, aspects that can hardly be expressed by facts and figures [1].

Overall, IONM has undoubtedly gained a solid place in various surgical disciplines today. Certainly, monitoring is not necessary for every surgical procedure in which nervous structures are affected. However, for certain interventions, IONM has proven to be definitely helpful. The selection of suitable patients, the proper selection of examination techniques, the expertise of the monitoring team, and effective communication in the operating room contribute decisively to the efficiency of neuromonitoring.

Safety

9.1 Introduction

Intraoperative neuromonitoring (IONM) is generally very safe but, like any medical procedure, can accidentally harm patients or staff. Understanding the possible and theoretical **hazards** and routinely applying **means of protection** are basic to safe practice. Therefore, in this chapter we explore electrical safety, procedure-specific safety, infection control, and essential performance, with the intention of explaining the rationale behind appropriate precautions. The information is from several key references [6–12], supplemented by some additional citations.

9.2 Electrical Safety

Neuromonitoring involves complex medical electric devices having multiple patient connections. Potential dangers include electric shock of patients or staff, hazardous stimulator output, electrode burns, and fire.

9.2.1 Electric Shock

An electric shock consists of stimulation of excitable tissues by current flowing between two or more body contacts. The effects range from benign perception or twitches to pain, muscle contractions, seizures, tissue necrosis, and cardiac failure due to **ventricular fibrillation** (VF) that is the usual cause of death by electrocution.

9.2.1.1 Ventricular Fibrillation

Neuromonitoring devices or connections could theoretically cause fatal VF and **we must protect against this hazard**. **Alternating current** of **10–200 Hz** is particularly dangerous, including 50 or 60 Hz power line frequency. Current from an **intracardiac** electrode is more dangerous than transthoracic current from limb, head, or trunk electrodes. At 50–60 Hz, the probability of VF is 100% with only 0.5 mA intracardiac current, but drops to 1% with 1000 mA transthoracic current because current strength dissipates with distance through the body.

Standard IONM stimulators generate ≤100 mA current applied locally between electrodes over neural targets. Inadvertent connection to an **intracardiac current pathway would be hazardous**, but normal stimulator use produces only negligeable transthoracic current. Even with accidental stimulation between limbs (e.g., cathode on one median nerve and anode on the other), 100 mA transthoracic current would have a low risk of VF.

However, **transcranial electric stimulation** (TES) for motor evoked potential (MEP) monitoring applies strong current of up to 250–1000 mA. Most flows between scalp stimulating electrodes, but **parasitic transthoracic current** can occur if TES current enters scalp recording electrodes, flows to leg electrodes via the **same headbox**, and then returns to the head through the thorax and heart [13]. This might partly explain rare cardiac arrhythmia during TES (0.03%); there are **no reports of VF**. Note that the parasitic pathway cannot arise if upper and lower body electrodes are in separate headboxes. Apart from stimulation current, there is also the danger that **leakage current** could cause electric shock or theoretically, trigger VF by reaching the heart.

9.2.1.2 Leakage Currents

All medical electric devices produce nonfunctional leakage currents. **Chassis** leakage current flows from device surfaces via the patient or operator to ground. **Auxiliary** leakage current flows between patient connections, such as impedance testing. **Patient** leakage current flows via patient connections to ground and may come from an extrinsic voltage source, including **accidental power mains connection** that is very hazardous and has actually occurred in the past with unprotected pin connectors [14].

Leakage currents are an important IONM safety issue because (1) multiple patient connections increase **total leakage current**, (2) other operating room electric device connections create **additional voltage sources** and **ground pathways**, and (3) intravenous **central lines** form **potential current pathways to the heart** that nearby IONM electrodes could contact, e.g., Erb's point is close to internal jugular or subclavian central lines. Central line tubing is not conductive but can leak, and blood can pool at the puncture site. Thus, the conductive fluids inside the tubing and in the fresh track around it are theoretical conductive pathways to the heart. This is the basis of a longstanding safety recommendation to avoid central line electric contact. For perspective, there are **no reports of VF** by this mechanism. Implanted cardiac pacemakers are not a leakage current issue because they are insulated and covered by intact skin.

9.2.1.3 Means of Protection Against Electric Shock

Considering the above, one must **never permit intracardiac connections** to IONM devices that are not designed for them. We should also prevent parasitic transthoracic current by using **separate upper and lower body head boxes** during TES. Manufacturers must design IONM devices to have at least **two means of protection**, such as grounding, insulation, or impedance. They also have to make devices **single-fault safe** so that failure of one protection does not create a hazard.

We must ensure **periodic biomedical inspection** to detect and repair single faults before a hazardous double fault arises. This important precaution should be done at manufacture, installation, every 6 months, and after any malfunction or damage. The engineer confirms that individual and total leakage currents are <0.1 and < 0.5 mA, and with simulated power mains connection, <5 mA. Inspection includes **power cords** that must be **heavy duty with strain relief**. We should **avoid extension cords,** but if used, they have to meet the same standards. We must use **touch-proof connectors** that cannot contact a voltage source when out of their receptacles. Finally, we should **avoid central line contact**; it is safest to omit Erb's point electrodes, although there are no reports of them causing cardiac arrhythmia so far. With these precautions, the chance of electric shock becomes very small.

> **Key Points: Protection Against Electric Shock**
> - *Never allow intracardiac connections.*
> - *Use separate upper and lower body headboxes during TES.*
> - *Ensure IONM devices have two means of protection.*
> - *Ensure IONM devices are single-fault safe.*
> - *Ensure periodic biomedical inspection.*
> - *Use heavy duty power cords with strain relief.*
> - *Avoid extension cords.*
> - *Use touch-proof connectors.*
> - *Avoid central line contact (safest to omit Erb's point).*

9.2.2 Hazardous Stimulator Output

Neuromonitoring normally applies safely controlled electric stimulation, but **excessive output** could possibly damage neural targets or other tissues. Consequently, we must understand stimulus parameters, strength–duration, injury mechanisms, and means of protection.

9.2.2.1 Stimulus Parameters

We apply monophasic or biphasic electric pulses for IONM (Fig. 9.1). Each phase has a width or **duration** D in seconds, **current** intensity I in amperes (A), **charge** Q in coulombs (C), and **energy** E in joules (J). Charge is the integral of current over phase duration, or the amount of electricity. Energy is the integral of current^2 over duration multiplied by **resistance** R in ohms (Ω). For a rectangular phase, $Q = I \times D$, and $E = I^2 \times D \times R$. In neuromonitoring, we express duration in ms or µs, current in mA, charge in µC, resistance in kΩ, and energy in mJ.

With **charge balancing**, the stimulus charge Q_S is followed by a reversal charge $Q_R = - Q_S$, so that net charge transfer is zero. With **asymmetric** balancing, the reversal charge has low current and decays slowly. Biphasic **symmetric** balancing follows the stimulus phase with an equally shaped but opposite-polarity reversal phase.

Trains are a series of pulses at a selected frequency in Hz or **interstimulus interval** (ISI) in ms, where ISI = 1000/frequency. For traditional "Penfield" cortical mapping, we apply 50–60 Hz trains lasting 1–4 s. For TES or direct cortical stimulation (DCS) muscle MEPs, we typically apply 5-pulse trains with a 4 ms ISI (250 Hz).

Constant-current stimulators adjust voltage V using Ohm's law $V = I \times R$ to maintain selected current. This compensates for resistance variations to promote **stable current and evoked responses**. However, if resistance is too high for the maximum available voltage, then output cannot reach selected current. The device must clearly indicate success or failure. Constant-current pulses are approximately rectangular.

Constant-voltage stimulators generate selected voltage. Consequently, resistance variations may cause **unstable current and evoked responses**. There should be a current read-out to aid interpretation. These pulses produce non-rectangular current, with an initial peak followed by exponential decay, or load distortion.

9.2.2.2 Strength–Duration and Injury Mechanisms

Threshold current (I_{th}), charge (Q_{th}), and energy (E_{th}) are continuous functions of D, so

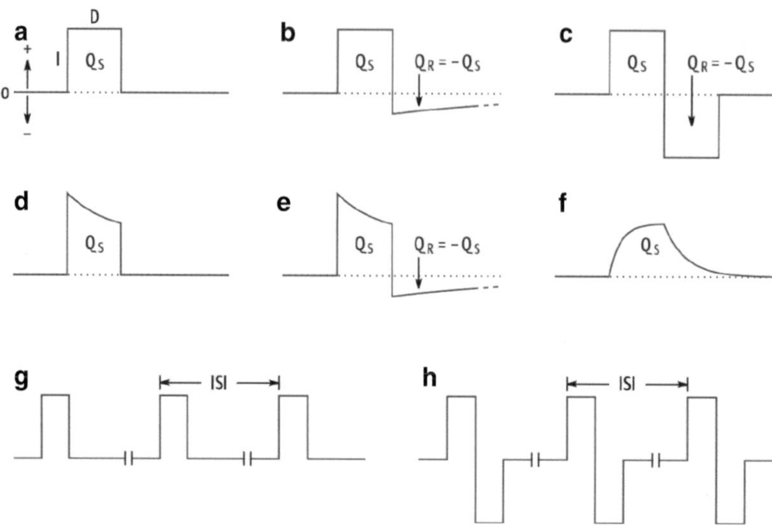

Fig. 9.1 Electric pulses of equal stimulus charge Q_S. (**a**) Monophasic constant-current with current I, duration D, and $Q_S = I \times D$. (**b**) Constant-current with asymmetric reversal charge Q_R. (**c**) Biphasic constant-current with symmetric reversal. (**d**) Monophasic constant-voltage with exponential decay. (**e**) Constant-voltage with asymmetric reversal. (**f**) Constant-voltage with load distortion. (**g**) Monophasic constant-current train. (**h**) Biphasic constant-current train. ISI, interstimulus interval. Modified from [10], with permission

pulse duration is the fundamental parameter. Thresholds also depend on the neural target's **rheobase** (*Rb*) defined as current threshold at infinite D and **chronaxie** (*Cx*) defined as the D at which threshold current is 2 × rheobase. If we know these excitability constants, then we can predict the neural target's thresholds at any D with strength–duration equations:

$$I_{th} = R_b \times \left(1 + \frac{Cx}{D}\right)$$

$$Q_{th} = R_b \times \left(1 + \frac{Cx}{D}\right) \times D$$

$$E_{th} = R_b^2 \times \left(1 + \frac{Cx}{D}\right)^2 \times D \times R$$

From short (0.05 ms) to long (1 ms) D, threshold current drops from high values and then levels off towards rheobase, while threshold charge increases linearly, and threshold energy drops to a minimum at the chronaxie and the rises again. Each has a different potential injury mechanism: energy generates heat that risks **thermal injury**, charge is an **excitotoxic** factor, and current risks **electrochemical toxicity**. These mechanisms are demonstrable in experimental animals, but are mostly theoretical in humans undergoing IONM. Still, we should try to minimize their likelihood.

The safest D will **minimize threshold strength** and thereby also suprathreshold and supramaximal strengths. However, using long D to minimize current causes high charge and energy, while using short D to minimize charge causes high current and energy. These choices are not necessarily unsafe, but the **safest pulse duration is the chronaxie** that minimizes energy while balancing modest current and charge (Fig. 9.2).

9.2.2.3 Means of Protection Against Thermal Injury

We can **set D to the chronaxie** to protect against thermal injury by minimizing energy. Unfortunately, the chronaxie is often unknown, although easy to determine (Fig. 9.2). There is good evidence that **mean DCS MEP chronaxie is 0.2 ms**, which is therefore generally the safest D for this modality [15]. Some evidence suggests

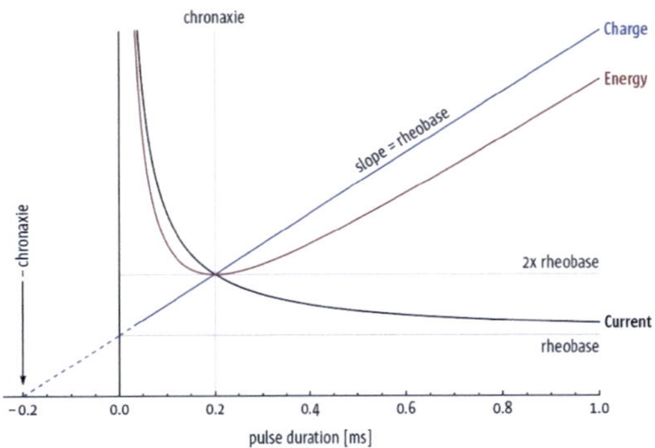

Fig. 9.2 Strength–duration. Threshold current, charge, and energy are functions of pulse duration. Since charge–duration is a straight line, one can determine the rheobase (slope) and chronaxie (X-intercept) from thresholds at two durations (e.g., 0.1 and 1.0 ms). Setting duration to the chronaxie is safest because this minimizes energy while balancing modest current and charge. Modified from [10], with permission

that the same may be true for TES MEPs, but most transcranial stimulators lack appropriate maximum output at 0.2 ms D. Fortunately, TES devices that adjust maximum output to selected D are starting to appear.

We can also **ensure ≥ 0.1 ms D for DCS**. This recommendation comes from animal experiments that showed cortical injury with highly energetic briefer pulses [16]. For most other applications where the chronaxie is unknown, we can **avoid stronger stimuli than needed**. For example, one can find supramaximal intensity for somatosensory evoked potentials (SEPs) with cubital and popliteal fossa recordings, rather than setting arbitrarily high strength.

Finally, we **ensure that energy is < 50 mJ**, the International Electrotechnical Commission safety limit assuming 1 kΩ resistance. There are no reports of thermal injury below this limit, and most neuromonitoring stimuli are far below. The exception is TES for MEP monitoring. Here the necessarily strong stimuli can reach or exceed 50 mJ. For example, 1000 mA at 0.05 ms D produces 50 mJ, and 250 mA at 1 ms D produces 62.5 mJ (1 kΩ resistance). Since there are rare observations of possible TES scalp burns (0.01%), **we should be particularly cautious with TES**.

> **Key Points: Protection Against Thermal Injury**
> - *Set pulse duration to the chronaxie, if known.*
> - *Set DCS MEP pulse duration to 0.2 ms.*
> - *Ensure ≥ 0.1 ms pulse duration for DCS.*
> - *Avoid stronger stimuli than needed.*
> - *Ensure < 50 mJ energy.*
> - *Be particularly cautious with TES.*

9.2.2.4 Means of Protection Against Excitotoxicity

In animal experiments, direct cortical stimulation can cause histologic neuron damage through excessive excitation, or excitotoxicity. **Charge** and **charge density** ($QD = Q$/electrode area) are **excitotoxic cofactors**: higher charge is tolerable with lower charge density and vice versa according to an **excitotoxic threshold** of $\log Q = 1.85 - \log QD$ [11]. From this, we see that **electrode area** is important for excitotoxicity.

Because the animal experiments studied 50–60 Hz pulse trains lasting hours or days, their relevance to much briefer IONM stimuli is unclear. Furthermore, there is **no clinical evidence of human excitotoxicity** so far. Nevertheless, the absence of a clinical deficit does not rule out histologic damage, and there is only one human study with histology [17], so **we must still consider the possibility of excitotoxicity**.

Charge and charge density values below the excitotoxic threshold are clearly safe, while those above it are theoretically dangerous. The good news is that due to skull dispersion, maximal TES for MEP monitoring falls below the threshold at the brain and is unlikely to cause excitotoxicity. Skull defects could increase brain Q/QD, which is why they are a relative contraindication for TES (see below Sect. 9.4.4, *Relative contraindications*). The bad news is that **commonly used DCS parameters are theoretically excitotoxic** even at threshold intensity because of small electrodes and/or long D (Fig. 9.3).

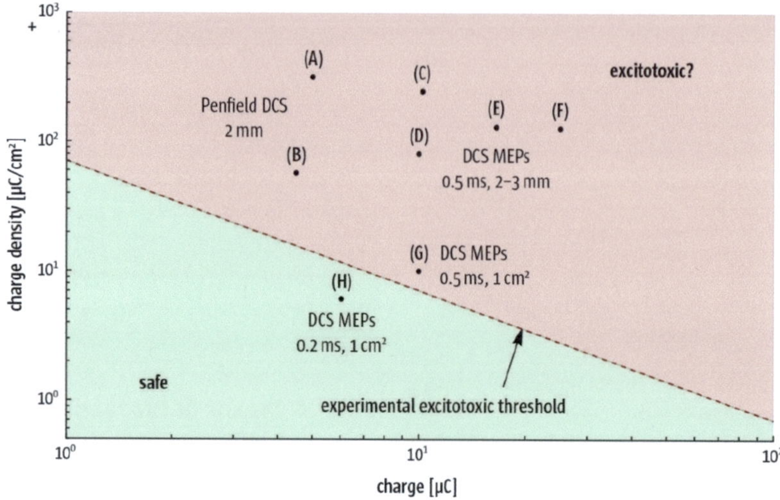

Fig. 9.3 Intraoperative direct cortical stimulation (DCS) vs. the experimental animal excitotoxic threshold. (**a**) and (**b**) 50–60 Hz Penfield stimulation with 2 mm probes. (**c**–**f**) DCS for motor evoked potentials (MEPs) using 0.5 ms pulses and 2–3 mm discs. (**g**) DCS MEPs with 0.5 ms pulses and a 1 cm² electrode. (**h**) DCS MEPs with 0.2 ms pulses and a 1 cm² electrode. Modified from [10], with permission

To explain, the first study of DCS MEPs used large 1 cm² cortical electrodes to limit charge density [18]. However, since then we often use small 2–3 mm diameter probes or subdural discs having only 0.03–0.07 cm² area and, therefore, high charge density. In addition, practitioners tend to use long 0.5–1 ms D to reduce threshold current, but this increases charge.

We could eliminate the theoretical risk of DCS excitotoxicity by keeping charge and charge density **below the experimental excitotoxic threshold**. To do so, we should use **1 cm² electrodes and 0.2 ms D**, which would produce safe mean charge and charge density values even at 2 × MEP threshold (Fig. 9.3), but is presently never done. In any case, one should **avoid stronger stimuli than needed** and **stay below published limits** that appear at least clinically safe.

Key Points: Protection Against Excitotoxicity
- *Consider keeping charge and charge density below the excitotoxic threshold.*
- *Consider 1 cm² DCS electrodes to limit charge density.*
- *Consider 0.2 ms pulse duration for DCS to limit charge.*

- *Avoid stronger stimuli than needed.*
- *Stay below published limits that appear clinically safe.*

9.2.2.5 Means of Protection Against Electrochemical Toxicity

An electrode on tissue forms an equilibrium potential. Cathodal pulses push electrons into the electrode, while anodal pulses pull electrons out of it. Both drive the electrode potential away from equilibrium. This normally induces **safe capacitive charge transfer** by attracting or repelling tissue anions and cations, making them flow within tissue fluid. However, if pulses drive the electrode potential beyond its capacitive limit, then **hazardous Faradic charge injection** forces electrons into or out of tissue (Fig. 9.4). This causes partially irreversible reductive or oxidative reactions producing toxic byproducts. While tissue buffering and blood flow remove some byproducts, animal experiments show that toxic accumulation can damage cortical neurons.

The risk of experimental animal electrochemical injury increases with $D > 1$ ms and especially with prolonged monophasic pulse trains that pro-

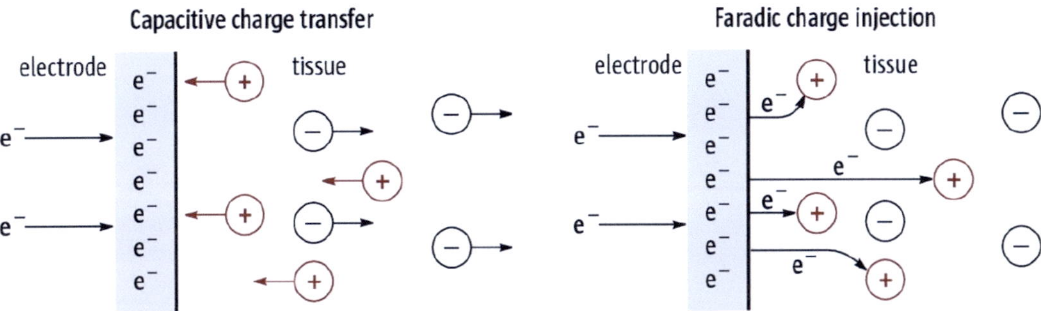

Fig. 9.4 A cathodal pulse producing safe capacitive charge transfer (left) or dangerous Faradic charge injection (right) at the electrode–tissue interface. Adapted from Merrill et al. [11], with permission

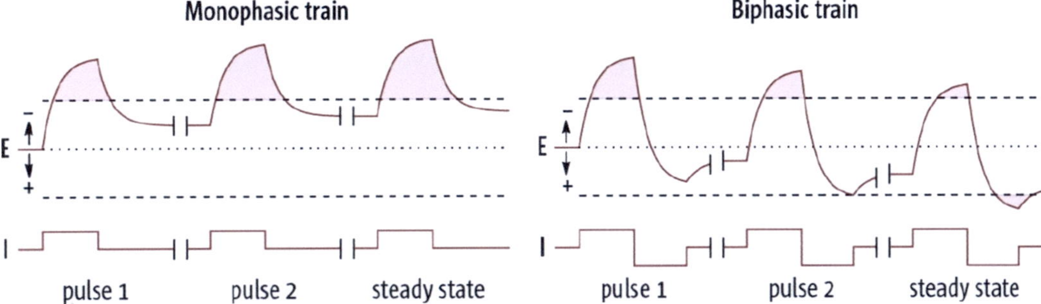

Fig. 9.5 Monophasic pulse trains (left) reach a steady state with mostly Faradic charge injection (shaded areas), while biphasic trains (right) reach a steady state with mostly capacitive charge transfer. E, electrode potential; dotted line, equilibrium potential; dashed lines, capacitive limits. Adapted from Merrill et al. [11], with permission

gressively shift the electrode potential beyond its capacitive limit until reaching a steady state with mostly Faradic injection. Biphasic trains avoid this by driving the electrode potential in opposite directions until a steady state with mostly capacitive transfer (Fig. 9.5). Therefore, we should **prefer $D \leq 1$ ms** for DCS and **use biphasic pulses for 50–60 Hz pulse trains** lasting seconds. Very brief 5-pulse monophasic trains are probably safe.

> **Key Points: Protection Against Electrochemical Injury**
> - *Prefer pulse duration ≤ 1 ms for DCS.*
> - *Use biphasic pulses for 50–60 Hz DCS.*

9.2.3 Electrode Burns

Burns at neuromonitoring electrodes are very infrequent, but can be painful or disfiguring and may require plastic surgery (Fig. 9.6). Consequently, **we must try to prevent them.** They range in severity from mild first-degree burns to full-thickness necrosis exposing bone and should be differentiated from other skin lesions such as abrasion, sustained-pressure necrosis, or allergic reaction. A confirmed burn calls for an investigation to find and correct the cause. Most burns are the result of **stray electrosurgery current**, some are caused by intraoperative **magnetic resonance imaging** (MRI), and a few are due to sustained **direct current** [19]. The American Society of

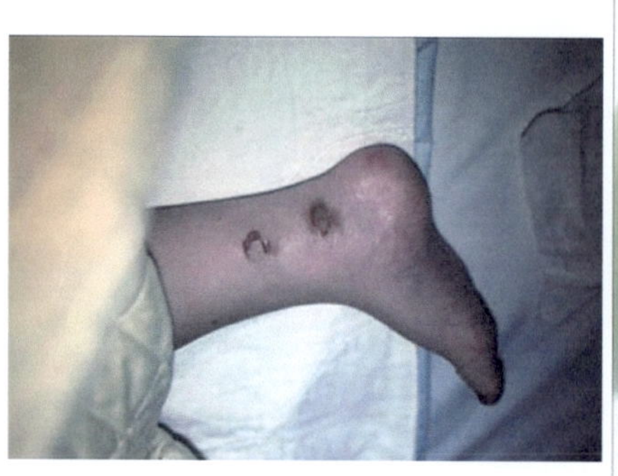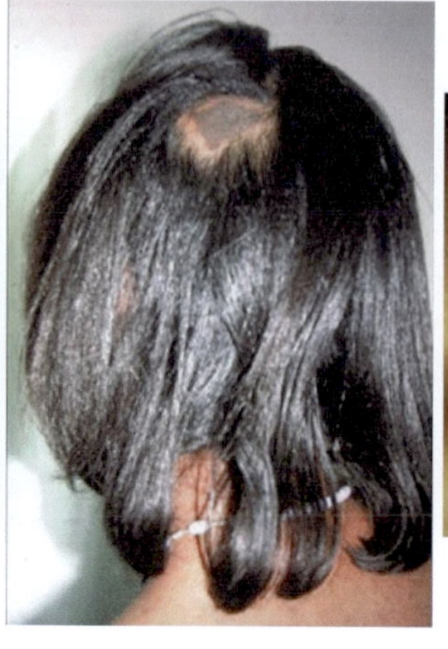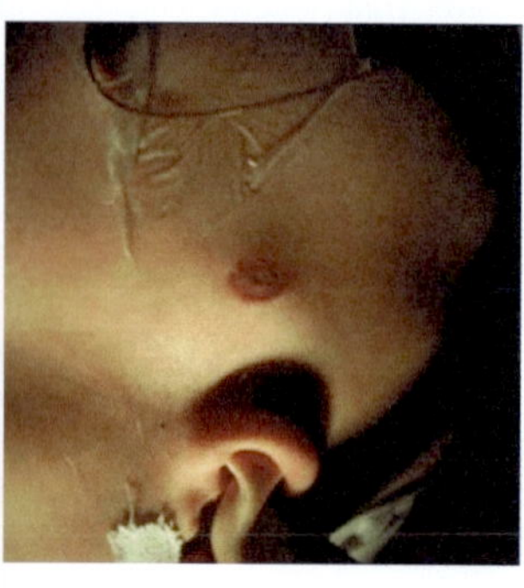

Fig. 9.6 Electrode burns. From MacDonald et al. [10], with permission

Electroneurodiagnostic Technologists is currently conducting a survey to estimate the incidence of IONM electrode burns.

9.2.3.1 Stray Electrosurgery Current Burns

The correct term is electrosurgery, not cautery. Cautery applies heat to tissue. Electrosurgery passes high-frequency 0.3–3 MHz current into tissue, where electric energy generates heat.

The **electrosurgery unit** (ESU) has bipolar or monopolar output. Bipolar mode passes current between the two tips of the surgical forceps, and the focal current cannot spread to cause IONM electrode burns. In contrast, monopolar mode passes current through one surgical blade into tissue. The blade's small area creates localized high energy density and heat. The current then spreads through the body and exits at all available contacts, including IONM electrodes. Under **normal conditions**, most current exits safely via the dispersive pad and its cable back to the ESU. The pad's large area creates low energy density and heat. Under **abnormal conditions**, more current exits through IONM electrodes and other contacts. Thus, **monopolar electrosurgery risks electrode burns**. Their frequency is unknown, but there are thousands of electrosurgery burn incidents annually, and some fraction involves IONM electrodes. The **risk increases with nee-dle electrodes** that have small surface area and, thus, high energy density and heat if they conduct electrosurgery current. **Surface electrodes have a lower risk** because their larger areas limit energy density.

Normal conditions consist of (1) circuit activation only when the blade contacts tissue, (2) full dispersive pad attachment on smooth dry skin close to the surgical site, (3) intact dispersive cable connection, and (4) a correctly functioning ESU (Fig. 9.7). Abnormal conditions arise with failure of any of these elements. **Open-circuit activation** when the blade is not contacting tissue promotes electromagnetic induction in IONM cables. Partial or complete **dispersive pad detachment** or **dispersive cable malfunction** forces more current to exit at IONM electrodes; repeated surgeon requests for more current can suggest malfunction. **Failure of periodic biomedical inspection** increases the likelihood of ESU malfunction.

Electrode burns can also occur in normal ESU conditions. This is because high-frequency currents exhibit prominent induction in nearby circuits. Monitoring device or cable **proximity to the ESU or its cables** and monitoring lead **loops or coils** facilitate electromagnetic induction. In addition, a monitoring **electrode between the surgical blade and dispersive pad** can pick up monopolar electrosurgery current.

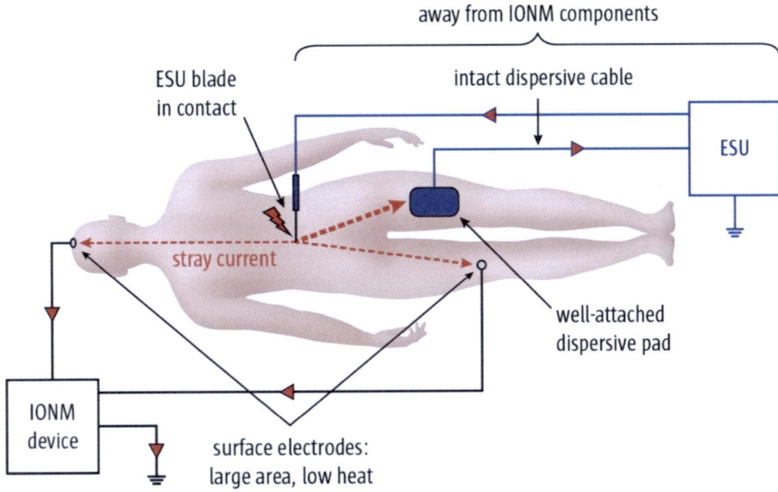

Fig. 9.7 Normal electrosurgery unit (ESU) conditions. © ARKANA Forum GmbH 2022. All Rights Reserved

9.2.3.2 Means of Protection Against Stray Electrosurgery Current Burns

Considering the above, we should **ensure normal ESU conditions**; **consider using surface electrodes** when effective; **consider limiting needle electrodes** to necessary purposes like muscle recording, keep monitoring devices, cables, and electrodes **away from ESU components**; keep monitoring cables **free of loops or coils**; and never place monitoring electrodes **between the ESU blade and dispersive pad**. Note that the common current practice of using mostly or entirely needle electrodes is not necessarily unsafe when all other precautions are in place.

> **Key Points: Protection Against Stray Electrosurgery Current Burns**
> - *Ensure full dispersive pad attachment.*
> - *Ensure dispersive cable integrity and connection.*
> - *Avoid open-circuit ESU activation.*
> - *Ensure periodic biomedical ESU inspection.*
> - *Consider using surface IONM electrodes when effective.*
> - *Consider limiting needle electrodes to necessary purposes.*

> - *Keep IONM devices and cables away from ESU components.*
> - *Avoid IONM cable loops or coils.*
> - *Never place IONM electrodes between the surgical blade and dispersive pad.*

9.2.3.3 Means of Protection Against Magnetic Resonance Imaging Burns

Intraoperative MRI creates strong magnetic fields that can induce current in monitoring cables and thereby cause burns at neuromonitoring electrodes or underneath their leads. The incidence is unclear, but 1/54 patients (1.9%) had a burn in a recent study [20]. There are no MRI-compatible IONM devices, so the instrument should be kept outside the relatively safe **5-Tesla line**. There are **MRI-compatible electrodes,** but if they are not available, then one may consider **disconnecting** before doing an MRI. Placing **insulation** between the skin and lead wires can avoid burns underneath electrode leads.

> **Key Points: Protection Against Magnetic Resonance Imaging Burns**
> - *Keep the IONM device outside the 5-Tesla line.*

> - *Use MRI-compatible electrodes if available.*
> - *Consider disconnecting non-compatible electrodes before doing an MRI.*
> - *Place insulation between the skin and lead wires.*

9.2.3.4 Means of Protection Against Direct Current Burns

Small but sustained direct current between electrodes can cause severe electrolytic skin burns. We should **avoid battery-powered devices** that facilitate direct current unless specifically engineered to prevent it. Fluid spills into an IONM headbox or amplifier can set up abnormal direct current circuits. Using **waterproof components** and **preventing fluid spills** by not mounting boxes underneath fluids on IV poles are protective measures.

> **Key Points: Protection Against Direct Current Burns**
> - Avoid battery powered devices unless specifically designed.
> - Use waterproof components.
> - Prevent fluid spills into monitoring device components.

9.2.4 Fire

There are about 100 operating room fires causing serious injury or death in the United States each year. The **ignition source** is electrosurgery sparking or medical device electrical fire. **Fuel** consists of flammable preparation liquids such as alcohol, collodion, or acetone; oxygen-rich gases near the patient's airway (e.g., supplemental oxygen through face mask or nasal cannula during awake craniotomy); and textiles such as surgical drapes.

To protect against fire, we should **prevent pooling of flammable liquids, ensure they are dry** before draping, and **never open them during electrosurgery**. The anesthesiologist should take care to limit oxygen concentration [21]. We should also ensure **biomedical inspection** of IONM devices exhibiting abnormally **hot surfaces or burning odors**. Finally, neuromonitoring personnel should undergo **fire and safety training**.

> **Key Points: Protection Against Fire**
> - *Prevent pooling of flammable liquids.*
> - *Ensure that flammable liquids are dry before draping.*
> - *Never open flammable liquids during electrosurgery.*
> - *Limit oxygen concentration around the patient's airway (anesthesiologist).*
> - *Ensure biomedical inspection of IONM devices with hot surfaces or burning odors.*
> - *Ensure fire & safety training.*

9.3 Procedure-Specific Safety

9.3.1 Invasive Electrodes

Invasive electrodes have a small but potentially serious risk of **hemorrhage, infection,** or **trauma**. Consequently, they are not merely an option and **we should justify their use** by the **lack of a suitable noninvasive method** to obtain the necessary information. Examples of justifiable invasive techniques include subdural strips for cortical mapping, probes for direct neural stimulation, and spinal epidural electrodes for D-wave monitoring during intramedullary spinal cord surgery. A less justifiable technique would be invasive spinal monitoring of extramedullary spinal surgery, for which noninvasive methods are normally sufficient.

9.3.2 Direct Cortical Stimulation

Direct cortical stimulation can incite **afterdischarges** consisting of repetitive spikes in the electrocorticogram (ECoG). They are actually focal seizure patterns since they evolve in frequency, amplitude, and distribution. Furthermore, they can build up to **clinical seizures** and rarely even **convulsions** possibly risking complications such as tongue laceration, shoulder dislocation, fracture, extubation, brain damage, and even death. For perspective, the incidence of serious complications is unknown and presumably very rare. There is also a theoretical risk of kindling postoperative epilepsy, although there are no reports of this so far.

Traditional **50–60 Hz pulse trains** for cortical mapping often incite afterdischarges that build to clinical **seizures in 5–15%** of patients. Afterdischarges could also cause **false localization** with this technique by spreading to unstimulated cortex to produce symptoms like tonic–clonic movement or speech arrest. Consequently, **ECoG is mandatory**: one tries to keep intensity below the afterdischarge threshold to avoid seizures and rejects apparent patient responses when there is an afterdischarge (Fig. 9.8).

The **DCS MEP** technique is **safer** for motor cortex mapping and monitoring since it causes fewer afterdischarges and incites **seizures in < 1–5%** of patients. Furthermore, it **does not**

risk false localization from afterdischarges because the response is a transient short-latency MEP. Consequently, ECoG is optional. Sustained muscle activity in MEP channels quickly indicates a motor seizure, often before it is clinically evident.

Seizures triggered by either method usually respond quickly to **cold irrigation** with 4 °C saline or Ringer's solution. If not, intravenous **anticonvulsants** may be indicated.

> **Key Points: Protection Against Direct Cortical Stimulation Seizures and False Localization**
> - *Use ECoG for the 50–60 Hz mapping technique.*
> - *Try to keep 50–60 Hz intensity below afterdischarge threshold.*
> - *Disregard 50–60 Hz patient responses in the presence of afterdischarges.*
> - *Prefer DCS MEPs for motor cortex mapping and monitoring.*
> - *Have cold irrigation and anticonvulsants ready.*

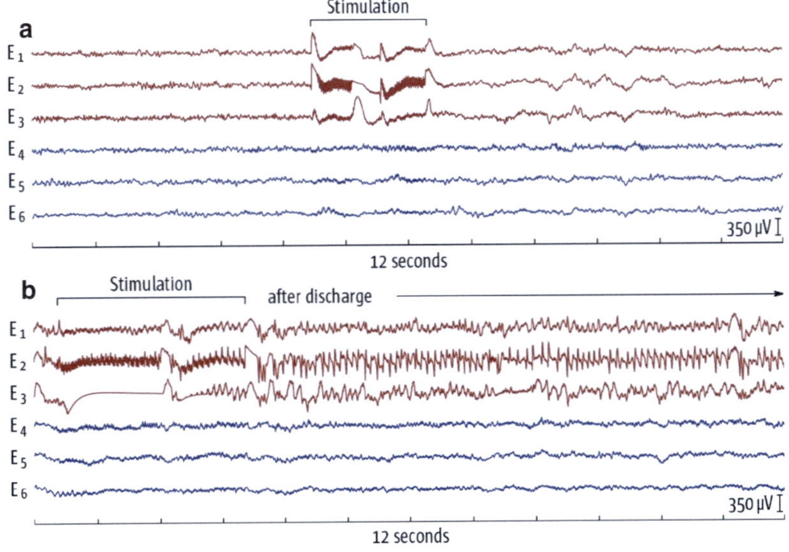

Fig. 9.8 Electrocorticography during 60 Hz cortical mapping. (**a**) Stimulation with no afterdischarge validates patient responses. (**b**) Stimulation with an afterdischarge invalidates patient responses. Modified from MacDonald et al. [10], with permission

9.3.3 Direct Subcortical Stimulation

The 1 mA/mm subcortical MEP threshold criterion for judging corticospinal tract proximity was developed with **0.5 ms pulse duration** that we should therefore use, pending further study. It could be misleading to use 0.2 ms duration as suggested for DCS because it would increase the threshold/distance ratio. Surprisingly, dynamic subcortical mapping induces **afterdischarges** in 4% of patients. Therefore, it may be advisable to record ECoG and have cold irrigation ready.

9.3.4 Transcranial Electric Stimulation

Bite injuries due to jaw muscle contractions are the most common (0.2%) and important TES complication. They include tongue or lip laceration, tooth or jaw fracture, and standard or even armored endotracheal tube rupture (Figs. 9.9 and 9.10). All reported incidents so far occurred with **C3/C4** TES. This may be due to direct stimulation of both temporalis muscles and to stronger twitching than with less potent C1/C2 or C3–Cz/C4–Cz circuits that are, however, not necessarily immune. Protective **soft bite blocks** are mandatory for any TES circuit, but do not prevent all bite injuries. They usually consist of rolled-up gauze between the molars on each side while keeping the tongue in the middle (Fig. 9.10). Do not use hard bite blocks that could promote tooth fracture.

Induced **movements** are a common issue. They are usually not problematic for orthopedic or aortic surgery, but can **interfere with neurosurgery**, especially when using the operative microscope. Unexpected movement when surgical tools are near neural or vascular structures could theoretically cause **neurologic injury**, although there are **no reports so far**. When movement concerns are likely, we can **avoid C3/C4**, prefer less potent TES circuits if effective, and consider **near-threshold intensity**. When movement is still an issue, we must apply **careful stimulus timing**, clear **communication** with the surgeon, and close observation of **surgical video**. Note that it can be dangerous if MEP acquisition becomes too infrequent for fear of movement because we could miss the onset of motor compromise. Thus, it may be important to **request stimulation** with sufficient regularity.

Seizures are very rare with TES (0.03%). If one occurs, we should **stop stimulating**, or possibly pause and try again after administering anticonvulsants if MEP monitoring is critical. There are also rare observations (0.03%) of **cardiac arrhythmia** or **hypertension** during TES. This might be explained by transthoracic parasitic current (see Sect. 9.3.1, *Ventricular fibrillation*) or TES current reaching brain autonomic centers. One must differentiate arrhythmia from TES artifact in the electrocardiogram (Fig. 9.11). We should use **separate upper and lower body headboxes** to avoid parasitic transthoracic TES

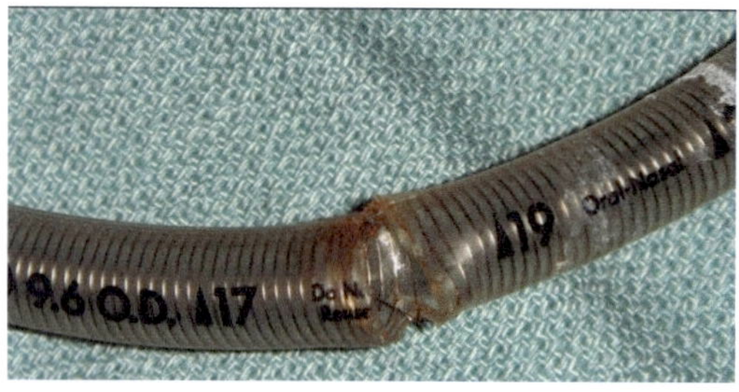

Fig. 9.9 Bitten-through armored endotracheal tube. This life-threatening bite complication requires emergency reintubation. Modified from [22], with permission

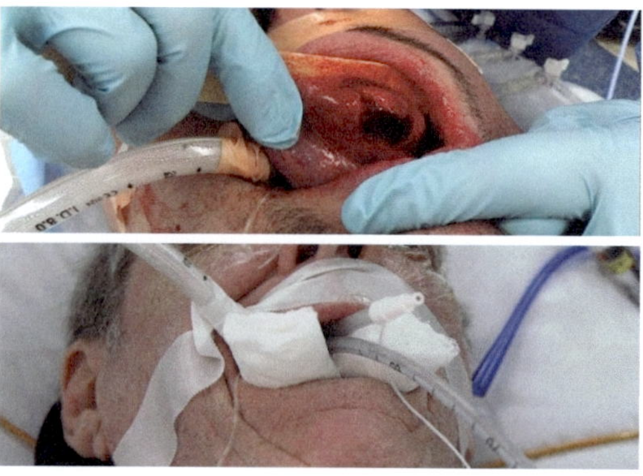

Fig. 9.10 Tongue laceration (top) and protective soft bite blocks (bottom). From [10], with permission

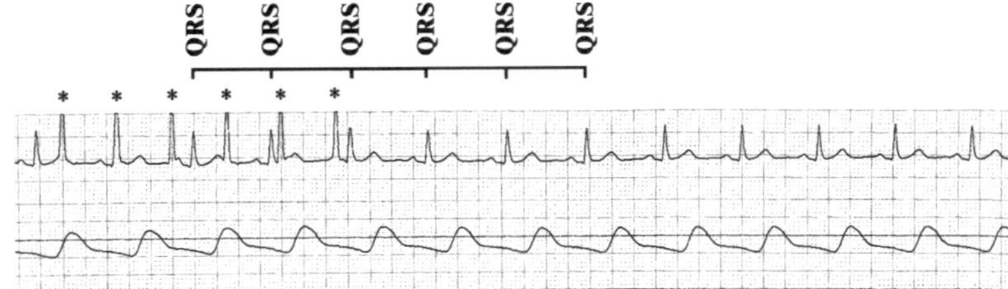

Fig. 9.11 Transcranial electric stimulation artifact (*) in an electrocardiogram. From [10], with permission

current and **suspend or pause stimulation** if significant cardiovascular disturbances arise.

Relative contraindications include epilepsy, skull defects, vascular clips or shunts, and biomedical implants. However, none are absolute, and many patients with one of these conditions have undergone uneventful TES MEP monitoring, with no reports of any complications so far. In particular, TES appears to be safe with cardiac pacemakers and cochlear implants. Nevertheless, we should obtain **specific informed consent** to proceed if there is a relative contraindication.

> **Key Points: Protection Against Transcranial Electric Stimulation Complications**
> - *Always use mandatory soft bite blocks.*
> - *Avoid C3/C4 and consider near-threshold intensity if movement would be problematic.*
> - *Use careful stimulus timing, clear communication, and surgical video.*
> - *Stop TES if it incites a seizure.*
> - *Suspend or pause TES if it causes cardiac arrhythmia or hypertension.*
> - *Use separate upper and lower body headboxes.*
> - *Obtain specific informed consent for a relative contraindication.*

9.3.5 Other Procedures

Direct brainstem stimulation can alter **heart rate** or **blood pressure**, presumably by stimulating autonomic centers. We should **interrupt stimulation** if this occurs.

For SEP monitoring, **do not use rigid bar stimulating electrodes** because they risk sustained-pressure skin necrosis in rare reports [23]. In addition, fibular or tibial nerve **stimulation at the knee risks anterior compartment syndrome** from repetitive leg muscle contractions. The incidence is unknown and presumably rare, but in one anecdotal report a patient needed surgical anterior compartment decompression [10]. For these proximal nerves, we should use **neuromuscular blockade** or **sub-motor threshold intensity**. Supramaximal stimuli are safe for distal nerves at the wrist and ankle.

With brainstem auditory evoked potential monitoring, excessively **deep earplug insertion** could possibly cause **tympanic membrane damage**. Again, the incidence is unknown and presumably rare. The outer boarder of the foam rubber should be flush with the external ear canal opening to ensure fixation, but no deeper.

Deep needle insertion for electromyography could possibly cause **hemorrhage**, **nerve damage**, **eyeball puncture**, or **pneumothorax** [24, 25]. For example, deep needle insertion into the iliopsoas muscle theoretically risks nearby femoral nerve or artery puncture. Therefore, either **ensure special expertise** or **avoid deep needle insertions** in iliopsoas, extraocular, intercostal, or diaphragm muscles. Special expertise could be from an appropriate specialist (e.g., electromyographer, ophthalmologist, etc.), or from specific training.

9.4 Infection Control

Infectious diseases are always a concern for patients and staff. We must observe standard precautions, minimize needlestick incidents, and apply additional precautions when indicated.

9.4.1 Standard Precautions

Standard precautions **assume that everyone is infectious**. **Handwashing** is basic between patient contacts, procedures, contact with body fluids, after removing gloves, and on entering or leaving the operating room. **Gloves** are essential for any potential body fluid contact, including head measurement, skin preparation, and needle insertion. Operating room **personal protective gear** is mandatory, including masks, caps, boots, and clothing. After the procedure, we must **safely discard single-use electrodes** by putting adhesive electrodes into a disposal bag and needles into a sharps box and ensuring invasive electrode destruction. In addition, we must **clean and disinfect** monitoring devices, boxes, cables, and reusable electrodes.

9.4.2 Needlestick

Needlesticks could theoretically transmit infectious diseases including hepatitis or human immunodeficiency virus and are a safety issue for IONM that employs multiple needle electrodes. Their incidence is about 0.34% of monitored surgeries, but with no reports of disease transmission so far [26]. To minimize needlesticks, we must **handle needles by their stems**, **never attempt recapping**, and **put them in a sharps box** after use. In the event of a needlestick, one should **encourage bleeding**, **wash the site** thoroughly, and **follow hospital procedures**.

9.4.3 Additional Precautions

Actively infected patients may need additional droplet, airborne, or contact precautions, but are unlikely to undergo surgery with IONM. Neuromonitoring staff should have all recommended **immunizations** and follow **post-exposure policies**. We must destroy electrodes used on patients with Creutzfeldt–Jakob disease, with the possible exception of EEG cups that autoclaving or hypochlorite can sterilize.

9.5 Essential Performance

Essential performance requires "correct output of diagnostic information that is likely to be relied upon to determine treatment, where incorrect information could lead to an inappropriate treatment that would present an unacceptable risk" [6]. It applies to neuromonitoring devices and practice.

9.5.1 Neuromonitoring Devices

Failures of monitoring device essential performance include **failure to monitor, data corruption or loss**, and **inaccurate display or output**. The manufacturer must demonstrate that the device has a **low probability** of loss of essential performance, so failures are presumably rare. Neuromonitoring staff should **avoid misuse or foreseeable accidents** that could degrade device performance.

9.5.2 Neuromonitoring Practice

Failures of neuromonitoring practice essential performance consist of **excessively slow surgical feedback** or **inaccurate interpretation** putting the patient at risk. Overly slow feedback risks neurologic injury that might have been reversible if detected earlier. Incorrect interpretation risks neurologic injury by prompting inappropriate surgical action or inaction. There is anecdotal information that such failures occur, but their incidence is unknown. To avoid failures of essential performance, we should **ensure adequate training**, individually **optimize surgical feedback rapidity**, use **selective methods**, and include **technical and systemic controls**.

> **Key Points: Means of Protection Against Essential Performance Failure**
> - *Devices must have a low probability of essential performance failure.*

- *Avoid misuse or foreseeable accidents that could impair device performance.*
- *Ensure adequate training.*
- *Individually optimize surgical feedback rapidity.*
- *Use selective neuromonitoring techniques.*
- *Include technical and systemic controls.*

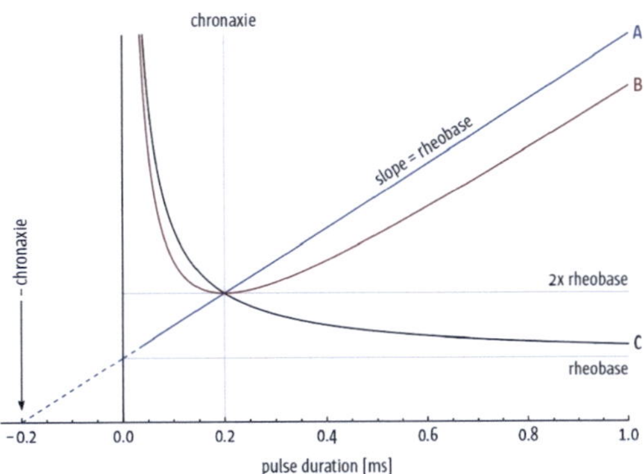

Fig. 9.12 Test question—Strength-duration. Modified from MacDonald et al. [10], with permission

9.6   Conclusion

Safety is fundamental to all aspects of medical care, including IONM. Understanding possible and theoretical neuromonitoring hazards and routinely applying means of protection against them makes IONM safe for clinical use in adequately trained hands.

9.7   Test Questions

1. Define electric shock and list the possible effects.
2. What is the usual cause of death from electric shock?
3. What current type and location is prone to cause ventricular fibrillation?
4. What is parasitic transthoracic current, and how can you prevent it?
5. Define the three types of leakage current and explain why they are a safety issue.
6. How can you prevent intracardiac leakage current?
7. Which two IONM device design features protect against electric shock?
8. Why is periodic biomedical inspection important, and when should it be done?
9. What are touch-proof connectors and why are they important?
10. What is the fundamental pulse parameter?
11. What is the charge in μC and energy in mJ of a rectangular pulse having 0.5 ms duration and 250 mA intensity with 1 kΩ resistance?
12. In Fig. 9.12, match threshold current, charge, and energy to labels A, B, and C.
13. What are rheobase and chronaxie?
14. What is the safest pulse duration choice and why?
15. List means of protection against thermal injury from stimulation.
16. What are the two excitotoxic cofactors?
17. List means of protection against excitotoxicity.
18. In Fig. 9.13, which panel illustrates Faradic charge injection?
19. Why is Faradic charge injection dangerous?
20. List means of protection against electrochemical injury.
21. What are the causes of IONM electrode burns?
22. List means of protection against stray electrosurgery current burns.
23. How can you protect against MRI and direct current electrode burns?
24. What are the ignition sources and fuels of an operating room fire?
25. List means of protection against operating room fire.
26. What do invasive electrodes risk, and when can you use them?
27. How would you interpret an apparent patient response to 60 Hz cortical mapping in panels (A) and (B) of Fig. 9.14?
28. List means of protection against DCS seizures and false localization.
29. What pulse duration should you use for subcortical MEP mapping and why?

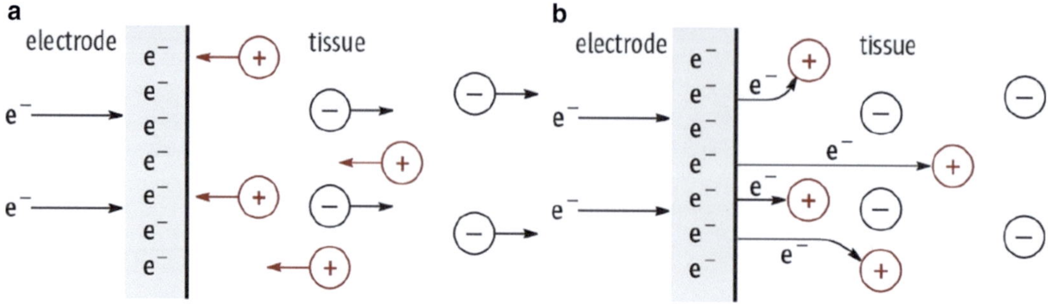

Fig. 9.13 Test question—Electrode-tissue interface. Adapted from Merrill et al. [11], with permission

Fig. 9.14 Test question—Electrocorticography during 60 Hz cortical mapping. Modified from MacDonald et al. [10], with permission

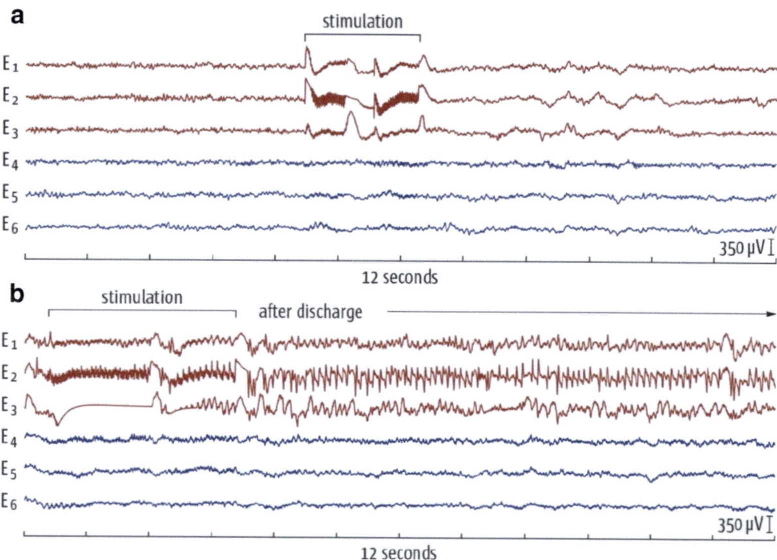

30. What is the most important complication of TES?

31. List means of protection against TES complications.

32. What is the risk of fibular or tibial nerve stimulation at the knee, and how can you prevent it?

33. How deeply should you inset earplugs for brainstem auditory evoked potentials and why?

34. What are the risks of deep needle insertion and how can you avoid them?

35. What standard precautions against infection must you follow?

36. How can you minimize needlesticks, and what should you do if you get one?

37. What does essential performance require of monitoring devices and practice?

38. List means of protection against essential performance failure.

References

1. Møller AR. Intraoperative neurophysiological monitoring. New York, NY: Springer New York; 2011. Available from: http://nbn-resolving.de/urn:nbn:de:1111-20101217303

2. López JR. The use of evoked potentials in intraoperative neurophysiologic monitoring. Phys Med Rehabil Clin N Am. 2004;15(1):63–84.

3. Wilson L, Lin E, Lalwani A. Cost-effectiveness of intraoperative facial nerve monitoring in middle ear or mastoid surgery. Laryngoscope. 2010;113(10):1736–45.

4. Kombos T, Suess O, Brock M. Kostenanalyse des intraoperativen neurophysiologischen Monitorings (IOM). Zentralblatt Für Neurochir. 2002;63(04):141–5.

5. Toleikis RJ. Neurophysiological monitoring during pedicle screw placement. In: Deletis V, Shils JL, editors. Neurophysiology in neurosurgery: a modern intraoperative approach. Amsterdam, Boston: Academic Press; 2002. p. 231–64. Available from: http://linkinghub.elsevier.com/retrieve/pii/B9780122090363500135.

6. International Electrotechnical Commission. IEC 60601-1 (Ed. 3.1): Medical electrical equipment—Part 1: General requirements for basic safety and essential performance [Internet]. 2012 [cited 2018 Apr 12]. Available from: www.iec.ch

7. International Electrotechnical Commission. IEC 60601-2-40 (Ed. 2.0): Medical electrical equipment – Part 2-40: Particular requirements for the basic safety and essential performance of electromyographs and evoked response equipment [Internet]. 2016 [cited 2018 Apr 16]. Available from: www.iec.ch

8. MacDonald DB. Safety of intraoperative transcranial electrical stimulation motor evoked potential monitoring. J Clin Neurophysiol. 2002;19(5):416–29.

9. MacDonald DB, Deletis V. Safety issues during surgical monitoring. In: Nuwer MR, editor. Intraoperative monitoring of neural function, Handbook of clinical neurophysiology, vol. 8. Amsterdam: Elsevier; 2008. p. 882–98.

10. MacDonald DB, Seidel K, Shils JL. Safety. In: Deletis V, Shils JL, Sala F, Seidel K, editors. Neurophysiology in neurosurgery a modern approach. 2nd ed. London: Academic Press; 2020. p. 581–96.

11. Merrill DR, Bikson M, Jefferys JGR. Electrical stimulation of excitable tissue: design of efficacious and safe protocols. J Neurosci Methods. 2005;141(2):171–98.

12. National Fire Protection Association. NFPA 99: Standards for health care facilities [Internet]. 2005 [cited 2005 Dec 2]. Available from: www.nfpa.org

13. Journée H. Electrical safety in intraoperative monitoring. In: Rodi Z, Deletis V, editors. Proceedings of the symposium on proceeding symposium on intraoperative neurophysiology 17–18 Oct 2003; 2003. p. 65–8.

14. Medical Device Safety Reports. Risk of electric shock from patient monitoring cables and electrode lead wires. 1993 [cited 2006 Jan 10]. Available from: www.mdsr.ecri.org

15. Abalkhail TM, MacDonald DB, AlThubaiti I, AlOtaibi FA, Stigsby B, Mokeem AA, et al. Intraoperative direct cortical stimulation motor evoked potentials: stimulus parameter recommendations based on rheobase and chronaxie. Clin Neurophysiol. 2017;128(11):2300–8.

16. Girvin J. A review of basic aspects concerning chronic cerebral stimulation. In: Cooper I, editor. Cerebellar stimulation in man. New York: Raven Press; 1978. p. 1–12.

17. Gordon B, Lesser RP, Rance NE, Hart J, Webber R, Uematsu S, et al. Parameters for direct cortical electrical stimulation in the human: histopathologic confirmation. Electroencephalogr Clin Neurophysiol. 1990;75(5):371–7.

18. Taniguchi M, Cedzich C, Taniguchi M, Cedzich C, Schramm J. Modification of cortical stimulation for motor evoked potentials under general anesthesia. Neurosurgery. 1993;32(2):219–26.

19. Russell MJ, Gaetz M. Intraoperative electrode burns. J Clin Monit Comput. 2003;18(1):25–32.

20. Sarnthein J, Lüchinger R, Piccirelli M, Regli L, Bozinov O. Prevalence of complications in intraoperative magnetic resonance imaging combined with neurophysiologic monitoring. World Neurosurg. 2016;93:168–74.

21. Jones TS, Black IH, Robinson TN, Jones EL. Operating room fires. Anesthesiology. 2019;130(3):492–501.

22. MacDonald DB. Intraoperative motor evoked potential monitoring: overview and update. J Clin Monit Comput. 2006;20(5):347–77.

23. Stecker MM, Patterson T, Netherton BL. Mechanisms of electrode induced injury. Part 1: theory. Am J Electroneurodiagnostic Technol. 2006;46(4):315–42.

24. Al-Shekhlee A, Shapiro BE, Preston DC. Iatrogenic complications and risks of nerve conduction studies and needle electromyography. Muscle Nerve. 2003;27(5):517–26.

25. Peake JB, Roth JL, Schuchmann GF. Pneumothorax: a complication of nerve conduction studies using needle stimulation. Arch Phys Med Rehabil. 1982;63(4):187–8.

26. Tamkus A, Rice K. Risk of needle-stick injuries associated with the use of subdermal needle electrodes during intraoperative neurophysiologic monitoring. J Neurosurg Anesthesiol. 2014;26(1):65–8.

Troubleshooting

10

Celine Wegner

Contents

C. Wegner (✉)
ARKANA Forum GmbH, Emmendingen, Germany
e-mail: c.wegner@arkana-forum.com

© The Author(s), under exclusive license to Springer Nature Switzerland AG 2024
J. Zentner et al. (eds.), *Intraoperative Neuromonitoring*,
https://doi.org/10.1007/978-3-031-46125-5_10

10.1 The Impedance of the Electrodes Is Too High

See Fig. 10.1.

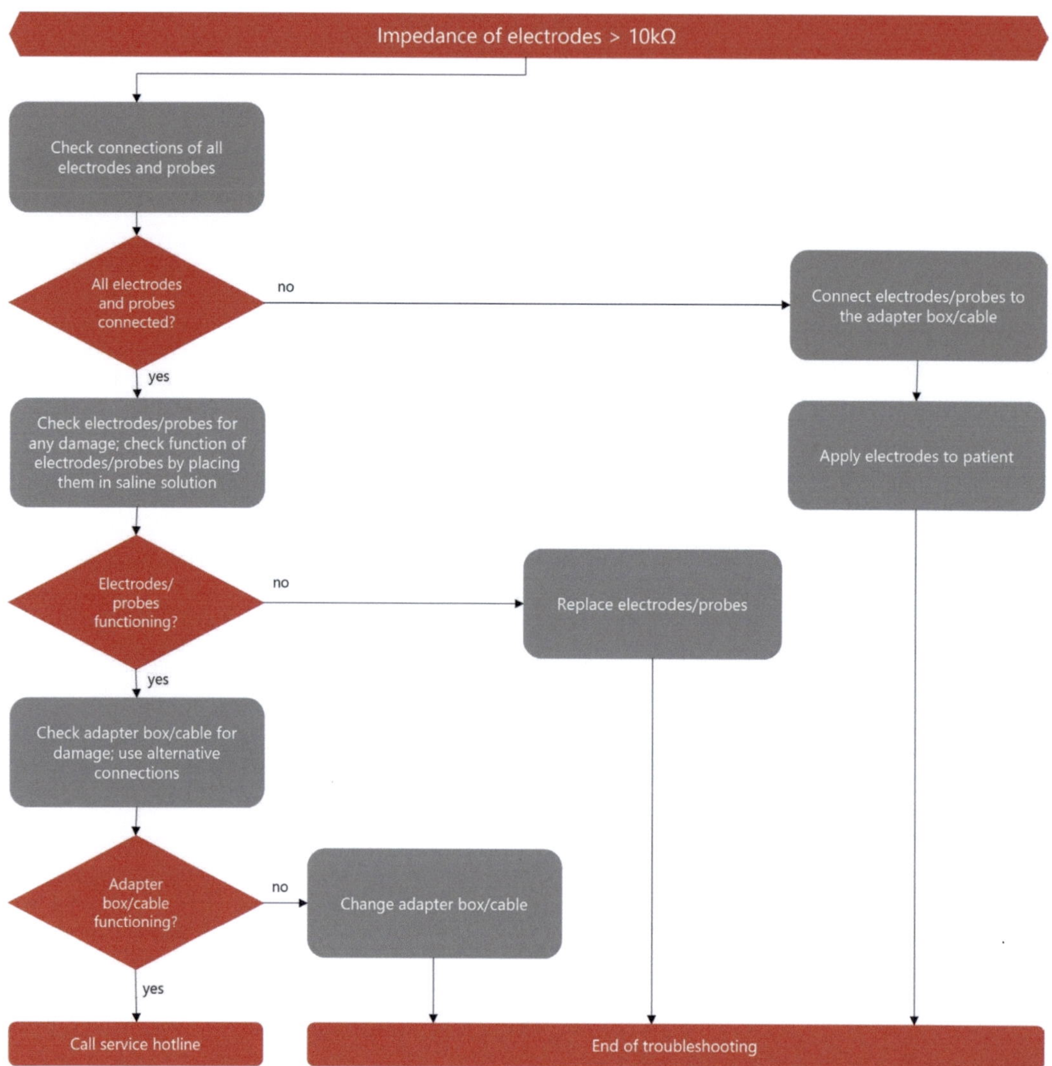

Fig. 10.1 Troubleshooting—The impedance of the electrodes is too high. © ARKANA Forum GmbH 2022. All Rights Reserved

10.2   There Is No Current Flow

See Fig. 10.2.

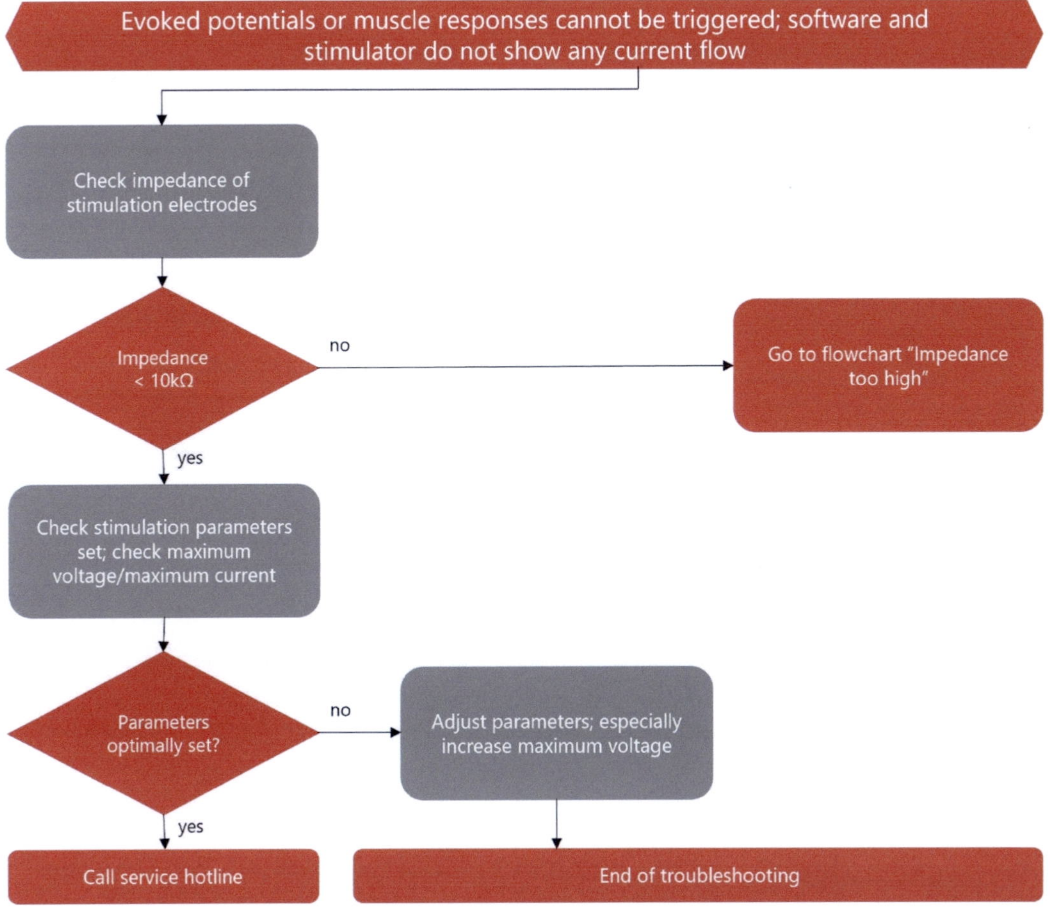

Fig. 10.2 Troubleshooting—There is no current flow. © ARKANA Forum GmbH 2022. All Rights Reserved

10.3 There Is No Response Signal Recordable

See Fig. 10.3.

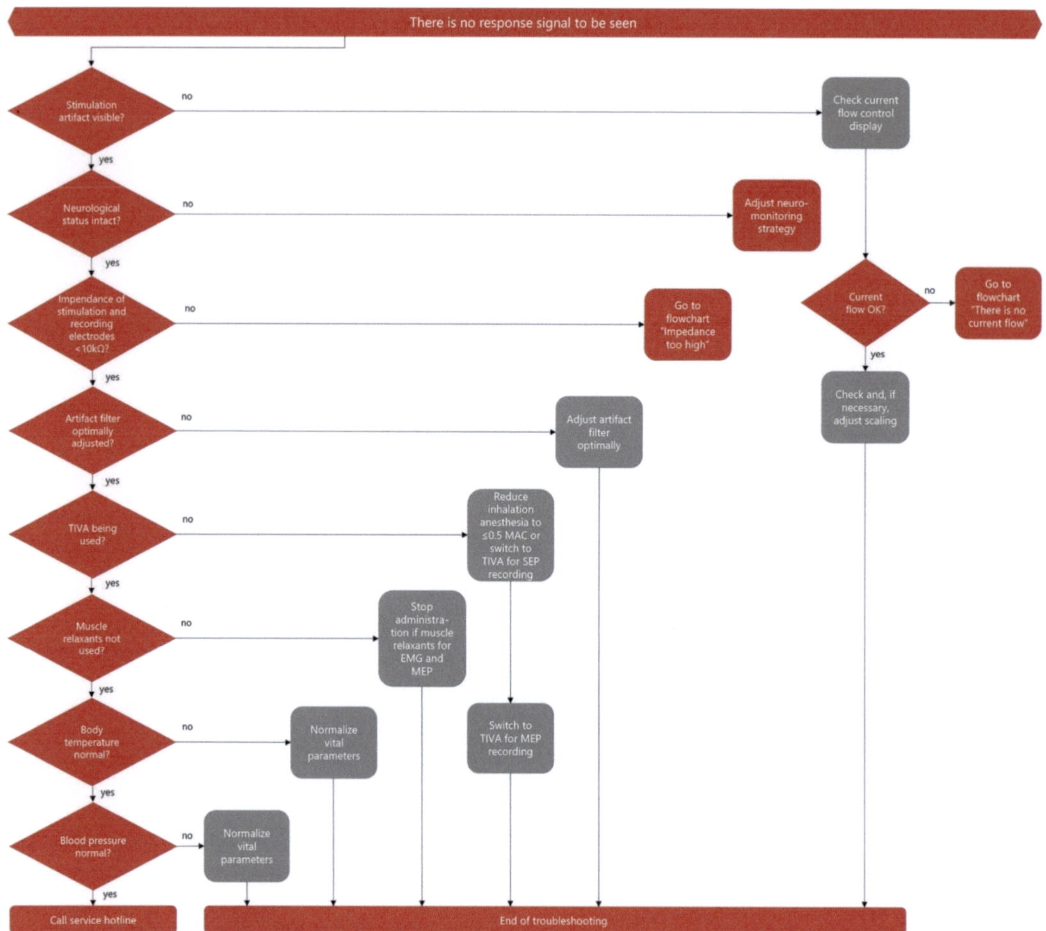

Fig. 10.3 Troubleshooting—There is no response signal recordable. © ARKANA Forum GmbH 2022. All Rights Reserved

10.4 The Response Signal Is Very Noisy

See Fig. 10.4.

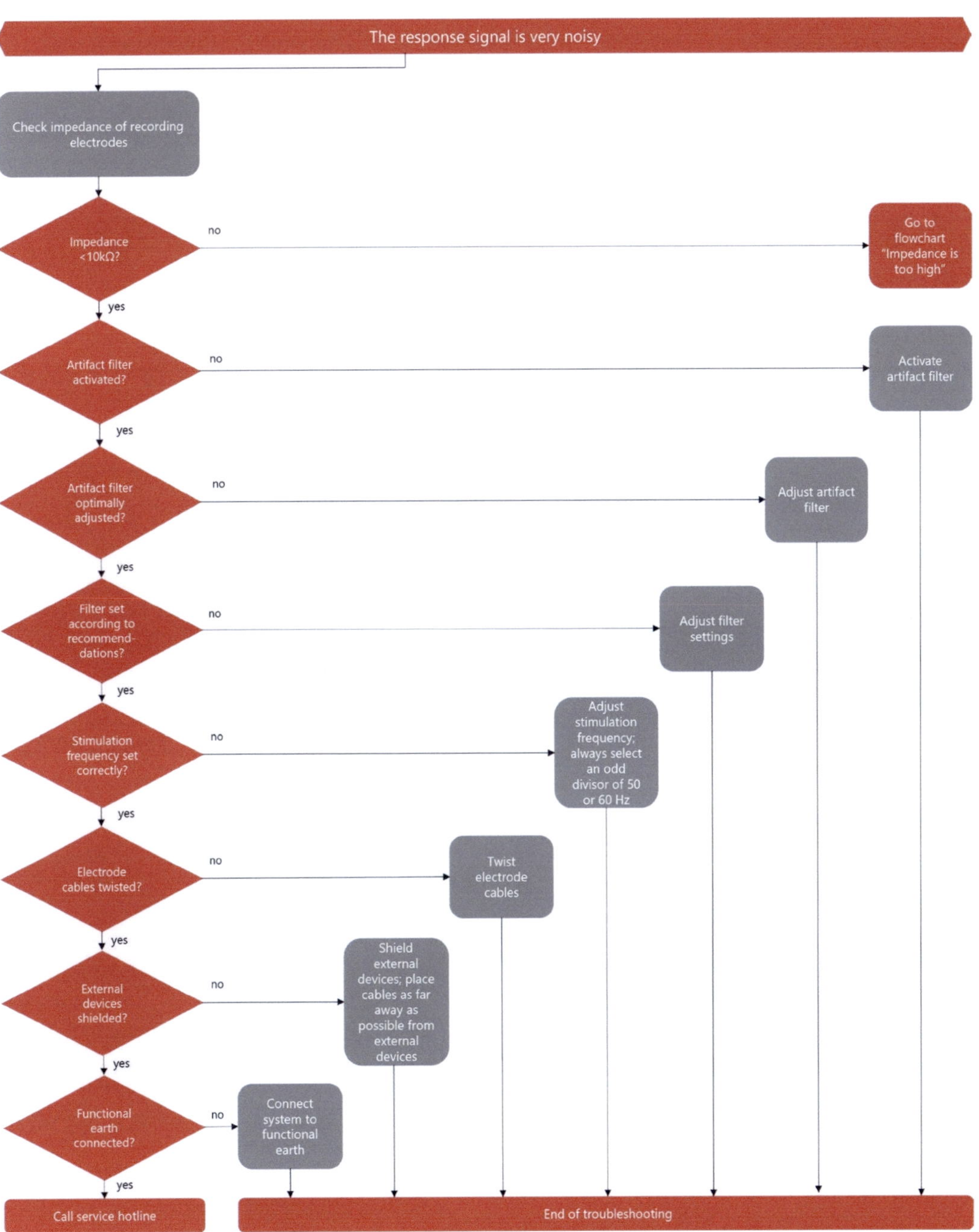

Fig. 10.4 Troubleshooting—The response signal is very noisy. © ARKANA Forum GmbH 2022. All Rights Reserved

10.5   The Response Signal Is Very Small

See Fig. 10.5.

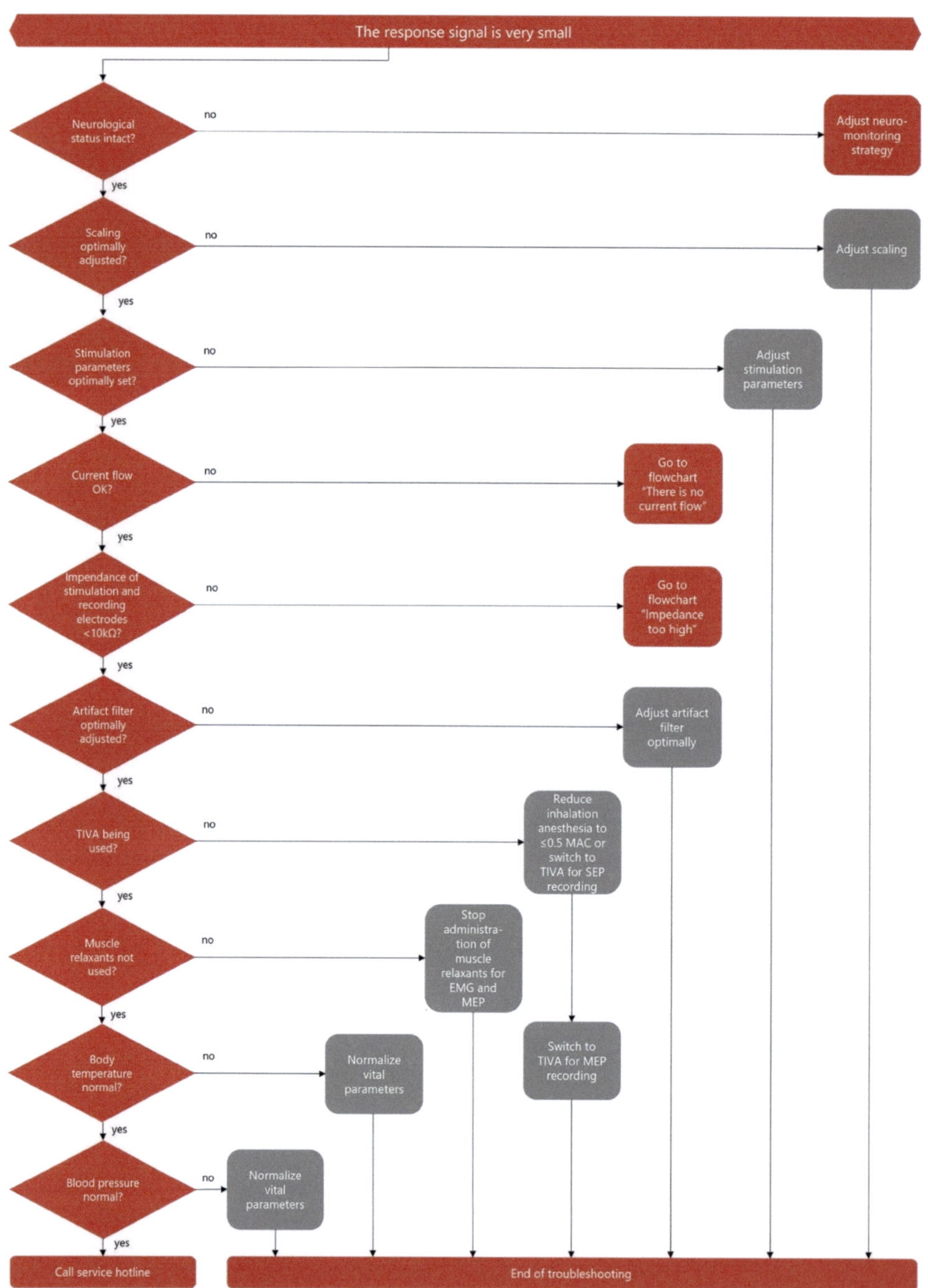

Fig. 10.5 Troubleshooting—The response signal is very small. © ARKANA Forum GmbH 2022. All Rights Reserved

10.6 The Response Signal Is Incompletely Displayed

See Fig. 10.6.

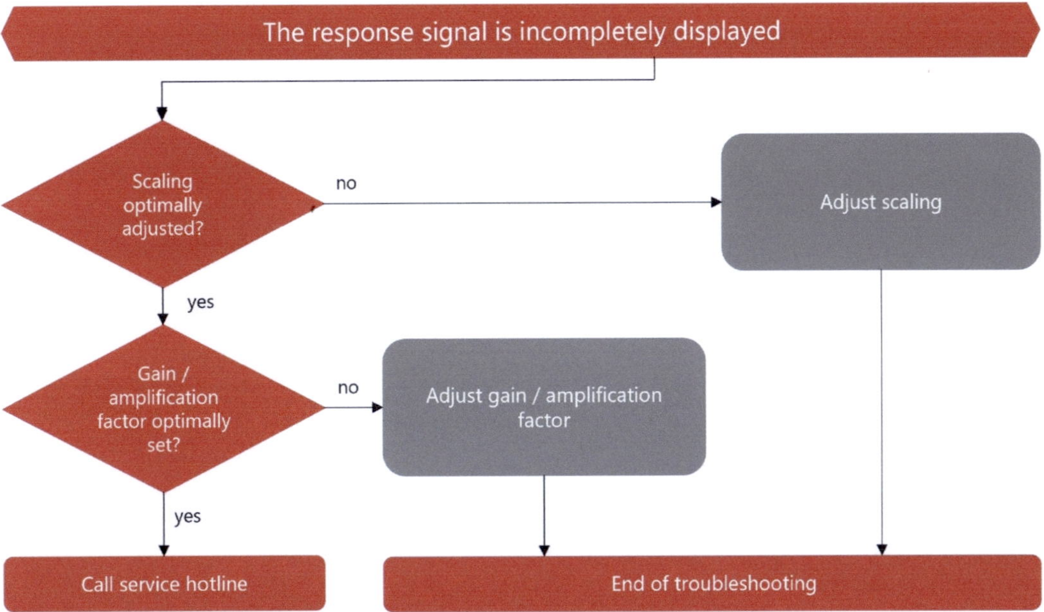

Fig. 10.6 Troubleshooting—The response signal in incompletely displayed. © ARKANA Forum GmbH 2022. All Rights Reserved

10.7 The Stimulation Cannot Be Triggered in the Software

See Fig. 10.7.

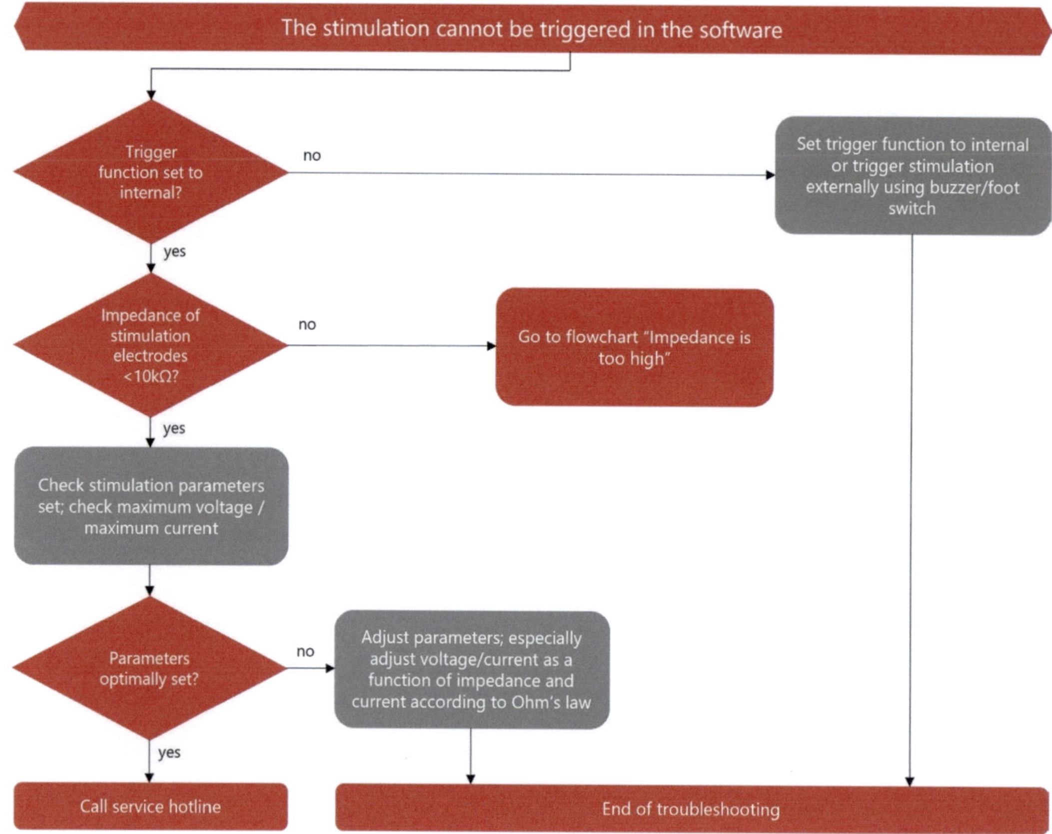

Fig. 10.7 Troubleshooting —The stimulation cannot be triggered in the software. © ARKANA Forum GmbH 2022. All Rights Reserved

Glossary

Abducens palsy Paralysis of the lateral rectus muscle supplied by the abducens nerve, which moves the eye outwards

Ablative Removing

Acoustic neuroma Benign tumor arising from Schwann cells of the vestibular portion of cranial nerve VIII (vestibulocochlear nerve)

Adjuvant Helpful, assistant

Affection Pathological condition

Afferent Towards the center; incoming (e.g., nerve tracts transmitting signals from the skin or internal organs to the brain)

Afferent disorder Disturbance of afferent (sensory) nerves

Agonist Unidirectional muscle strength (opposite: antagonist)

Alpha rhythm EEG rhythm in the alpha frequency range of 8–13 Hz, occurs occipitally in an awake, relaxed adult with eyes closed

Alveoli Functional units of the lung in which gas exchange takes place

Amplitude Maximum deflection of a signal, measured from its lowest to highest level

Analgesia Insensitivity to pain stimuli

Anamnesis History of illness; consists of a description of the development of current complaints as well as previous symptoms, examinations and treatments

Anastomosis Connection between two anatomical structures; in a broader sense, the artificially created connection between hollow organs

Anesthesia Loss or elimination of sensations and absence of pain with or without preservation of consciousness (local versus general anesthesia)

Anesthetics Drugs used to produce anesthesia

Angioma Malformation of arterial and venous vessels with pathological short circuits of different architecture

Anocutaneous line Transition between the lower margin of the internal anal sphincter and external skin

Anterior Lying in front

Anterior horn Part of the gray matter in the spinal cord

Antidromic Against the physiological direction (e.g., impulse propagation)

Apical Referring to the tip of an organ

Artery (Arteria, A., Arteriae, Ae.) Blood vessel that carries blood from the heart to the periphery of the body, resp. lungs

Ataxia Disorder of coordination of body movements; inability to fine-tune body movements such as walking, standing, or grasping

A-train Pattern in EMG showing a high-frequency sequence of spikes

Audiometry Hearing test

Auditory evoked potentials (AEPs) Sequence of voltage fluctuations in the EEG triggered by series of short sounds presented via headphones or earplugs; after averaging and amplification, these voltage fluctuations can be recorded from the scalp and assigned to different brain structures; usually only the early brainstem auditory evoked potentials (BAEPs) are recorded

Autonomic nervous system Part of the peripheral nervous system that is not subjected to consciousness and voluntary control; serves the automatic regulation of vital functions such as respiration or digestion

Barbiturates Group of drugs with sedative, hypnotic, and narcotic effects

© Arkana Forum GmbH 2024
J. Zentner et al. (eds.), *Intraoperative Neuromonitoring*,
https://doi.org/10.1007/978-3-031-46125-5

Basal Lying at the base, low down

Baseline Electrophysiological recordings before surgical measures are commenced; serves as a reference for signal interpretation during surgery

Benign Good-natured; slowly growing (e.g., brain tumor)

Bilateral On both sides

Binocular With both eyes

Biooccipital On both sides of the occipital lobes

Bipolar recording Registration of the voltage difference between two nearby electrodes

Bipolar stimulation Triggering a pulse by two adjacent electrodes

Blink reflex Eye closure reflex circuited in the brainstem that can be triggered by sensory, visual, auditory, or electrical stimuli

Bolus Singular rapid administration of a drug in order to quickly achieve a high serum drug level

Brainstem Part of the brain connecting the cerebrum with the spinal cord, through which all nerve impulses travel in both directions

Brainstem seizure Rare motor and/or and sensory phenomena of a seizure-like pattern generated in the basal ganglia and brainstem

Bulbocavernosus reflex A reflex with few synapses involving the pudendal nerve and the sacral area of the spinal cord

Bulbus oculi Eyeball

Burst Series of spikes in EMG as a result of spontaneous activity

Calotte Bony roof of the skull (skullcap or calvarium)

Capsula interna White substance between the basal ganglia through which the bundled nerve tracts run from the cerebrum to the spinal cord and vice versa

Carcinoma Cancer

Caudal Towards the tail; downwards

Central Inside; located in the center

Central nervous system Brain and spinal cord; responsible for the reception, processing, storage and output of information

Cerebellar Relating to the cerebellum

Cerebellum Part of the brain located below the tentorium which is mainly responsible for balance and coordination of movements

Cerebral Relating to the brain

Cerebral cortex Gray matter located at the surface of the brain; location of higher (mental) functions

Cerebrospinal Relating to the brain and spinal cord

Cerebrospinal fluid (CSF) Fluid in the cavities of the brain (ventricles) and around the brain and spinal cord (subarachnoid space)

Cerebrovascular Relating to the blood supply and venous drainage of the brain

Cerebrum Brain

Cervical Relating to the neck

Chordotomy Transection of the pain-conducting nerve bundles in the anterolateral tract of the spinal cord for the treatment of pain

Cingulotomy Transection of the cingulate gyrus; in the past used to treat severe psychological diseases

Coagulation Blood clotting, hemostasis (e.g., by electric current)

Colorectal Relating to the colon (large intestine) and rectum

Compound muscle action potential (CMAP) Summated motor unit potential response to stimulation of a nerve or nerve root supplying the recorded muscle

Concentric Arranged around a common center

Contraindicated Not indicated under any circumstances; not to be used

Contralateral At the opposite side

Conus medullaris Cone-shaped lower end of the spinal cord

Convalescence Recovery phase

Convulsion Involuntary muscle spasm; epileptic seizure

Corneal reflex Eyelid reflex (blink reflex)

Cortex Outer layer of the cerebrum and cerebellum containing nerve cells

Cortical Relating to the cortex

Corticobulbar Relating to the cortex and brainstem

Corticospinal Relating to the cortex and spinal cord

Cranial Towards the skull; upwards

Craniocervical Concerning the skull and the neck

Creutzfeldt-Jacob disease Infectious brain disease due to atypical protein formation and degeneration of the central nervous system; leads to rapidly progressive dementia and ultimately to death

Cryotherapy Cold therapy; treatment with application of cold

Decompression Surgical relief of a space-occupying lesion

Dendrite Projection of a nerve cell

Denervation Loss of nerve supply, e.g., by injury or disease

Denervation potential Potential occurring after functional loss of a nerve that can be recorded, for example, from the associated muscle

Dermatome Skin area supplied by the sensory fibers of a spinal nerve root

Desflurane A volatile anesthetic

Dexmedetomidine Intravenous anesthetic with sedative effect; can be used for general anesthesia in combination with propofol

Dexter Right from the patient's view

Diencephalic Relating to the diencephalon

Diencephalon Part of the brain between the telencephalon and the mesencephalon

Disobliteration Surgical removal of obstructions, for example, blood clots or plaques, from a stenosed or occluded blood vessel (e.g., carotid endarterectomy)

Dissection Targeted exposure and visualization of anatomical structures

Dissociated Separated; not connected with each other

Distal Away from the center of the body

Dorsal Backward

Dorsal column-medial lemniscus pathway Nerve tract in the posterior part of the spinal cord and brainstem for transmission of sensory signals from the skin and internal organs to the sensory cortex

Dysfunction Functional disorder

Dyskinesia Involuntary movement disorder

Dysmetria Uncertainty with targeted movements

Dysphasia Language disorder

Dysraphic malformation Congenital malformation of the spinal cord due developmental disorders or incomplete closure of neural tube

Dysrhythmia Irregularity of a rhythm

Dystonia Disorder of muscle tone with involuntary spasms

Efferent Towards the periphery, outgoing (e.g., nerve tracts transmitting signals from the brain to muscles)

Electrocorticography (ECoG) Recording of voltage fluctuations of the cerebral cortex, e.g., by means of strip or grid electrodes

Electroencephalography (EEG) Recording of voltage fluctuations of the brain from the surface of the scalp

Electromyography (EMG) Recording of muscle potentials, e.g., by a needle electrode inserted into the muscle

Electroneurography Electrodiagnostic method to determine the functional state of a peripheral nerve

Electronystagmography (ENG) Diagnostic test to record involuntary (or rarely voluntary) eye movements (nystagmus)

Electrophysiology Investigation of the electrical excitability and function of neural and muscular structures

Electrotherapy Treatment of paralyzed muscles by electrical stimulation

Encephalitis Inflammation of the brain

Encephalomyelitis Inflammation of the brain and spinal cord

Encephalon Brain

Encephalopathy A general, nonspecific term for a functional disorder or disease of the brain

Endocrine Relating to the function of endocrine glands that secrete hormones into the blood

Endogenous Arising within the body

Epidural Located in the epidural space (between bone and dura mater)

Erb's point Topographic point just above the mid-clavicle, from which stimulus responses from the brachial plexus can be recorded

Erythrocytes Red blood cells

Evoked potential Time-locked signal conducted partly or entirely through the central nervous system in response to a specific stimulus; can be recorded from different parts of the central and peripheral nervous system or the musculature; used for testing various neural pathways, e.g., visual evoked potentials (VEPs), auditory evoked potentials (AEPs), somatosensory evoked potentials (SEPs), and motor evoked potentials (MEPs)

Extracranial Outside the skull

Extrameatal Outside the ear canal

Extremities Limbs (arms and legs)

Facet joints Small joints between the articular processes of neighboring vertebrae

Facial paralysis Paralysis of the facial musculature due to impairment or failure of the facial nerve

Femur Bone of the thigh

Flash VEP Visual evoked potential (VEP) elicited by flash stimuli

Focal Affecting only a circumscribed area (e.g., pathological EEG pattern)

Fracture Broken bone

Frontal At the front of the head, located at the forehead

Ganglion cell Nerve cell in the central nervous system

Gap junction Tight cell-cell connection, consisting of a series of channels through which ions and small molecules can directly and rapidly transfer to the other cell by diffusion; thus, an action potential can be transmitted to the next cell with almost no time delay, facilitating synchronization of the cells

Generalized Affecting all parts (e.g., brain areas)

Glia Supporting and nourishing cells of the central nervous system located between the nerve cells and blood vessels; forms the myelin sheaths of the nerve cells

Gliosis Nonspecific reactive changes of glial cells in response to damage to the central nervous system

Granulocytes Large white blood cells; among others responsible for immune defense

Hemiataxia Movement and coordination disorder of one half of the body; mainly caused by damage to one cerebellar hemisphere

Hemifacial spasm Involuntary contractions of the facial muscles on one side

Hemiparesis Incomplete loss of motor function of one half of the body

Hemisphere One half of the cerebrum

Hemithyroidectomy Unilateral surgical removal of the thyroid gland

Histology Microscopic tissue analysis

Hyperthyroidism Overactivity of the thyroid gland; excessive secretion of thyroid hormones

Hypnagogia Transitional state from wakefulness to sleep

Hypnopompia Transitional state from sleep to wakefulness

Hypoacusis Hearing impairment

Hypoesthesia Reduction in the sensation of touch and pressure on the skin; often accompanied by a disturbance in pain perception

Hypothalamus Brain area located below the thalamus; seat of many regulatory centers, e.g., for thirst and hunger

Hypoxia Deficient oxygen supply to tissue

Idiopathic Arising by itself; without any ascertainable cause

Ileostoma Artificial outlet for the bowel at the ileum (third section of the small intestine)

Incision Surgical cut into a tissue

Incubation period Time between infection with a pathogen and the appearance of clinical signs of illness

Indication Reason/necessity/motivation to perform a procedure

Induction Initiation (e.g., of anesthesia)

Infarction Tissue death (necrosis) due to inadequate blood supply

Inferior Lying below

Infiltration Circumscribed penetration of non-local cells into the tissue

Inhibitory Hindering, impeding

Inion The palpable prominence on the back of the occipital bone

In situ In site; in place

Intracerebral Within the brain

Intracranial Inside the skull

Intrameatal Within the auditory canal

Intramuscular Within the musculature

Intraspinal Within the spinal canal

Intrathecal Within the cerebrospinal fluid space

Intravenous Within the veins

Intraventricular Within the cerebral ventricles

Intubation Insertion of a tube through the mouth or nose for ventilation

Invasive Introduction of an object into the body or body cavities

In vitro In the test tube; in the laboratory

In vivo In the living organism

Ipsilateral On the same side

Isoelectric line Horizontally running line with no deflections in an electrophysiologic recording; absence of electrical activity

Jannetta American neurosurgeon who introduced microvascular decompression to treat trigeminal neuralgia

Ketamine Intravenous anesthetic that has narcotic and analgesic effects but preserves reflex activity; it can be used for general anesthesia in conjunction with propofol

Laminectomy Permanent removal of a vertebral arch

Laminoplasty Reconstruction of a vertebral lamina to decompress the spinal cord

Laminotomy Temporary removal of a vertebral arch

Language areas Parts of the brain responsible for language; in right-handed and the majority of left-handed persons, located in the posterior first temporal gyrus for language comprehension (Wernicke's area), and in the posterior and inferior frontal lobe for language production (Broca's area), each on the left (dominant) side

Latency Time delay between stimulus and response

Latent Hidden, dormant

Lateral Sideways

Lateral lemniscus Nerve pathway in the brainstem that transmits acoustic signals from the cochlear nucleus to various brainstem nuclei and ultimately the contralateral inferior colliculus in the midbrain

Lesion Causally unspecified damage or disturbance of a tissue structure

Lethal Leading to death; deadly

Leukocytes White blood cells

Lobe A relatively well-defined part of an organ (e.g., brain lobe)

Macroscopic Analysis by the naked eye

Malignant Fast and invasive growing (e.g., tumor)

Masseter reflex Brainstem reflex triggered by a light blow on the chin

Mastoid process Posterior part of the temporal bone behind the ear

Mastoidectomy Surgical removal of the mastoid process

Mayfield clamp A clamp for fixation of the head during surgery

Medial Towards the middle

Medulla oblongata Most inferior part of the brain connecting the brainstem with the spinal cord

Meninges Triple membrane surrounding the brain and spinal cord

Meningitis Inflammation of the meninges

Mesencephalic Relating to the midbrain

Mesencephalon Midbrain; upper part of the brainstem associated with vision, hearing, motor control, alertness, and temperature regulation

Metastasis Secondary tumor by hematogenous or lymphogenous spreading of the primary tumor

Monopolar recording Registration of the voltage difference between a recording electrode and a distant reference

Monopolar stimulation Stimulation between an active electrode near the target tissue and a distant reference electrode

Muscle relaxant Drug to reduce or eliminate muscle tension

Muscle (Musculus, M., Musculi, Mm.) Bundle of muscle cells and fibers surrounded by protective tissue which are able to contract and produce a force. Depending on the histological structure and function, three different muscle types are distinguished: skeletal or striated muscle, smooth muscle (non-striated) and cardiac muscle

Myelin sheath Lipid-rich substance surrounding and insulating axons; facilitates fast nerve conduction

Myelopathy Disease or damage of the spinal cord (e.g., due to compression or ischemia)

Myelotomy Cutting of certain tracts in the spinal cord (e.g., for the treatment of therapy resistant pain)

Myopathy Muscle disease

NaCl Sodium chloride; isotonic saline solution

Nasal Towards the nose

Nasion Point on the skull where the frontal bone meets the two nasal bones

Nerve (Nervus, N., Nervi, Nn.) Cable-like bundle of nerve fibers (axons) in the peripheral nervous system

Nervous system Complex system of nerve cells and their connections, consisting of the brain, spinal cord, and peripheral nerves

Neurinoma Benign tumor of the peripheral nervous system

Neurological Relating to the nervous system

Neurolysis Surgical detachment of adhesions in a peripheral nerve

Neuron Nerve cell

Neurophysiology Branch of physiology and neuroscience that focusses on the functioning of the nervous system

Neuropsychology Branch of psychology that focuses on the relationships between brain and behavior/cognition (e.g., perception, memory, language)

Neurotomy Surgical transection of a peripheral nerve

Neurotropic Acting on the nervous system

Nociceptive pain Pain, triggered by special nerve endings (nociceptors), to warn the organism of impending danger and to provide information about injuries

Nucleus Local accumulation of neurons in the central nervous system

Nystagmus Involuntary movements of the eyeballs with a rapid and a slow component

Occipital Towards the back of the head

Opioid Natural or synthetic drug with analgesic, depressant, and sedative properties

Optical Relating to vision

Optokinetic Relating to the vision of moving objects

Oral In the mouth

Orbit Bony boundary of the eye; eye socket

Orthodromic In the physiological direction (e.g., impulse propagation)

Oscillation Time-periodic deviations of a signal from the resting state

Palpation Examination by touching

Paralysis Complete or almost complete loss of function of one or more muscles

Paramedian Aside the middle

Parasympathetic nervous system Part of the autonomic nervous system counteracting the sympathetic system; responsible for metabolism and the recovery of the body

Paresis Partial loss of function of one or more muscles

Parietal Towards the vertex

Parotidectomy Surgical removal of the parotid gland

Paroxysmal Sudden attack or recurrence; seizure-like

Pedicle Connection between vertebral body and vertebral arch in the spine

Percutaneous Through the skin

Perforation Rupture or penetration of a tissue

Periaqueductal Around the aqueductus mesencephali (canal connecting the third and fourth cerebral ventricles)

Peripheral Outside, located at the boundary

Peripheral nervous system (PNS) Parts of the nervous system that are outside the brain and spinal cord

Periradicular therapy Percutaneous application of drugs to a nerve root, e.g., for pain treatment

Perivascular Located around blood vessels

Perivenous Located around veins

Periventricular Located around the brain ventricles

Phylogenetic Biological evolution of new tribes from earth-historically older ones

Physical Relating to the body, bodily

Physiological Corresponding to the normal processes of the body

Physiology Science of normal processes in the healthy body

Pituitary gland Endocrine gland located at the brain base; produces a variety of hormones that in turn control many glands in the body

Placebo Sham drug without active ingredients; used for control purposes in tests on the efficacy and tolerability of new drugs

Plantar At the sole of foot

Plegia Complete loss of function of a skeletal muscle

Polyspikes Spikes occurring in short sequence in the EEG

Posterior Backward

Postinfectious After infection

Postoperative After surgery

Preauricular Located in front of the ear

Propofol Short-acting anesthetic for intravenous use

Proximal Towards the center of the body

Pyramidal tract Double-sided pathway in the central nervous system; runs from the cerebral cortex along the spinal cord and mediates movements

Radial Towards the radius

Radicular Relating to nerve roots

Radiculitis Inflammation of a nerve root

Receptor Structure that is sensitive or responsive to specific stimuli

Reclination Dorsal extension of the spine

Rectal Relating to the rectum; administration of a drug through the anus

Recurrence Relapse

Recurrent nerve palsy Failure of the function of the recurrent laryngeal nerve

Redon drainage Closed tube system for draining wound secretions to the outside with negative pressure

Reference Base value; control value

Reflex Involuntary but regular reaction of the body that can be triggered by an appropriate stimulus

Refractory Insensitive; cannot be influenced

Remifentanil Ultra-short-acting opioid; often used as an analgesic during anesthesia

REM sleep Rapid Eye Movement sleep; sleep stage in which rapid irregular eye movements occur and which does not appear until 40–100 min after falling asleep, also called dream sleep

Renal Related to the kidneys

Respiration Breathing

Restitution Restoration of function; recovery

Reticular formation Reticular arrangement of gray and white matter that traverses the brainstem and consists of widespread nuclear areas; contains functionally important control centers, such as the respiratory and circulatory centers

Retrobulbar Located behind the eye

Retrobulbar neuritis Inflammation of the optic nerve behind the eye

Retrograde Directed backward

Retrospective Looking back

Reversible Capable of being reversed

Rhizotomy Surgical transection of a spinal nerve root

Rocuronium Drug for muscle relaxation; used during anesthesia

Root ganglionectomy Transection of the sensory root and excision of the sensory ganglion for the treatment of pain

Rostral At the front of the head

Rupture Tearing of a tissue structure (e.g., of an aneurysm)

Saccade Jerky eye movement

Sacral Relating to the sacral spine (os sacrum)

Sagittal In the longitudinal axis of the body (anteroposterior or posteroanterior)

Sagittal plane Representation of the body in the longitudinal anteroposterior or posteroanterior axis

Saltatory Jumping excitation conduction in myelinated nerves facilitated by the nodes of Ranvier

Scintigraphy Nuclear medical examination technique in which radioactive markers are injected that accumulate in certain organs or tissues and can be detected with the aid of a gamma camera

Screening Diagnostic check

Sedate Make sleepy

Selective dorsal rhizotomy Surgical method for the treatment of spasticity by cutting dorsal nerve roots

Sensitivity Measure of the ability to detect abnormalities in examination or test procedures

Sensory Relating to sensorial perceptions (vision, smell, taste, hearing)

Sensory neuron Nerve cell responsible for the perception of sensations

Sequential In uninterrupted order

Sharp waves Steeply rising or falling waves in the EEG, which are slightly longer than spikes and are considered to be epilepsy-typical potentials

Significant Differences that can be calculated and not explained by random fluctuations

Simulation Pretense; imitation; modeling

Simultaneous Concurrent; at the same time

Sinister On the left side from patient´s view

Skull base Lower part of the skull with openings for entry and exit of the spinal cord, cranial nerves and blood vessels

Soma Cell body

Somatic Physical

Somatoform Appearing physical, but having mental causes

Somatomotor Relating to the motor system

Somatosensory Relating to the sensory system

Somatosensory evoked potentials (SEPs) Evoked potentials reflecting the functional status of sensory pathways; can be recorded from nerves, plexuses, the spinal cord, and the scalp after averaging

Spikes (EEG) Short sharp and spiky waves in the EEG, which are considered to be epilepsy-typical potentials

Spikes (EMG) Bi- or triphasic waves in EMG as a result of spontaneous activity

Spike-and-wave complex Initial spike followed by a slow wave in the EEG; considered to be an epilepsy-typical potential

Spinal Relating to the spine

Spondylodesis Surgery to stabilize two or more vertebrae in the cervical, thoracic and/or lumbar spine

Stenosis Narrowing of a hollow organ (e.g., a blood vessel)

Stereotyped Uniform; constant

Stroke Sudden interruption of blood flow to a part of the brain (ischemic stroke), or hemorrhage (hemorrhagic stroke), resulting in focal neurological deficits, e.g., hemiparesis, dysphasia, etc.

Struma (goiter) Palpable, visible and measurable enlargement of the thyroid gland

Subcortical Located below the cerebral cortex

Subcutaneous Under the skin

Sulcus Furrow between two cerebral convolutions (gyri)

Superior Lying above

Suppression Elimination (e.g., of artifacts)

Suprapubic Above the pubic bone (os pubis); in the case of a bladder catheter, this means that the catheter is inserted through the abdominal wall into the urinary bladder

Sweep One epoch of a recorded signal at the selected time base; averaging a number of sweeps is often used to extract an evoked potential from random noise

Sympathectomy Surgical removal of individual ganglia of the sympathetic nervous system to treat excessive sweating in certain parts of the body (focal hyperhidrosis)

Sympathetic nervous system Part of the autonomic nervous system counteracting the parasympathetic nervous system; it leads to an increase in the performance of the body, e.g., to stimulate the body's fight or flight response

Symptomatic Relating to the symptoms and signs of disease; treatment acting only on the symptoms, but not on the cause of a disease

Synapse Contact area between nerve cells at which the electrical excitation is passed on from one nerve cell to the next by means of chemical transmitters

Systemic Affecting the whole body

Tactile Relating to the sense of touch, tactile perception

Temporal Towards the temple region

Temporary Transient

Terminal boutons Distal terminations of an axon at a synapse

Tethered cord Attachment of the caudal (lower) portions of the spinal cord causing increased traction on the nerve fibers and corresponding disorders

Thalamotomy Coagulation of nuclear areas of the thalamus for the surgical treatment of severe pain

Thalamus Gray matter in the dorsal part of the diencephalon from which nerve fibers project to the cerebral cortex; relays sensory and motor signals to the cerebral cortex and regulates consciousness, sleep and alertness

Thoracic Belonging to the chest area

Thrombocytes Blood platelets

Thrombosis Partial or complete occlusion of an artery or vein by a thrombus

Thrombus Blood clot

Thyroidectomy Complete surgical removal of the thyroid gland

Tonic Relating to continuous muscle contraction

Tractus corticobulbaris Pathway that runs from the cortex to the motor nerve nuclei of the brainstem

Train Complexes of spikes or bursts in the EMG as a result of spontaneous activity; repetitive stimulus pulses at fixed frequency

Transcranial Through the skull

Transcutaneous Through the skin

Transurethral Through the urethra

Trigeminal neuralgia Facial pain, typically with episodes of severe and sudden pain attacks one side of the face lasting for seconds to a few minutes in the area supplied by the affected branch of the trigeminal nerve

Trocar Instrument used in minimally invasive surgery to create access to the abdominal cavity and keep it open with a tube

Tube Flexible hose for ventilation

Tympanoplasty Operation to close the tympanic membrane (eardrum)

Ulnar Towards the ulna

Ultrasound aspirator Device for tissue destruction and removal (e.g., of a tumor) by means of sound waves with frequencies from 20 kHz to several gigahertz

Unilateral One-sided

Vascular Relating to blood vessels

Vegetative Unconscious; involuntary (e.g., vegetative or autonomic nervous system)

Vein (Vena, V., Venae, Vv.) Blood vessel that carries deoxygenated blood from the periphery to the heart

Ventral Relating to the abdomen; on the front of the body; relating to the bottom portion of foot (plantar) and/or hand (palmar, volar)

Ventricle Cavity in the brain that contains cerebrospinal fluid

Vestibular Relating to the vestibular system

Vestibular system Fluid-filled semicircular canals and receptors located in the petrous bone at the skull base; detects movement and body position

Visual evoked potentials (VEPs) Evoked potentials reflecting the functional status of the visual pathways; can be recorded from the scalp over the visual cortex after averaging

Visual field defect A blind area (scotoma) within the normal visual field of one or both eyes

Visual pathway Course of the nerve tracts responsible for vision from the retina through the brain to the visual cortex

Vitality Viability; vital force

Vital signs Measures of the most important body functions (e.g., heart rate, respiratory rate, blood pressure, body temperature)

Volar Palm, palmar

Volatile Gaseous, vaporous (e.g., volatile anesthetics delivered by inhalation)

White matter Part of the central nervous system consisting mainly of medullary nerve fibers

WHO World Health Organization